Outcome Assessment in Advanced Practice Nursing

SECOND EDITION

Ruth M. Kleinpell, PhD, RN-CS, FAAN, FAANP, FCCM, is currently the Director of the Center for Clinical Research and Scholarship at Rush University Medical Center and a Professor at Rush University College of Nursing in Chicago, Illinois. In addition, she is a nurse practitioner at Our Lady of the Resurrection Medical Center in Chicago, Illinois. She received her diploma in nursing from Lutheran Medical Center School of Nursing, Cleveland, Ohio, and her baccalaureate, master's, and doctoral degrees in nursing from the University of Illinois College of Nursing, Chicago, Illinois. She received her Acute Care Nurse Practitioner certification at Rush University College of Nursing. Dr. Kleinpell is known for her work on outcomes research and has presented and published in the areas of assessing outcomes of advanced practice nursing, outcomes research, and other areas of nursing practice. She is a fellow of the American Academy of Nursing, the American Academy of Nurse Practitioners, the Institute of Medicine of Chicago, and the American College of Critical Care Medicine. Most recently, she received the 2007 Society of Critical Care Medicine's Norma J. Shoemaker Award for Critical Care Nursing Excellence and the 2007 Clinical Scholarship Award from Sigma Theta Tau International.

Outcome Assessment in Advanced Practice Nursing

SECOND EDITION

Ruth M. Kleinpell, PhD, RN-CS, FAAN, FAANP, FCCM
Editor

SPRINGER **PUBLISHING COMPANY**
New York

Springer Publishing Company, LLC
11 West 42nd Street
New York, NY 10036
www.springerpub.com

Acquisitions Editor: Allan Graubard
Production Editor: Jean Hurkin-Torres
Cover design: Steve Pisano
Composition: International Graphic Services
Ebook ISBN: 978-0-8261-2583-5

09 10 11 12 13 / 5 4 3 2

Library of Congress Cataloging-in-Publication Data

Outcome assessment in advanced practice nursing / Ruth M. Kleinpell, editor. — 2nd ed.
    p. ; cm.
    Includes bibliographical references and index.
    ISBN 978-0-8261-2582-8
    1. Nurse practitioners. 2. Nursing assessment. 3. Outcome assessment (Medical care)
I. Kleinpell, Ruth M. [DNLM: 1. Nurse Clinicians—standards. 2. Outcome Assessment
(Health Care) 3. Nurse Practitioners—standards. WY 128 094 2009]
RT82.8.O89 2009
610.7306'92—dc22   2008052497

Printed in the United States of America by Bang Printing.

The author and the publisher of this Work have made every effort to use sources believed to be reliable to provide information that is accurate and compatible with the standards generally accepted at the time of publication. Because medical science is continually advancing, our knowledge base continues to expand. Therefore, as new information becomes available, changes in procedures become necessary. We recommend that the reader always consult current research and specific institutional policies before performing any clinical procedure. The author and publisher shall not be liable for any special, consequential, or exemplary damages resulting, in whole or in part, from the readers' use of, or reliance on, the information contained in this book. The publisher has no responsibility for the persistence or accuracy of URLs for external or third-party Internet Web sites referred to in this publication and does not guarantee that any content on such Web sites is, or will remain, accurate or appropriate.

Contents

Contributors

Rhonda Arthur, DNP, CNM, WHNP-BC, FNP-BC
Course Coordinator
Frontier School of Midwifery and Family Nursing
Hyden, Kentucky

Denise Bryant-Lukosius, RN, PhD
Assistant Professor, Nursing and Oncology
Clinical Nurse Specialist, Juravinski Cancer Program
  Hamilton Health Sciences
McMaster University, Faculty of Health Sciences, School of Nursing
Hamilton, Ontario, Canada

Suzanne M. Burns, MSN, RRT, ACNP, CCRN, FAAN, FCCM, FAANP
Professor of Nursing and APN2
Director, PNSO Research Program—UVA Health System
University of Virginia
Charlottesville, Virginia

Nancy E. Dayhoff, EdD, RN, CNS
Associate Professor Emeritus
Indiana University School of Nursing
Managing Partner, Clinical Solutions LLC
Indianapolis, Indiana

Jan Buffo Dempsey, MLS
Retired Reference Librarian, Assistant Director
Naval Medical Center
San Diego, California

Alba DiCenso, RN, PhD
Professor, Nursing and Clinical Epidemiology and Biostatistics
CHSRF/CIHR Chair in Advanced Practice Nursing
Director, Ontario Training Centre in Health Services and Policy
    Research
McMaster University, Faculty of Health Sciences, School of Nursing
Hamilton, Ontario, Canada

Margaret Faut-Callahan, CRNA, PhD, FAAN
Dean and Professor
Marquette University School of Nursing
Milwaukee, Wisconsin

Kevin D. Frick, PhD
Director of the Interdepartmental Health Economics Program and
    Associate Professor
Johns Hopkins Bloomberg School of Public Health
Department of Health Policy and Management
Baltimore, Maryland

Anna Gawlinski, RN, DNSc, CS-ACNP, FAAN
Director, Evidence-Based Practice and Adjunct Professor
Ronald Reagan UCLA Medical Center and
University of California, Los Angeles School of Nursing
Los Angeles, California

Mary Jo Goolsby, EdD, MSN, NP-C, CAE, FAANP
Director of Research and Education
American Academy of Nurse Practitioners
Austin, Texas

Roger Green, DNP, FNP, FAANP
Regional Manager of Operations, The Little Clinic
Phoenix, Arizona
Lecturer, Department of Nursing
California State University Dominguez Hills
Carson, California

Michael J. Kremer, PhD, CRNA, FAAN
Associate Professor and Chair, Nurse Anesthesia Department
Rosalind Franklin University of Medicine and Science
North Chicago, Illinois

Brenda L. Lyon, DNS, CNS, FAAN
Professor, Indiana University School of Nursing
Indianapolis, Indiana

Julie A. Marfell, DNP, BC, FNP
Chairperson, Department of Family Nursing
Frontier School of Midwifery and Family Nursing
Hyden, Kentucky

Kathy McCloy, RN, MSN, ACNP
Acute Care Nurse Practitioner
Division of Cardiology
UCLA Santa Monica Cardiology Center
University of California
Los Angeles, California

Ann F. Minnick, PhD, RN, FAAN
Senior Associate Dean for Research
Julia Eleanor Chenault Professor of Nursing
School of Nursing, Vanderbilt University
Nashville, Tennessee

Patricia W. Stone, PhD, MPH, RN, FAAN
Associate Professor of Nursing, Columbia University
New York, New York

Marilyn Wolf Schwartz, MLS
Retired Medical Library Director
Naval Medical Center, San Diego, California and
Rocky Mountain University of Health Professions
Provo, Utah

Suzan Ulrich, DrPh, CNM, FACNM
Chair of Midwifery and Women's Health
Frontier School of Midwifery and Family Nursing
Hyden, Kentucky

Julie Vohra, MSc
Research Coordinator
McMaster University, Faculty of Health Sciences, School of Nursing
Hamilton, Ontario, Canada

Foreword

Outcomes assessment is essential to the survival and success of advanced practice nursing. Health care entities, employers, insurers, consumers, and others are requesting that advanced practice nurses (APNs) justify their contribution to health care and demonstrate the value they add to patient care. And although a growing body of literature demonstrates that APNs deliver high-quality care that is comparable or superior to that of other care providers, the need persists for well-designed outcome evaluation studies that provide reliable and valid data to substantiate the impact of APN care. As a result, it is essential for APNs in all specialty areas of practice to have a good understanding of the field of outcomes assessment and to play a proactive role in demonstrating the outcomes of APN care.

This book serves as an ideal tool for assisting APNs in gaining an understanding of the process of outcomes assessment, including findings from the literature that showcase APN outcomes and the process of measuring APN impact. The approach used to address outcome assessment in all of the APN practice roles, including nurse practitioner, clinical nurse specialist, certified nurse midwife, and certified registered nurse anesthetist, offers a direction for APNs undertaking the process of outcomes measurement and management. By discussing outcomes specific to APN role(s) and the methods used to measure them, the book also serves as a useful resource for APN students, researchers, educators, and administrators who have an interest in further understanding issues related to APN outcomes assessment. In addition, the incorporation of examples from clinical practice assists in making the concepts real and in highlighting the ways in which APN practice can influence care delivery processes and outcomes.

As the field of outcomes assessment and evaluation grows, APNs will receive the recognition they deserve and will be seen as critical members of the health care team. The authors in this book have provided insights into and recommended actions for making that happen.

Gail L. Ingersoll, EdD, RN, FAAN
Director, Center for Outcomes Measurement
and Practice Innovation
Loretta Ford Professor of Nursing
University of Rochester Medical Center
Rochester, New York

Preface

Assessing outcomes of advanced practice nursing care is an important aspect of bringing recognition to the multifaceted roles of advanced practice nurses (APNs) and of their impact on outcomes. Since 2001, when the first edition of this book was published, the field of outcomes research has further grown and developed. The second edition of *Outcome Assessment in Advanced Practice Nursing* has been written to provide APNs with updated resources and information on measuring outcomes of practice. The chapters within this book focus on presenting an overview of advanced practice nursing outcomes research and discussing outcome measurement in all areas of advanced practice nursing, including clinical nurse specialist, nurse practitioner, certified registered nurse anesthetist, and certified nurse midwife. Examples of outcome studies are presented from actual research in APN practice. Additional chapters provide sources of outcome measures and instruments that can be used by APNs to establish the effectiveness of the role. New chapters added to this second edition include discussion of outcomes assessment of APN practice in community primary care and ambulatory settings, additional information on locating instruments and measures for APN outcome assessment, and information on an ongoing international initiative focusing on the development of an APN research data collection toolkit. The contributors to this second edition are recognized expert practitioners, educators, and researchers, and collectively they offer invaluable insights into the process of conducting outcomes assessments in APN practice.

The ever-expanding field of outcomes measurement can make conducting an outcomes assessment complex. *Outcome Assessment in Advanced Practice Nursing* provides APNs with up-to-date resources and examples of outcome measures, tools, and methods that can be used by APNs in their quest to measure outcomes of care. This second edition of the book was written to serve as a resource for assessing outcomes for APNs, regardless of specialty area of practice or practice setting. Having knowledge of the APN outcome literature as well as the process of assessing outcomes of practice is important for all APNs. The true impact of APN care can only be established through continued focus on outcomes assessment and evaluation—something that this book encourages readers to actively pursue.

1

Measuring Outcomes in Advanced Practice Nursing

RUTH M. KLEINPELL

Assessing the outcomes of advanced practice nursing (APN) has become essential, due in part to the emphasis on outcomes that has become a component of the majority of health care initiatives. The demands for measuring outcomes of care have been emphasized by federal and state regulatory agencies, practice guidelines, employers, and consumer groups. Health care organizations are now actively monitoring patient outcomes as a means of evaluation as well as for requirements for accreditation and certification. In addition, health care restructuring continues to change the way in which care is delivered, and as APN roles change, the measurement of outcomes is an important parameter by which APN care can be evaluated. Moreover, as advanced practice nurses (APNs) are involved in providing care to a variety of patient groups and in various settings, they are often the most familiar with the clinical problems that need to be studied and are therefore the ideal practitioners to participate in the development of outcome-based initiatives (Resnick, 2006).

For APNs, outcomes are the result of interventions based on the use of clinical judgment, scientific knowledge, skills, and experience (Byers & Brunell, 1998). As APNs have traditionally been involved in unique and diverse aspects of patient-focused care, outcomes measure-

1

ment enables the significant contributions of APNs to be delineated. However, the field of outcomes measurement is expanding rapidly, making the conduct of an outcomes assessment even more complex. Knowledge of the process of outcomes measurement and available resources is essential for all APNs regardless of practice specialty or setting. This chapter reviews important issues in measuring outcomes in advanced practice nursing, including a discussion of the state of the science on APN outcomes research.

OUTCOMES RESEARCH

Patient outcomes are the end results of medical care treatments or interventions (Jennings, Staggers, & Brosch, 1999; Lohr, 1988). Outcomes describe the responses, behaviors, feelings, or results of care provided. Outcomes are used to evaluate the effectiveness of care, to describe the effects of care on patients' lives, to identify areas for improvement in care, and to establish a basis for clinical decision making (Davies et al., 1994). Important outcome goals related to patient care include improving physical and functional status, maintaining well-being, symptom relief, avoiding or decreasing adverse effects of care, and achieving patient satisfaction (Davies et al., 1994).

The field of outcomes research is expanding and the literature on outcomes is extensive. Although it is clear that measuring outcomes is important, selecting which outcome measures to include in an outcomes assessment remains challenging. The selection of outcome measures should be based on a clear sense of what is to be measured, and why (Kane, 2004). The process of outcomes research involves outlining how to evaluate an aspect of care and choosing specific parameters to be monitored that may provide an accurate assessment of the impact of that care.

Outcome Measurement in Advanced Practice Nursing

Measuring outcomes of APN practice involves identifying and choosing indicators to be monitored and selecting a methodology to conduct the outcomes assessment. Yet, the process of monitoring outcomes of APN practice is complex, as time needs to be allocated to the planning and conduct of the outcome assessment. The chapters in this book outline several examples of practice-based outcome assessments related to APN practice, including indicators monitored and how an outcome assessment was conducted, as well as sources for identifying outcome-related tools.

A review of the literature on outcome measurement in APN provides specific examples of outcome parameters influenced by APN care (see Table 1.1). A MEDLINE, PubMed, or OvidMed search with the words "outcomes" and "advanced practice nursing" results in over 500 citations. A review of those citations reveals over 200 completed and published studies, including several synthesis reviews, that examine outcomes related to APN care. Several synthesis reviews have critiqued early studies on APN practice, including studies comparing nurse practitioner (NP) and physician assistant (PA) care with physician (MD) care (Sox, 1979), studies comparing NP and MD practice (Horrocks, Anderson, & Salisbury, 2002; Prescott, Duncan, & Driscoll, 1979), and studies on APN effectiveness (Bourbonnier & Evans, 2002; Cunningham, 2004; Edmunds, 1978; Feldman, Ventura, & Crosby, 1987; Fulton & Baldwin, 2004; McGrath, 1990). Other explorations have included integrative reviews on the effect of APN care in specialty areas of practice such as heart failure management (Benatar, Bondmass, Ghitelman, & Avitall, 2003; Osevala, 2005). An ongoing technical evaluation of the quality, safety, and effectiveness of APN care, currently being conducted by investigators at Johns Hopkins University (Newhouse et al., 2009, in progress), should provide updated information on the state of the science related to outcomes research on APN care.

Early studies assessing the outcomes of APN care examined process and client-outcome variables, including client management, activities, cost of care, problem identification, physician acceptance, and disease- or condition-specific outcomes. Other studies measuring outcomes of APN care have explored a variety of factors, including the impact of APN care on patients, on patient satisfaction with care, on quality of care provided by APNs as compared with MDs, and on outcomes of care provided by APNs in comparison with other practitioners, including PAs, medical residents, and MDs (Brooten & Naylor, 1995; Brown & Grimes, 1995; Carzoli, Martinez-Cruz, Cuevas, Murphy, & Chiu, 1994; Crosby, Ventura, & Feldman, 1987; DiGirol & Parry, 1983; Lombness, 1994; Moody, Smith, & Glenn, 1999; Mundinger et al., 2000; Rudy et al., 1998; Sakr et al., 1999; Seale, Anderson, & Kinnersley, 2006; Sears, Wickizer, Franklin, Cheadle, & Berkowitz,

Table 1.1

EXAMPLES OF OUTCOME MEASURES FOR ADVANCED PRACTICE NURSES

Blood glucose control
Symptom management
Patient length of stay
Hospital care costs
Smoking cessation
Adverse events (e.g., accidental extubation)
Patient and family knowledge
Staff nurse knowledge
Staff nurse retention rates
Nosocomial infection rates
Readmission rates
Nutritional intake
Skin breakdown rates
Restraint use
Hand-hygiene compliance
Patient and family satisfaction rates
Nurse satisfaction rates
Rates of adherence to best practices

Source: Adapted from Kleinpell and Gawlinski (2005).

2007, 2008; Sidani et al., 2006; Simborg, Starfield, & Horn, 1978; Sox, 1979; Spisso, O'Callaghan, McKennan, & Holcroft, 1990). Additional studies have explored characteristics of APNs that affect outcomes, such as provider proficiency, complication rates, clinical competency, and personal activities (Buchanan & Powers, 1997; Mundinger et al., 2000; Rudy et al., 1998; Stetler, Effken, Frigon, Tiernan, & Zwingman-Bagley, 1998).

Identifying outcome measures that are "nurse-sensitive" has been identified as a way of linking nursing roles to specific health care outcomes. A number of nurse-sensitive outcome measures have been proposed, including clinical outcomes such as symptom control and health status indicators; prevention of complications such as prevention of infection and prevention of complications of immobility; knowledge of disease and its treatment, including patient knowledge of the illness process and knowledge of medications; and functional health outcomes, including physical and social functioning (Irvine, Sidani, & Hall, 1998).

Table 1.2

NURSE-SENSITIVE OUTCOMES OF ADVANCED PRACTICE NURSING

Patient satisfaction
Symptom resolution or reduction
Compliance/adherence
Patient/family knowledge
Collaboration among care providers
Functional status
Patient self-esteem
Knowledge and skill of other care providers
Length of time in hospital
Staff satisfaction with work
Costs of care
Patient preparedness for interventions

Source: Adapted from Ingersoll, McIntosh, and Williams (2000).

Specific nurse-sensitive outcomes of advanced practice nursing have also been identified (see Table 1.2) (Ingersoll, McIntosh, & Williams, 2000).

Studies focusing on APN care in specialty areas of practice such as acute care have examined several aspects of patient care outcomes, including ventilatory weaning (Burns & Earven, 2002; Burns et al., 2003), rates of urinary tract infection and skin breakdown (Russell, Vorder-Bruegge, & Burns, 2002), use of laboratory tests (Gawlinski, 2001), length of stay (LOS) (Burns & Earven, 2002; Burns et al., 2003; Meyer & Miers, 2005; Miller, 1979; Russell et al., 2002; Spisso et al., 1990), readmission rates (Venner & Steelbinder, 1996), mortality (Burns et al., 2003; Venner & Steelbinder, 1996), and costs of care (Burns & Earven, 2002; Burns et al., 2003; Carzoli et al., 1994; Cintron, Bigas, Linates, Aranda, & Hernandez, 1983; Dahle, Smith, Ingersol, & Wilson, 1998; Meyer & Miers, 2005; Paul, 2000), discharge instructions (Kleinpell & Gawlinski, 2005), smoking cessation (Kleinpell & Gawlinski, 2005), use of angiotensin converting enzyme inhibitors, beta-blockers, and anticoagulation for cardiac patients (Kleinpell & Gawlinski, 2005), X-ray interpretation skills (Freij, Duffy, Hackett, Cunningham, & Fothergill, 1996), thoracostomy tube performance (Bevis et al., 2008), intracranial pressure monitor placement (Kaups, Parks, & Morris, 1998), epilepsy care outcomes (Sarkissian & Wennberg, 1999), and time savings for MD staff (Spisso et al., 1990) (see Table 1.3). It is evident that a number of studies have evaluated APN outcomes, yet, because APN roles are diverse, information on APN outcomes remains needed, especially for new and evolving APN roles.

Classifying APN Outcome Studies

Organizing studies related to APN outcomes according to categories can facilitate discussion and evaluation. Outcomes have been categorized as care related, patient related, and performance related (Jennings et al., 1999). These groupings, although not mutually exclusive, can be used to examine outcome studies of APN care and can aid both in summarizing important findings and in highlighting areas needing further study. Table 1.4 outlines outcome measures used in APN-effectiveness research grouped according to these areas.

Care-Related Outcomes of APN

Care-related outcomes are those outcomes that result from APN involvement in care or from an APN intervention. Studies assessing the impact of APN care have ranged from those exploring its effects on quantitative indices such as lab values, on physiological values such as weight gain, on clinical symptoms such as dyspnea or pain, and on aspects of health such as physical function and mobility (Jennings et al., 1999; Poduri, Palenski, & Gibson, 1996; Ziemer et al., 1996). Other studies in this category have measured the effect of APN care on length of patient hospitalization, hospital readmission rates, costs, appropriateness of prescribing decisions, timeliness of consultations, and mortality and morbidity rates (Batey & Holland, 1985; Boville et al., 2007; Burns et al., 2003; Cowan et al., 2006; Delgado-Passler & McCaffery, 2006; Dellasega & Zerbe, 2002; Ettner et al., 2006; Gawlinski et al., 2001; Lindberg et al., 2002; Litaker, Mion, Planavsky, Kippes, Mehta, & Frolkis, 2003; McCauley, Bixby, & Naylor, 2006; Meyer & Miers, 2005; Moody et al., 1999; Monroe, Pohl, Gardner, & Bell, 1982; Naylor, Brooten, & Campbell, 2004; Naylor et al., 1999; Neff, Madigan, & Narsavage, 2003; Neidlinger, Scroggins, & Kennedy, 1987; Quenot et al., 2007; Rideout, 2007; Rosenaur, Stanford, Morgan, & Curtin, 1984; Russell et al., 2002; Schultz, Liptak, & Fioravanti, 1994; Simborg et al., 1978; Vanhook, 2000).

Table 1.3

EXAMPLES OF OUTCOME MEASURES USED IN APN EFFECTIVENESS RESEARCH

CARE RELATED	PATIENT RELATED
Costs of care	Patient satisfaction
Length of stay	Patient access to care
In-hospital mortality	Patient compliance
Morbidity	Symptom resolution or reduction
Readmission rates	Health maintenance
Occurrence of drug reactions	Return to work
Procedure success rate/complications	Stress levels
Clinic wait time	Knowledge
Time spent with patients	Blood pressure control
Number of visits per patient	Diet and weight control
Number of patient hospitalizations	Blood glucose levels
Use/ordering of lab tests	Clinic wait time
Rate of drug prescription	Emergency room wait time
Management of common medical problems	Patient self-esteem
Number of consultations	Patient/family knowledge
Infant immunizations	Functional status
Diagnoses made	
Diagnostic screening tests ordered	**PERFORMANCE RELATED**
Acute care home visits	Quality of care
Intravenous fluid volume	Interpersonal skills
Total parenteral nutrition use	Technical quality
Number of blood transfusions	Completeness of documentation
Prenatal/postpartum visits	Time spent in role components
Low-birthweight rates	APN job satisfaction
Rates of cesearean section	Clinical competence
Number of induced labors	Performance ratings
Analgesia/anesthesia used	Collaboration
Quality of life	Procedure complication rates
Time to readmission	Revenue generation
Length of time between discharge and readmission	Physician recruitment & retention
	Time savings for house staff MDs on MD workload
	Resuscitation outcomes
	Clinical examination comprehensiveness
	Adherence to best-practice guidelines

Source: Adapted from Kleinpell (2001).

Table 1.4

SAMPLE LISTING OF OUTCOMES MEASURES USED TO ASSESS OUTCOMES OF APN PRACTICE IN ACUTE CARE

Ventilatory weaning (Burns & Earven, 2002; Burns et al., 2003)

Pneumonia (Russell et al., 2002)

Emergency room care (Cooper et al., 2002; Sakr et al., 1999)

Use of laboratory tests (Gawlinski, 2001)

Trauma care (Sole et al., 2001; Spisso et al., 1990)

Time savings for physicians (Spisso et al., 1990)

Rates of urinary tract infection and skin breakdown (Russell et al., 2002)

Length of stay (Burns & Earven, 2002; Burns et al., 2003; Cowan et al., 2006; Lombness, 1994; Meyer & Miers, 2005; Russell et al., 2002; Spisso et al., 1990)

Readmission rates (Meyer & Miers, 2005; Paul, 2000; Venner & Steelbinder, 1996)

Implementation of quality improvement initiatives such as rapid response team (Morse et al., 2006)

Compliance with practice guidelines (Bargardi et al., 2005; Gawlinski et al., 2001, Gracias et al., 2008)

Unplanned ICU readmissions (Morse et al., 2006)

Inpatient cardiac arrests (Morse et al., 2006)

Mortality (Burns et al. 2003; Venner & Steelbinder, 1996)

Costs of care (Burns & Earven, 2002; Burns et al., 2003; Carzoli et al., 1994; Cintron et al., 1983; Dahle et al., 1998; Meyer & Miers, 2005; Paul, 2000)

Discharge instructions (Kleinpell & Gawlinski, 2005)

Use of ACE-I, beta blockers, and anticoagulation for cardiac patients (Kleinpell & Gawlinski, 2005)

Intracranial pressure monitor placement (Kaups et al., 1998)

Epilepsy care outcomes (Sarkissian & Wennberg, 1999)

X-ray interpretation skills (Freij et al., 1996)

Thoracostomy tube placement (Bevis et al., 2008)

Source: Adapted from Kleinpell, Ely, & Grabenkort (2008).

These studies have concluded that APNs perform a comprehensive range of activities that include both expanded nursing practice activities and collaborative physician-related activities (physical assessment and diagnosis, ordering diagnostic tests, prescribing treatments, seeking and giving consultations, case management). In general, these studies have found a variety of results related to APN care, ranging from no effect to a significant impact on outcomes. Studies reporting significant results of APN care have cited such parameters as decreased length of hospitalization stay, annual cost savings, time savings per day for house staff, and decreased outpatient clinic waiting times (Bergeron, Neuman, & Kinsey, 1999; Burns et al., 2003; Cintron et al., 1983; Cowan et al., 2006; Dahle et al., 1998; Lombness, 1994; McCauley et al., 2006; Meyer & Miers, 2005; Morse, Warshawsky, Moore, & Pecora, 2006; Paladichuck, 1997; Paul, 2000; Rideout, 2007; Russell et al., 2002; Venner & Steelbinder, 1996). Table 1.5 outlines selected studies in this category of APN outcomes, including outcome measures explored.

Patient-Related Outcomes of APN

Patient-related outcomes of care are those outcomes that affect patient perceptions, preferences, or knowledge. Studies in this category have measured the effect of APN care on patient satisfaction, quality of life, patient access to care, use of health services, patient compliance, patient complaints, patient knowledge, symptom management, social function, and psychological function. Findings from these studies have revealed that APN care results in increased patient satisfaction, patient compliance with treatment plans, cost savings in terms of annual costs and hospital charges, decreased length of hospital stay, decreased readmission rates, changes in patient clinical parameters such as lipid levels (Andrus & Donaldson, 2006; Paez & Allen, 2006) and blood pressure control (Benkert, Buchholz, & Poole, 2001), and improvement in patient care practices such as pneumococcal vaccine administration (Mackey, Cole, & Lindenberg, 2005), cervical cancer screening (Kelley, Daly, Anthony, Zausniewski, & Stange, 2002), and increased patient education, among others (Blue et al., 2001; Brooten & Naylor, 1995; Bryant & Graham, 2002; Buchanan & Powers, 1997; Cooper, Lindsay, Kinn, & Swann, 2002; Curran & Roberts, 2002; De Jong, 1981; Gracias et al., 2003; Graveley & Littlefield, 1992; Hankins, Shaw, Cruess, Lawrence, & Harris, 1996; Hanneman, Bines, & Sajtar, 1993; Miller, 1997; Mundinger et al., 1999; Sears et al., 2007; Sinuff et al., 2007; Sole, Hunkar-Huie, Schiller, & Cheatham, 2001; Spitzer et al., 1974; Sulzbach-Hoke & Gift, 1995; Thompson, 1980). Table 1.6 outlines studies in this category of APN outcomes, including outcome measures explored.

Table 1.5

STUDIES ASSESSING CARE-RELATED OUTCOMES OF ADVANCED PRACTICE NURSING (APN)

STUDY	APN ROLE	OUTCOME INDICATORS	FINDINGS
Albers-Heitner et al. (2008) Impact of nurse practitioner (NP) care in primary care for adult patients with urinary incontinence	NP	Urinary incontinence, quality of life, costs	Ongoing clinical trial.
Rideout (2007) Evaluation of pediatric NP care coordinator model for hospitalized children, adolescents, and young adults with cystic fibrosis	NP	Timeliness of inpatient consultations; weight gain, length of stay (LOS), patient/family satisfaction, change in forced expiratory volume in first second (FEV1)	In 21 patients, there was a significant decrease in time to complete consultations, a decrease in LOS by 1.35 days ($p = .06$); patient/parent satisfaction was high.
Boville et al. (2007) Impact of NP care in chronic disease management care of 110 patients with diabetes	NP	Glycemic control, lipid management, blood pressure control	NP care with the use of clinical algorithms for medication intensification resulted in improved glycemic control, lipid management, and control of hypertension.
Hamilton & Hawley (2006) Impact of CNS care for patients with chronic renal failure in an outpatient anemia management program	CNS	Quality of life	CNS-managed patients had a statistically significant increase in quality-of-life indicators.
Morse et al. (2006) Assessment of an NP-led rapid response team (RRT)	NP	Codes outside the intensive care unit (ICU), staff perceptions of the RRT, in-hospital mortality rates	An NP-led RRT resulted in ↓ in-house codes, ↓ in-hospital mortality rates, and high satisfaction ratings from staff.
Cowan et al. (2006) Analysis of impact of acute care NP care for medical inpatients comanaged with medical doctor (MD) compared to hospitalist managed care	NP	LOS, hospital costs, readmission rates 4 months after discharge ($p <.001$)	Average LOS was lower in NP-MD comanaged patients (5 vs 6 days); costs of care were less; there were no differences in readmission rates.

Table 1.5 (continued)

STUDY	APN ROLE	OUTCOME INDICATORS	FINDINGS
Cragin et al. (2006) Impact of nurse-midwifery care on patient outcomes	CNM	Perinatal outcomes	Midwifery patients had more optimal care processes with no differences in neonatal outcomes.
Ettner et al. (2006) Impact of NP on costs of care for medical inpatients	NP	Costs of care	The addition of an NP to general medicine teams was cost-effective; NP care reinforced medical compliance, follow-up plans, & symptom management.
McCauley et al. (2006) Impact of APN care on elderly patients with heart failure	APN	Length of time between hospital discharge and readmission, hospital readmission LOS, costs	APN care resulted in reduced hospital readmission, reduced LOS of readmissions, and decreased overall health care costs.
Shebasta et al. (2006) Impact of pediatric NP on staff nurse satisfaction	NP	Staff nurse satisfaction	Involvement of a pediatric NP in patient care resulted in higher staff nurse satisfaction.
Reigle et al. (2006) Impact of acute care NP on cardiology patients	NP	LOS, prescription of appropriate discharge medications; documentation of patient education	NP-managed patients undergoing cardiac catheterization or percutaneous coronary intervention resulted in ↓ LOS, more prescription of indicated medications, and more documentation of patient status and patient education.
Stolee et al. (2006) Impact of NP role for long term care residents	NP	Ratings of effectiveness and satisfaction of NP role	NP care significantly impacted the primary care of residents in long term care.

(continued)

Table 1.5 (continued)

STUDY	APN ROLE	OUTCOME INDICATORS	FINDINGS
Kutzleb & Reiner (2006) Prospective quasi-experimental study assessing the impact of NP care on patients with heart failure	NP	Quality of life; functional status	NP-directed care resulted in increased patient quality of life, health, and functioning ($p = .0003$) over a 12-month period.
Forster et al. (2005) Impact of CNS care on medical patients	CNS	Readmission, risk of adverse events, mortality, quality of care	CNS-managed patients had higher overall quality of care; no differences were observed in readmission rates, adverse events, or mortality rates compared to usual care-managed patients.
Meyer & Miers (2005) Acute care NP in cardiovascular (CV) surgery	NP	LOS, costs of care	Care given by ACNPs on the CV team resulted in ↓ LOS by 1.91 days and ↓ cost of care by $5,038.91 per patient.
Neff et al. (2003) Impact of APN care for homecare patients with chronic obstructive pulmonary disease	APN	Dyspnea, activities of daily living, rehospitalizations, ER visits	APN-directed pulmonary disease management resulted in shorter rehospitalization LOS and fewer rehospitalizations; a significantly higher number of patients in the APN group were discharged and remained at home compared to the control group ($p < .05$).
Ahrens et al. (2003) Impact of CNS-led communication intervention with families of ICU patients	CNS	ICU LOS, hospital LOS, hospital costs	A structured CNS initiative resulted in shorter ICU LOS and lower costs of care.

Table 1.5 (continued)

STUDY	APN ROLE	OUTCOME INDICATORS	FINDINGS
Burns et al. (2003) ACNP care for mechanically ventilated patients in ICU	NP	Ventilator duration, LOS in ICU, mortality, costs of care	An outcomes management model of ACNP care resulted in ↓ ventilator duration ($p = .0001$), ↓ ICU LOS ($p = .0008$), ↓ hospital LOS ($p = .0001$), ↓ mortality rates ($p = .02$), and > \$3,000,000 cost savings.
Litaker et al. (2003) Impact of NP-physician team in managing patients with chronic disease	NP	Glycosylated hemoglobin, high-density-lipoprotein (HDL) cholesterol, satisfaction with care, health-related quality of life	Patients randomized to the NP-MD team care experienced significant improvements in mean hemoglobin A_{1c} (HbA_{1c}), HDL-cholesterol, and satisfaction with care.
Tijhuis et al. (2002) Impact of CNS care for patients with rheumatoid arthritis	CNS	Functional status, quality of life, disease activity, health utility, satisfaction with care	CNS-managed patients had a significant improvement ($p < 0.05$) in functional status, quality of life, health utility, and patient satisfaction.
Russell et al. (2002) ACNP care for neuroscience ICU patients	NP	LOS, rates of urinary tract infection (UTI), skin breakdown, Foley catheter time, mobilization out of bed	Patients managed by ACNPs had shorter LOS ($p = .03$), shorter ICU LOS ($p < .001$), lower rates of UTI and skin breakdown ($p < .05$), and shorter time to discontinuation of Foley catheter and mobilization out of bed.

(continued)

Table 1.5 (continued)

STUDY	APN ROLE	OUTCOME INDICATORS	FINDINGS
Lindberg et al. (2002) Impact of asthma NP care for 347 patients	NP	Asthma symptoms, quality of documentation, patient self-management	NP-managed patients reported less asthma symptoms and more self-management; documentation quality of NP care was high.
Dellasega & Zerbe (2002) Impact of APN intervention on caregivers of frail rural older adults	APN	Caregiver physical health, well-being, and perceived stress	Caregivers who received APN intervention had higher self-rated emotional health scores, fewer depressive symptoms, and lower stress scores.
Gawlinski et al. (2001) ACNP care for cardiac ICU patients using extubation protocols	NP	Mechanical ventilation time, reintubation events, LOS	Decreased mean time to extubation, decreased rates of ventilator-associated pneumonia, shorter LOS, and decreased use of arterial blood gases.
Ley (2001) Impact of CNS care for cardiac surgery patients	CNS	Cardiac surgical bleeding	A quality improvement initiative resulted in decreased preoperative exposure to clopidogrel and decreased postoperative bleeding.
Larsen et al. (2001) Impact of CNS care for adult sickle cell patients	CNS	Pain consultations, patient-controlled analgesia use, patient education	Implementation of a clinical pathway resulted in increased pain consultations, patient-controlled analgesia use, and increased patient education.
Brooten et al. (2001) Impact of CNS care for women with high-risk pregnancies	CNS	Preterm infant, prenatal hospitalizations, infant rehospitalizations, costs of care, LOS, mortality	CNS managed patients had fewer preterm infants, fewer infant deaths, fewer prenatal hospitalizations, decreased LOS.

Table 1.5 (continued)

STUDY	APN ROLE	OUTCOME INDICATORS	FINDINGS
Carroll et al. (2001) Impact of APN care for unpartnered elders following acute myocardial infarction	APN	Patient education, self-efficacy; functional status	APN-led intervention resulted in increased self-efficacy and improved function.
Dobscha et al. (2001) Effectiveness of a CNS-led intervention to improve primary care provider recognition of depression	CNS	Recognition and management of depression	A CNS-led intervention resulted in improved recognition and initial management of depression in a VA primary care setting
Barnason et al. (2000) Impact of CNS-led recovery program for cardiac surgery patients	CNS	Factors facilitating and inhibiting adherence to cardiac therapy program	CNS-managed patients required less oxygen use on day 2.
Vanhook (2000) Analysis of effect of the implementation of acute stroke team facilitated by NP	NP	Mortality rate, length of stay, hospital charges, time to arrival after symptom onset	Mortality rate ↓ from 5.7% to 3.8%, LOS ↓ from 10 days in 1995 to 3.2 days in 1998. Hospital charges ↓ 50% and time to arrival after symptom onset ↓ from 22 hours to 7 hours.
Paul (2000) Retrospective review of impact of NP-managed heart failure clinic for 15 patients with congestive heart failure	NP	Hospital readmissions, emergency room (ER) visits, LOS, charges, reimbursement	6 months after implementation of heart failure clinic, hospital admissions ↓ (from 151 hospital days to 22); mean LOS ↓ (from 4.3 days to 3.8 days) and mean inpatient hospital charges ↓ from $40,624 per patient admission to $5,893; % of recovered charges from reimbursement ↑ from 73% to 87%.

(continued)

Table 1.5 (continued)

STUDY	APN ROLE	OUTCOME INDICATORS	FINDINGS
Jacavone et al. (1999). Impact of CNS care for cardiac surgery patients	CNS	Extubation time, ambulation time, postoperative nausea, decreased postoperative pneumonia	Implementation of a clinical pathway resulted in earlier extubation, earlier ambulation, decreased nausea, and postoperative pneumonia.
White (1999) Impact of CNS care on pain-management practices for postoperative patients	CNS	Pain documentation	Implementation of a pain-management program resulted in improved pain documentation.
Naylor et al. (1999) Impact of APN discharge planning and home follow-up of 363 hospitalized elders in randomized control trial	APNs	Readmissions, time to first readmission, acute care visits after discharge, costs, functional status, patient satisfaction	APN follow-up resulted in significant decreases in readmissions, fewer days of hospitalization when readmitted and decreased costs.
Bergeron et al. (1999) Survey data from 285 rural hospitals awarded a Rural Health Care Transition Grant; use and benefit of APN care were assessed	APNs	APN duties, effect of APN on MD workload, benefit of APN in terms of revenues, reduced operating costs	APNs benefit rural hospital care: 20% of hospitals used NPs, 30% used physician assistants (PAs), and 20% used both. APNs were used to visit hospital inpatients, educate patients, visit nursing home patients, and cover the ER. Reported benefits of APNs were $\downarrow$ costs, $\downarrow$ revenues, $\downarrow$ operating costs, $\downarrow$ patient volume, $\downarrow$ staffing needs and improved physician recruitment and retention.

Table 1.5 (continued)

STUDY	APN ROLE	OUTCOME INDICATORS	FINDINGS
Barnason et al. (1998) Impact of CNS intervention for clinical pain management	CNS	Patients' pain ratings; nurse's cognitive knowledge of pain management	CNS intervention for clinical pain management resulted in consistency in patient's ability to rate pain intensity; and a significant improvement of staff nurse knowledge of pain management.
Dahle et al. (1998) Study on impact of acute care NP on cost of managing 215 inpatients with heart failure	NP	Hospital costs, LOS, 30-day readmission rate, cost savings	Total hospital costs and length of stay were significantly lower, with an estimated annual total cost savings of $133,000.
Sechrist & Berlin (1998) Literature review related to role of clinical nurse specialist (CNS)	CNS	CNS contributions to patient and family outcomes, cost of care	Measurement of impact of CNS practice on care outcomes is difficult because of the indirect nature of much of CNS practice. There is a lack of effective documentation for CNS outcomes. There is a need for selection of appropriate nurse-sensitive patient outcome indicators.
Alexander et al. (1998) Impact of CNS-managed program for children with chronic asthma	CNS	ER visits	CNS-managed patients had a significant decrease in ER visits ($p < 0.0001$).

(continued)

Table 1.5 (continued)

STUDY	APN ROLE	OUTCOME INDICATORS	FINDINGS
Paladichuk (1997) Evaluation of effect of CNS and NP in outpatient chronic disease clinic for congestive heart failure patients	CNS & NP	Quality of life, cost savings, annual readmission rate	APN-run clinic resulted in the prevention of 160 readmissions a year (cost savings of $1.2 million); ↓ in annual readmissions from 11% to 1%, and a ↑ in quality of life at 6 months after initial visit.
Ziemer et al. (1996) 6-month prospective study of 325 type II diabetes patients at 2, 4, 6, and 12 months at hospital-based clinic	NP	Metabolic profiles, HbA_{1c} weight loss	Significant decreases in HbA_{1c}: 52% of obese patients lost weight; 59% of patients were maintained on diet control alone; 35% of patients using pharmacologic agents discontinued oral agents or insulin by 1 year.
Mitchell-Dicenso et al. (1996) Randomized controlled study comparing outcomes of NP-CNS team with pediatric resident team in a neonatal ICU	NP-CNS	LOS, mortality rates, complication rates, parent satisfaction, quality of care, costs	No significant differences were found between NP-CNS team and resident staff in all outcome measures.
Hooker & McCaig (1996) Comparisons of emergency room NP and PA care with physician care using data from the National Ambulatory Medical Care Survey	NP	Type of ER patient cared for, drugs prescribed, diagnostic screening tests ordered, diagnoses made	No differences between the services of the NP-PA group and physicians.

Table 1.5 (continued)

STUDY	APN ROLE	OUTCOME INDICATORS	FINDINGS
Venner & Steelbinder (1996) Evaluation of impact of case management and implementation of CNS-led clinical path in 40 congestive heart patients compared to 40 nonpath patients	CNS	30-day readmission rate, LOS, cost of care	Average hospital charges, LOS, readmission rate and mortality rate ↓ in clinical path patients compared to nonpath patients. Patients followed in the outpatient congestive heart failure clinic ($n = 84$) had 0% hospital readmission rate at 2 years.
Mahoney (1994) National random-sample comparison of prescribing decisions of NPs ($n = 298$) and MDs ($n = 373$) using 3 standardized geriatric case vignettes	NP	Index of appropriateness of prescribing decisions	NPs scored higher on the index of appropriateness than physicians ($p < 0.001$), a difference that remained whether or not the NP had prescriptive authority. NPs made more recommendations for nondrug therapeutic interventions, compared to MDs ($p < .001$).
Hylka & Beschle (1995) Retrospective chart reviews of surgery patients and general discussion of impact of NP care	NP	Cost savings, inservice teaching to RNs, patient education literature, review of practice guidelines	Implementing NP care into neurosurgery and general surgery resulted in cost savings related to patient care orders and creation of practice guidelines. NPs also contributed to patient and RN education.
Brooten & Naylor (1995) Review article on effect of APNs in a variety of settings, including rehabilitation, home care, nursing homes, and hospitals	NPs-CNSs	Variety of indicators used, including return-to-work rates, patient education, hospital admission rates, ER visits, hospital length of stay, and others	Substantiated the positive impact of APN care in: ↓ LOS, ↓ health care costs, ↓ hospital admissions, ↓ readmission rates, ↓ patient education, and others.

(continued)

Table 1.5 (continued)

STUDY	APN ROLE	OUTCOME INDICATORS	FINDINGS
Langner & Hutelmyer (1995) Patient satisfaction survey to 52 patients with HIV, comparing NP to physician provider care in an ambulatory care services clinic	NP	Clinic wait time, patient perceptions of provider knowledge, continuity of care, social service support, patient education	Overall satisfaction with patient care was high. NP ratings were higher in areas of provider knowledge, continuity of care, patient education, and clinic wait time.
Sulzbach-Hoke & Gift (1995) Quality assessment of implementation of nutritional support guidelines for intubated patients for 51 patients over a 12-month time period	CNS	Length of time to institute nutrition, presence of complications	Intubated patients were fed sooner after initiation of nutritional guidelines by CNS; days to institute feedings was reduced by 6.4 days; average time from start of intubation to decision to feed was reduced from 11 to 4.6 days.
Carzoli et al. (1994) 6-month retrospective chart-review comparison of neonatal NP, PA, and resident physician care	NP	LOS, use of total parenteral nutrition; blood transfusions, procedure complication rate, infant mortality	No differences in outcomes of NPs, PAs, and resident MD staff; NP-PA care was associated with an overall cost savings in terms of annual costs and hospital charges.
Lombness (1994) Descriptive study using retrospective chart audits of 105 randomly selected CABG patients cared for by PA and CNS teams comanaged with cardiac surgeons	CNS	LOS; complications, including dysrhythmias, abnormal lab values, infections, labile blood pressure, urinary retention, pneumothorax, thrombus	CNS-managed group had a statistically significant shorter length of stay. Complication rates were similar.

Table 1.5 (continued)

STUDY	APN ROLE	OUTCOME INDICATORS	FINDINGS
Hanneman et al. (1993) Retrospective chart audits pre- ($n = 79$ patients) and post-implementation ($n = 81$ patients) of a unit-based CNS (formal workshops and daily rounds) examining indirect patient care effects on reducing incidence of pulmonary complications	CNS	Preventable pulmonary complications, including malpositioned endotracheal tube and inadvertent extubation	Incidence rates of malpositioned endotracheal tubes was significantly reduced ($p < .001$) and inadvertent extubations were decreased ($p = .021$) after 6 months of implementation of unit-based CNS interventions.
Neidlinger et al. (1987) Experimental study evaluating discharge planning activities of gerontological CNS for hospitalized elderly patients ($n = 39$) verus control group ($n = 41$)	CNS	Costs of care, gross excess revenues	Hospital costs for CNS-managed patients averaged $60 less per patient per day; gross excess revenues were higher for CNS-managed patients by $911 per patient ($35,529 difference between groups).
Cintron et al. (1983) Chart review of 15 patients with congestive heart failure in a cardiology clinic before and after introduction of NP in a heart failure clinic	NP	In-hospital time, medical costs, patient satisfaction	Decrease in number of hospitalizations from 2.8 to 0.7 per patient; decrease in number of hospitalized days from 62 to 9; decrease in in-hospital costs of $8,009 per patient; patient satisfaction and reports of better care, rapport, and less wait.
DiGirol & Parry (1983) Comparison of frequency of consultation and similarities in treatment plans of pediatric CNS and pediatrician in pediatric acute emergency clinic	CNS	Comparison of treatment on eye and throat cultures, cough protocols, antibiotics used, ABD and X-ray studies and referrals	In 83% of cases, CNS was able to independently manage care. Overall agreement on treatment plans was high (69%).

(continued)

Table 1.5 (continued)

STUDY	APN ROLE	OUTCOME INDICATORS	FINDINGS
Weinberg et al. (1983) Chart review of 25 inpatients in a rehabilitation hospital comparing NP care to internist care	NP	LOS, laboratory, and X-ray costs, consultations, index scores on management of common medical problems, including UTI, congestive heart failure, anemia, diabetes, hypertension, and hypokalemia	No significant differences were found between the patient groups managed by the NP supervised by an internist and 3 independent internists.
Simborg et al. (1978) Chart review of 1,369 patient-practitioner encounters to compare MD ($n = 109$) to NP ($n = 35$) in primary care practices	NP	Diagnoses, tests, non-drug therapies	MDs prescribed more drug therapies ($p < .05$); NPs recorded more signs and symptoms; NPs emphasized patient education more than MDs.
Runyan (1975) Experimental study of care provided by NP to 1,006 patients, compared to MD care to 498 ambulatory patients with diabetes, hypertension, and CV disease	NP	Clinic visits, blood glucose, diastolic blood pressure, hospital inpatient days, mortality	Patients with hypertensive disease experienced greater reductions in diastolic blood pressure. Patients with diabetes had greater reductions in blood glucose levels and patients had fewer hospitalization days ($p < .05$).

Table 1.6

STUDIES ASSESSING PATIENT-RELATED OUTCOMES OF ADVANCED PRACTICE NURSING (APN) CARE

STUDY	APN ROLE	OUTCOME INDICATORS	FINDINGS
Sears et al. (2007) Impact of 3-year pilot program to expand nurse practitioner (NP) care in state workers' compensation system	NP	Medical costs and disability outcomes	Likelihood of work–time loss was less for NP claims; duration of lost work time and medical costs did not differ with medical doctors (MDs).
Paez & Allen (2006) NP management of hypercholesterolemia following coronary revascularization	NP	Low-density-lipoprotein (LDL) cholesterol change	Case management by an NP resulted in significant reduction in LDL cholesterol levels.
McCabe (2005) Impact of CNS care for patients with atrial fibrillation	CNS	Patient self-care management complications of treatment, care fragmentation	CNS care resulted in improved patient functioning and self-care management, reduced complications of treatment and decreased fragmentation of care.
Tsay et al. (2005) Impact of CNS care for patients with end-stage renal disease	CNS	Perceived stress, depression, quality of life	CNS-managed patients had less perceived stress ($p = 0.0005$), depression ($p = 0.001$), and improved quality of life ($p = 0.02$).
Krein et al. (2004) Randomized clinical trial of NP care for patients with diabetes	NP	Glycemic control, patient satisfaction	There were no differences in glycemic control; patients managed by NPs had higher satisfaction.
Gracias et al. (2003) NP care in surgical intensive care unit (ICU) for 900 patient days	NP	Influence on compliance with clinical practice guideline use for deep vein thrombosis/pulmonary embolism (DVT/PE), stress ulcer and anemia	Compliance was significantly higher for NP team for all 3 clinical practice guidelines (DVT/PE $p < .001$, stress ulcer $p < .001$, anemia $p < .02$).

(continued)

Table 1.6 (continued)

STUDY	APN ROLE	OUTCOME INDICATORS	FINDINGS
Cooper et al. (2002) NP care in emergency room (ER) for 199 patients	NP	Patient care, patient satisfaction, clinical documentation	Patients reported higher levels of satisfaction with NP care compared to MD care ($p < .001$), and NP clinical documentation was rated of higher quality ($p < .001$). There were no differences in level of symptoms, recovery times, or unplanned follow-up between the groups.
Corner et al. (2003) Longitudinal study assessing impact of palliative care APN on cancer patients over 28 days	APN	Quality of life, anxiety scores	Significant improvements were found in emotional ($p = .03$) and cognitive functioning ($p = .03$) and a decrease in anxiety scores ($p = .003$).
Kelley et al. (2002) Impact of NP preventative care for cervical cancer screening	NP	Cervical cancer screening	NP preventative care for cervical cancer resulted in a significant increase in documentation of cervical cancer screening (from 2% to 69%).
Bryant & Graham (2002) Client satisfaction of 506 patients who received care by 36 APNs at 26 different practice sites	APN	Client satisfaction scores	Client satisfaction scores were high, indicating patients were very satisfied with APN care.
Dellasega et al. (2002) Impact of APN intervention for caregivers of frail rural older adults	APN	Caregiver physical health and well-being, stress, burden	Caregivers in the APN-managed group experienced more positive physical and emotional health outcomes, and fewer depressive symptoms.

Table 1.6 (continued)

STUDY	APN ROLE	OUTCOME INDICATORS	FINDINGS
Moore et al. (2002) Randomized clinical trial of APN care for patients with lung cancer	APN	Quality of life, patient satisfaction, resource use, costs of care	APN-managed patients reported less dyspnea at 3 months ($p = 0.03$), better care for emotional functioning ($p = 0.03$), and higher quality of life ($p = 0.01$).
Rantz et al. (2001) CNS care for nursing home patients	CNS	Resident assessment measures, falls, activity behavior, presssure ulcers	CNS care resulted in trends in improvement in quality improvement measures including falls, behavior symptoms, activity, and pressure ulcers.
Sole et al. (2001) NP care on trauma service during a 6-month period	NP	Types of patients cared for; diagnoses; orders; patient disposition	NPs identified new diagnoses in 53% of patients; they were also more likely to order rehabilitation and discharge planning, bowel management, and nutrition-based orders.
Benkert et al. (2001) Assessment of blood pressure control for patients with hypertension in a nurse-managed center	NP	Blood pressure control	Insured and uninsured patients managed by NPs had comparable blood pressure control; uninsured patients averaged 3.2 more visits per year.
Willoughby & Burroughs (2001) Descriptive study of impact of CNS care for skin care of diabetic patients	CNS	Foot-care practices	CNS-managed patients were more likely to use appropriate foot-care practices.
Blue et al. (2001) Randomized controlled trial of NP care for 165 heart failure patients	NP	Readmission, length of stay (LOS)	Compared with usual care, patients in NP group had fewer readmissions for heart failure ($p = .018$) and spent fewer days in hospital for heart failure ($p = .0051$).

(continued)

Table 1.6 (continued)

STUDY	APN ROLE	OUTCOME INDICATORS	FINDINGS
Diesch et al. (2000) Impact of CNS guided imagery intervention for coronary artery bypass surgery patients	CNS	Pain, fatigue, anxiety, narcotic use, LOS, patient satisfaction	CNS guided imagery intervention resulted in ↓ pain, fatigue, anxiety, narcotic use, and LOS and ↑ patient satisfaction.
Lacko et al. (2000). Quasi-experimental study assessing impact of APN education intervention for staff nurses	APN	Delirium-screening abilities of staff nurses	An APN educational intervention resulted in improved delirium-screening abilities of staff nurses.
Wheeler (2000). Quasi-experimental comparative study of CNS managed care for patients with total knee replacement	CNS	LOS, complications	CNS-managed patients received more nursing care interventions, had ↓ LOS, and fewer complications
Ryden et al. (2000). Randomized controlled trial of APN intervention for long-term-care residents.	APN	Incontinence, pressure ulcers, aggressive behavior	APN-managed patients experienced greater improvement or less decline in incontinence, pressure ulcers, and aggressive behavior.
Ritz et al. (2000) Randomized clinical trial of APN intervention for newly diagnosed patients with breast cancer	APN	Well-being, mood states, uncertainty, costs of care	Uncertainty decreased significantly in the intervention group at 1, 3, and 6 months with the strongest effect on subscales of complexity, inconsistency, and unpredictability. There were no differences in costs.

Table 1.6 (continued)

STUDY	APN ROLE	OUTCOME INDICATORS	FINDINGS
Bargardi (1999) Chart review of documentation and adherence to best practice guidelines for 180 patients undergoing cardiac catheterizations or percutaneous coronary interventions	NP	Indicators of best practice, including lipid management, smoking cessation counseling, nutrition/diet recommendations, physical activity recommendations, control of blood pressure, diabetes/glucose control, medication therapy	NP care significantly increased adherence to best-practice guidelines. The use of all best-practice indicators increased; LOS decreased, 12-month LDL goals achieved in 91% to 94% of NP-managed patients compared to 10% to 17% of patients managed by primary care physician.
Topp et al. (1998) Quasi-experimental retrospective review of CNS care for patients with congestive heart failure	CNS	LOS, hospital charges	CNS-managed patients demonstrated ↓LOS and reduced costs.
Buchanan & Powers (1997) Study of NP-staffed minor ER regarding aspects of patient care	NP	Visit time, patient satisfaction, patient complaints, laceration care, NP job satisfaction	Visit times for NPs were shorter in minor emergency than main emergency area; patients' and NPs' satisfaction were high. Laceration care audits showed appropriate care.
Miller (1997) Retrospective analysis of care to nursing home elderly patients admitted to a hospital by NP and PA–physician teams	NP	LOS	Comanagement of NP and physician team resulted in shorter LOS in 17 of 20 diagnostic groups; overall mean decrease in stay of 2.78 days, compared to PA-physician teams.

(continued)

Table 1.6 (continued)

STUDY	APN ROLE	OUTCOME INDICATORS	FINDINGS
Crimslick et al. (1997) Impact of CNS on endotracheal intubation rates	CNS	Unplanned extubation, reintubations	CNS intervention resulted in ↓ reintubation rate ($p = .005$).
Pozen et al. (1997). Prospective randomized study assessing impact of CNS on rehabilitation of patients with myocardial infarction	CNS	Return-to-work rate, smoking cessation, patient knowledge	CNS-managed patients had increased return-to-work rates ($p < .05$), decreased smoking ($p < .05$), increased patient knowledge of heart disease ($p < .01$).
York et al. (1997). Randomized clinical trial of CNS managed care for high-risk childbearing women	CNS	Rehospitalizations, hospital charges, low-birth-weight infants	CNS-managed patients had fewer rehospitalizations, were less likely to have infants with a low birth weight (< 2500 g), and less costs of care.
Hankins et al. (1996) Cross-sectional patient satisfaction survey of 3,257 women from 10 collaborative obstetrical-gynecological practices comparing collaborative practice versus physician-only practice	NP	Patient satisfaction, practice efficiency, provider qualities, wait time	Higher percentage of patients in collaborative practices reported shorter wait times ($p = .001$), more time with provider ($p = .001$), more individualized care ($p = .001$), more health information ($p = .05$), better preventive care ($p = .001$), and more specific diet information ($p = .017$).
Patton & Schaerf (1995) Impact of teaching plan on patients with thoracotomy	CNS	LOS, ancillary resource use, recidivism after surgery, costs of care	Over a 2-year period a CNS-led coordinated teaching plan resulted in ↓ LOS, less use of ancillary resources, less recidivism, and reduced costs of care.

Table 1.6 (continued)

STUDY	APN ROLE	OUTCOME INDICATORS	FINDINGS
Haddock (1994) Impact of CNS-led discharge planning intervention	CNS	LOS, readmissions postdischarge service use	CNS intervention resulted in shorter LOS, fewer readmissions, and higher rate of postdischarge service use.
Damato et al. (1993) Impact of CNS-directed care for very low-birth-weight infants	CNS	Acute care visits; infant rehospitalizations	CNS-managed care resulted in $\downarrow$ acute care visits ($p < .01$) and infant rehospitalizations ($p < .01$).
Russell (1989) Retrospective audit of impact of CNS care on modified radical mastectomy patients	CNS	LOS, costs of care	CNS-managed patients had $\downarrow$ LOS and $\downarrow$ costs of care ($p < .001$).

Performance-Related Outcomes of APN Care

Performance-related outcomes include those outcomes that reflect the quality of care provided by APNs. Other studies in this category have compared APN care with care provided by other midlevel providers, such as PAs, or other health care providers, such as medical residents and MDs. Studies in this category have also measured the effect of APN care on quality of care, interpersonal skills, technical quality, completeness of documentation, time spent in role components, patient perceptions of care, and clinical examination comprehensiveness (Aubrey & Yoxall, 2001; Avorn, Everitt, & Baker, 1991; Bevis et al., 2008; Considine, Martin, Smit, Winter, & Jenkins, 2006; Hoffman, Miller, Zullo, & Donahoe, 2006; Kirkwood, Pesudovs, Loh, & Coster, 2005; Lambing, Adams, Fox, & Divine, 2004; Lenz, Mundinger, Hopkins, Lin, & Smolowitz, 2002; Mundinger et al., 2000; Pioro et al., 2001; Reveley, 1998; Rhee & Dermyer, 1995; Seale et al., 2006; Sidani et al., 2006; Spisso et al., 1990; Stetler et al., 1998; Sullivan-Marx & Maislin, 2000; Vazirani, Hays, Shapiro, & Cowan, 2005; Woods, 2006). Clinical outcomes, processes of care, use of services, and cost-effectiveness have been found to be equivalent or superior to MD, PA, and medical resident care (Batey & Holland, 1985; Brown & Grimes, 1995; Hall et al., 1990; Monroe et al., 1982; Moody et al., 1999; Mundinger et al., 1999; Ockene, Adams, Gurley, Wheeler, & Hebert, 1999; Poduri et al., 1996; Prescott & Driscol, 1979; Rudy et al., 1998; Sakr et al., 1999; Sox, 1979; Spitzer, 1997; Sullivan-Marx & Maislin, 2000; U.S. Congress Office of Technology Assessment, 1986).

Table 1.7 outlines studies in this category of APN outcomes, including outcome measures explored. Of those studies conducted and published in the literature, those categorized as assessing performance-related outcomes of APN practice represent the largest number of studies.

Although categorization of APN studies facilitates analysis and critique, the categories are not mutually exclusive. Several studies combined measures of care-related, patient-related, and performance-related outcome measures. As APNs are evaluated on several levels, including clinical aspects of care, productivity, resource use, and patient satisfaction, multiple measures may be needed to establish the impact of the APN role (Buppert, 1999).

Table 1.7

STUDIES ASSESSING PERFORMANCE-RELATED OUTCOMES OF ADVANCED PRACTICE NURSING (APN) CARE

STUDY	APN ROLE	OUTCOME INDICATORS	FINDINGS
Bevis et al. (2008) Comparison of outcomes of thoracostomies performed by nurse practitioners (NPs) vs medical doctors (MDs)	NP	Insertion complications, (length of stay) LOS, morbidity	There were no differences in insertion complications, LOS, or morbidity.
McCorkle et al. (2007) Randomized clinical trial of a an APN intervention for patients with a radical prostatectomy	APN	Quality of life, depressive symptoms	Patients experienced more moral distress related to sexual functioning while spouses experienced marital interaction distress; both patients and spouses reported decreased depression.
Considine et al. (2006) Comparison of NP care with emergency room (ER) MD care for patients with hand/wrist wounds, hand/wrist fractures and cast removal	NP	ER wait times, treatment time, LOS in ER	There were no differences in median wait times, treatment times, and LOS in ER.
Hoffman et al. (2006) Comparison of NP and MD care for 192 intensive care unit (ICU) mechanically ventilated patients	NP	LOS, days of mechanical ventilation, readmissions, mortality	There were no differences in LOS, days of mechanical ventilation, critical care fellow care readmissions, weaning status or mortality.
Krichbaum et al. (2005) Impact of APN intervention to reinforce protocols for long-term-care residents	APN	Urinary incontinence, pressure ulcers, depression, aggression	An APN-directed intervention resulted in improved resident outcomes for urinary incontinence, pressure ulcers, depression, and aggression.

(continued)

Table 1.7 (continued)

STUDY	APN ROLE	OUTCOME INDICATORS	FINDINGS
Seale et al. (2006) Comparison of treatment advice of primary care NP vs general MD practitioners	NP	Treatment advise during same-day appointments	A statistically significant greater proportion of NP's talk concerned treatments, with discussion of how to use treatments and of side effects.
Sidani et al. (2006) Comparison of processes of care (roles and coordination of services) of acute care NPs and physician residents	NP	Patient perceptions of care	NPs engaged in management and informal coordination activities more than MDs while MDs engaged in more formal coordination activities. NPs encouraged more patient participation in care and provided more patient education.
Woods (2006) Comparison of neonatal NP and MD care for neonates	NP	Assessment and clinical examination comprehensiveness, completeness of management plan, procedures performed, medications ordered, quality of record keeping	Management and care were found to be similar; there were no statistically significant differences in the standard and quality of care; however NPs did not perform as well as MDs in terms of overall completeness or comprehensiveness of care.
Vazirani et al. (2005) 2-year review of NP care for inpatients	NP	Perceptions of NP role by 156 MDs and 123 staff nurses	Physicians reported greater collaboration ($p < .001$) and better communication ($p = .006$); nurses reported better communication with NPs than with MDs ($p < .001$).

Table 1.7 (continued)

STUDY	APN ROLE	OUTCOME INDICATORS	FINDINGS
Hoffman et al. (2005) Comparison of acute care NP care with critical care fellows care for 526 ICU patients	NP	Readmission, duration of mechanical ventilation, LOS	There were no differences in readmission, mortality, duration of mechanical ventilation, LOS or disposition.
Kleinpell (2005) 5-year longidutinal study of 437 acute care NPs	NP	Role and role components	Acute care nurse practitioners (ACNPs) reported spending a majority of time in direct patient care management (85% to 88%). Other aspects of the role include teaching, research, program development, quality assurance and administrative components.
Lambing et al. (2004) Comparison of NP and MD care for geriatric inpatients	NP	Time spent in activities including patient care, documentation, care planning, charges per LOS, readmission and mortality rates	Readmission and mortality rates were similar. NPs spent more time doing progress notes and care planning; MDs spent more time on literature reviews. Charges per LOS were lower for MDs.
Aigner et al. (2004) Comparison of NP and MD care for nursing home residents	NP	ER visits, hospitalizations, LOS, costs, annual history and physical exams	No differences were found between the groups for the outcomes; NP-managed patients were seen more often, reflecting increased patient access to care.
Lenz et al. (2004) Comparison of NP and MD care for primary care patients	NP	Health status, disease specific physiologic measures, ER visits satisfaction	No differences were found between the groups in any measure.

(continued)

Table 1.7 (continued)

STUDY	APN ROLE	OUTCOME INDICATORS	FINDINGS
Scisney-Matlock et al. (2004) Comparison of hypertension care by physicians versus physician–APN care	NP	Blood pressure control, patient knowledge of hypertension	NP–MD-managed patients had lower bp readings and higher scores for discussion of blood pressure readings.
Hoffman et al. (2003) ACNP care in comparison to pulmonary critical care fellows in ICU	NP	Activities and roles in the ICU	ACNPs and fellows spent a similar proportion of time performing required tasks. Physicians spent more time in nonunit activities such as education while ACNPs spent more time interacting with patients and patients' families and collaborating with health care team.
Lenz et al. (2002) Comparison of NP and MD care for adults with type 2 diabetes	NP	Processes of care, HbA_{1c} testing, documentation	NPs were more likely than MDs to document HbA_{1c} levels, general education, patient height, urinalysis results and education about nutrition, weight, exercise and medications.
Aubrey & Yoxall (2001) Comparison of neonatal NP vs MD care in resuscitation of 245 preterm infants at birth	NP	Resuscitation outcomes	Resuscitation teams led by neonatal NPs provided the same interventions as those led by MDs. Babies resuscitated by NPs were intubated more quickly, received surfactant sooner ($p = .0001$) and were less likely to be hypothermic on admission to the ICU ($p = .013$).

Table 1.7 (continued)

STUDY	APN ROLE	OUTCOME INDICATORS	FINDINGS
Pioro et al. (2001) Comparison of NP and MD care for 381 general medical patients	NP	LOS, costs, consultations, complications, transfers to ICU	There were no significant differences between NP and MD care.
Sullivan-Marx & Maislin (2000) Exploratory comparison study of NP ($n = 43$) and family MD ($n = 46$) relative work values in the Medicare fee schedule for 3 office visit codes	NP	Relative work values and intensity for 3 current procedural terminology (CPT) codes for office visits: 99203 (office visit for new patient), 99213 (office visit for established patient with low complexity medical decisions), and 99215 (office or outpatient visit of established patient with high-complexity medical decisions)	No significant differences between NPs and MDs were found in the 3 CPT codes for relative work values and intensity. NPs estimated higher intraservice (face-to-face) time with patients ($p < .01$); MDs estimated higher pre-service time (reviewing health records, lab data) and post-service time ($p < .05$) (documentation, coordination of care, contact with family and insurer).
Mundinger et al. (2000) Randomized trial of NP and physician care in primary care in 4 community-based and 1 hospital-based clinic; care delivered to 806 NP patients was compared to care given to 510 physician patients	NP	Patient satisfaction, health status, physiologic test results, 1 year use of services	No significant differences found in patient's health status at 6 months; no differences in health service use at 6 months or 1 year; no differences in satisfaction ratings following initial appointment; satisfaction with provider attributes was higher for physician at 6 months; for patients with hypertension, diastolic value was lower.
Karlowicz &McMurray (2000) Comparison of neonatal NP and pediatric residents' care of 201 low-birth-weight infants	NP	LOS, survival to discharge, costs	There were no significant differences between NP and MD care.

(continued)

Table 1.7 (continued)

STUDY	APN ROLE	OUTCOME INDICATORS	FINDINGS
Moody et al. (1999) Survey research study of random sample of 115 NPs practicing 20 or more hours per week in primary care in Tennessee during one selected day of care involving 680 clients compared to physician practices based on the National Ambulatory Medical Care Survey	NP	Client health status, diagnostic tests ordered, therapeutic interventions, client disposition	NPs tended to care for more younger and female clients, perform fewer office surgical procedures (1.5% versus 6.1%), and provide more health teaching/counseling interventions, including nutrition counseling (19% versus 15%), exercise (12% versus 7%), weight reduction (15% versus 4%), smoking cessation (7% versus 2.5%), and family planning counseling (5% versus 0.1%).
Chang et al. (1999) Comparison of NP care and MD care in ER setting for 232 patients	NP	Wound care management, treatment of blunt limb trauma, patient satisfaction	No significant differences were found between NP and MD care.
Ockene et al. (1999) Randomized study of patient-centered counseling to 530 high-risk drinkers by NPs, attending MDs and resident MDs	NP	Change in alcohol use from baseline to 6 months as measured by weekly alcohol consumption and frequency of binge drinking episodes	Brief (5–10 minute) advice and counseling by NP or MD as part of routine primary care significantly reduced alcohol consumption by high-risk drinkers. There were no differences in provider characteristics by treatment condition for NP, attending physicians or resident physicians.

Table 1.7 (continued)

STUDY	APN ROLE	OUTCOME INDICATORS	FINDINGS
Sakr et al. (1999) Randomized control trial in United Kingdom of ER patients cared for by NP ($n = 704$) or by MD ($n = 704$) compared to junior doctor ($n = 749$ patients)	NP	Adequacy of care, history taking, examination of patient, interpretation of X-rays, treatment decisions, advice, follow-up	There were no differences in the % of NPs and junior doctors making clinically important errors (9.2% for NPs versus 10.7% for MDs); NPs were better at recording medical history and fewer patients seen by NP had to seek unplanned follow-up advice about their injury; there were no differences between NPs and MDs in accuracy of exams, adequacy of treatment, planned follow-up, or requests for or interpretation of X-rays.
Rudy et al. (1998) Study comparing outcomes of 16 ACNPs and PAs, 16 resident physicians at 2 academic medical centers for 187 patients treated by the ACNP-PA team and 202 patients treated by the resident physicians	NP	Number of patients cared for, completeness of admission note, readmission rates, occurrence of drug reactions, in-hospital mortality rate, LOS, personal activities, care-related activities, activities during rounds	No difference in patient-related outcomes; ACNP-PA group was more likely to include social history in patients admission note and to take a more active role in discussing patient outcomes with the bedside nurse and family.
Stetler et al. (1998) Program evaluation of acute care NP role in medical, neonatal and cardiothoracic ICUs	NP	Performance ratings by adminstrators, physicians, nursing staff and patients; role performance, clinical competency, process of care, including continuity of patient care, timely orders, collaboration, prevention of complications, cost of care	Positive performance ratings were given by clinicians, patients and families; ACNPs had positive impact on patient care quality and process of care.

(continued)

Table 1.7 (continued)

STUDY	APN ROLE	OUTCOME INDICATORS	FINDINGS
Reveley (1998) 2-year evaluation study comparing care given by MD (*n* = 173 patients) and NP care (*n* = 113 patients) in general medical practice group in England	NP	Patient satisfaction, work analysis	All patients were satisfied with length of time spent with either NP or MD. Both MD and NP gave advice along with a prescription, but NP was more likely to examine the patient; NPs' consultations averaged 15 minutes compared to 7.5 for MDs; 93.3% of patients waited less than 1 day to see the NP.
Spitzer (1997) Evaluation of 4 models of nurse faculty practice: primary care, physician partnership, outsourcing of NPs and employee-based health care	NP	Quality of health care, access to care, communication among health care team members, job satisfaction	NPs delivered health care at 23% below average cost of other providers; NP inpatient rate was 21% below average, lab utilization was 24% below average, prescription drug use was 42% below average and 82% of patients reported being very satisfied with the quality of care.
Freij et al. (1996) Retrospective analysis comparison of NP and senior house MDs for ability to request and interpret X-rays of patients in a minor injury unit in the United Kingdom	NP	X-ray request and interpretation	There were no statistically significant differences in the ability of NPs and MDs in requests or interpretation of X-rays. In both groups, an X-ray was considered appropriate in 70% of patients; sensitivity of X-ray interpretation was 93% in both groups.

Table 1.7 (continued)

STUDY	APN ROLE	OUTCOME INDICATORS	FINDINGS
Poduri et al. (1996) 3-year comparison of outcomes in stroke patients based on admission to an inpatient unit by an NP or physiatrist	NP	Appropriateness of admission, discharge to home versus nursing home, functional gains, LOS	No significant differences were found in LOS or appropriateness of admissions. 96% of patients in each group were discharged home. Functional goals were reported higher in the physician-treated group; however, the total gain was equal.
Brown & Grimes (1995) Meta-analysis of 53 studies on NPs and certified nurse midwives (CNMs) in primary care roles	NP CNM	Interpersonal skills, process of care, utilization, cost-effectiveness, patient satisfaction	Interpersonal skills of APN were better than physicians; outcomes of NPs and CNMs were equivalent to physicians' outcomes; NPs and CNMs facilitated continuity of patient care and improved access to care in rural and other settings.
Rhee & Dermyer (1995) Prospective telephone survey of 30 patients treated by NP and 30 patients treated by 4th-year medical students or house staff in an emergency department	NP	Patient satisfaction, satisfaction with technical and humanistic care aspects, satisfaction with aspects of ER service	No difference among NP, medical student, and house staff care; overall satisfaction was good in both groups of patients.
Kearnes (1994) Chart review of impact of NP and MD collaborative practice on 110 hospitalized frail elderly compared to 31 matched patients managed by MD only	NP	LOS, timeliness of discharge, number of consultants used, number of treatments	Collaborative practice group had significantly ↓ LOS (32% lower); had significantly ↓ time from admission to first discharge planning visit; had ↓ number of consultant physicians involved.

(continued)

Table 1.7 (continued)

STUDY	APN ROLE	OUTCOME INDICATORS	FINDINGS
Hill et al. (1994) Randomized clinical study comparing NP and MD care in rheumatology clinic	NP	Patient knowledge, physical functioning, lab test results, pain, morning stiffness, mobility, referrals, patient satisfaction	NP-managed patients had significant improvements in mobility, less pain, had acquired greater knowledge and were more satisfied with their care.
Safriet (1992) Synthesis review of APN care studies for NPs and CNMs	NP CNM	Quality of care, relative cost and access, patient satisfaction	NPs and CNMs substantially ↑ access to basic health care and are cost-effective; patients are satisfied with APN care; concluded that significant barriers exist to effective utilization of NPs and CNMs, including scope of practice reimbursment and prescriptive authority restrictions.
Graveley & Littlefield (1992) Descriptive study of 156 women receiving prenatal care at 3 clinics comparing CNS and PA care with physician care	CNS	Adequacy of prenatal visits; physiologic variables, including weight gain, lab values, birth complications; maternal satisfaction, costs of care	No differences on maternal physiological variables; no differences on neonatal variables; no differences in complications; no differences in satisfaction with accessibility and affordability; CNS care had better cost-per-client ratio.
Avorn et al. (1991) Telephone survey of 54 internists (family practice and general practice MDs) and 298 office-based NPs regarding case vignette of a patient with epigastric pain and endoscopy showing gastritis	NP	History taking, treatment recommendations, drug-prescribing practice	NPs more likely to collect more historical information before deciding on therapy, less likely to prescribe prescription drug (12% vs 46%), more likely to ask about diet, less likely to take a drinking history, and more likely to suggest nonprescription treatment approach.

Table 1.7 (continued)

STUDY	APN ROLE	OUTCOME INDICATORS	FINDINGS
Spisso et al. (1990) Retrospective study of use of NPs as part of a trauma service team at a tertiary care center 12 months before and after NP implementation	NP	Cost of care, quality of care, documentation time, clinic wait time, patient complaints, time savings for house staff	Use of NPs was associated with ↓ average LOS, ↓ outpatient clinic wait time, ↓ patient complaints, ↑ documentation of quality of care; time savings of 352 minutes per day for house staff physicians.
Hall et al. (1990) Comparison of care between MDs and residents and NPs and PAs from 8 general medicine and 8 pediatric group practices	NP	Care for 8 conditions evaluated: cancer screening (breast exams and Pap smears), adult glucose, hemoglobin levels, well-child, UTI, otitis media, and gastroenteritis	Comparable or superior performance was found for NPs for all tests except for cancer screening in women.
James & Pyrgos (1989) Comparison of theoretical management of NP and middle-grade physician of walking wounded patients in an accident and emergency department in the United Kingdom	NP	Management of patient, X-ray requests, waiting time savings for patients	Out of 400 patients seen, 332 were assessed by NPs; management of 298 patients was satisfactory; 12 patients were mismanaged by NPs based on local practice; NPs requested X-rays in 22 more patients than MDs. The waiting time savings for patients was 11 minutes.
Crosby et al. (1987) Synthesis of 248 documents that examined NP effectiveness	NP	Use of services, delivery of care, patient satisfaction, access to care, cost effectiveness, patient compliance, health maintenance	NPs had a positive impact on outcomes; NPs performed a comprehensive range of activities.

(continued)

Table 1.7 (continued)

STUDY	APN ROLE	OUTCOME INDICATORS	FINDINGS
Feldman et al. (1987) Synthesis review of 56 studies of NP effectiveness	NP	Ambulatory care prescribing practices, mortality and morbidity, health outcomes, saved MD time, volume of care, technical quality, referrals, administrators' ratings, patient satisfaction	NPs effectively delivered care of equal quality to that of MDs; NP use increased volume of care; utilization of NPs saved MD time, decreased costs; health outcomes similar to MD; patients had more discussion and satisfaction with NPs; NPs more likely to provide patient education than MD.
Office of Technology Assessment (1986) Review of outcomes of NPs, PAs, CNM in primary care setting compared to physician care	NP CNM	Quality of care, access to care, productivity of providers, costs of care	Care provided by APNs was of equivalent quality to physicians; APNs were more adept at providing services that depended on communication and preventive actions; APNs increased access to primary care for underserved populations; increased total practice output by 20% to 50%.
Batey & Holland (1985) Review of log recordings of 89 NPs from 5 states in adult/family practice on 7,086 prescriptions issued during 890 clinical days and comparison to physician practices based on the National Ambulatory Medical Care Survey	NP	Number of prescriptions, average number of drugs prescribed per client visit	Drug utilization of NPs was similar to physican prescribing; intensity of prescribing of NP was less than MD; MD consultation prior to prescribing occurred with the highest incidence for health problems treated with the least frequently prescribed drugs; MD consultation or referral was reported for 14.3% of prescriptions.

Table 1.7 (continued)

STUDY	APN ROLE	OUTCOME INDICATORS	FINDINGS
Thompson et al. (1982) Comparison of NP care (to 735 patients) in HMO to MD-run clinic (to 685 patients)	NP	Quality of examinations, waiting times, costs, patient satisfaction	NP-managed patients had ↓ clinic wait time for appointments (14 days vs 35 for MD group); NP total costs were 36% less, patient satisfaction was higher for NP group; MDs reported ↑ complexity of workload working with NPs but there was no quantitative change in workload.
Monroe et al. (1982) Six-month evaluation of prescribing patterns (1,000 prescriptions randomly analyzed and a detailed audit of 100 cases) of APNs in urban university-affiliated ambulatory care facility	NP & CNS	Prescription practices for primary prevention, secondary prevention, chronic disease maintenance regarding: (1) indication, (2) consistency with formulary and protocol, (3) drug safety	Study demonstrated effective and appropriate use of prescription drugs by APNs; 98% of drugs prescribed were indicated according to evidence in the record; 99% of drugs ordered were consistent with protocol; all audited records were deemed appropriate in relation to safety.
Salkever et al. (1982) Participant observation comparing efficiency of MD and NP in treating otitis media (409 cases) and sore throat (390 cases) in pediatric medicine department	NP	Cost of episode of care for otitis media and sore throat	NP per-episode costs were 20% below MD costs; NP care was less costly but not less effective.
De Jong (1981) Retrospective chart reviews of 444 patients of a women's health clinic comparing CNS and PA care with resident care	CNS	Frequency of consultation, identification of surgical candidates, discovery of malignancies, patient compliance to seek follow-up for abnormal Pap test	Care delivered by CNSs and PAs was not different than that delivered by resident physicians; patient compliance was increased for the CNS and PA provider patients.

(continued)

Table 1.7 (continued)

STUDY	APN ROLE	OUTCOME INDICATORS	FINDINGS
Thompson (1980) Contrast of effectiveness of neonatal transport NPs with MDs	NPs	Neonatal survival rates, stabilization, and transport management	No difference in overall survival rates; NPs demonstrated equal ability to assess, manage, stabilize, and transport ill newborns.
Brown et al. (1979) Evaluation of patient satisfaction with NP and MD care	NP	Attitude scale of health appraisal, clinic wait time	Although both groups received favorable patient evaluations, NPs received significantly more; NPs had shorter wait time and more new problems identified; equal patient satisfaction ratings were found for both groups concerning patient compliance, existing health problems undetected, confidence in and cost of the exam.
Sox (1979) Synthesis review of 21 studies comparing NP and PA care with MD care in office-based practice	NP	Quality of care including disease control, symptom relief, satisfaction, triage of acute illness, accuracy of clinical diagnosis	Concluded that NPs and PAs provide office-based care equal in quality to care provided by physicians.
Prescott & Driscoll (1979) Synthesis review of 31 studies comparing NP and MD practice in primary health care	NP	Patient satisfaction, disease- or condition-specific outcomes, global functioning, hospitalizations, mortality, discharge from care	Reviewed studies with the intent of assessing comparison criteria and research methods. Concluded NPs are at least as capable as MDs in performing primary care functions. Recommended that random sampling use of multiple data sources and evaluations of NP effectiveness should represent the full range of the NP role.

Table 1.7 (continued)

STUDY	APN ROLE	OUTCOME INDICATORS	FINDINGS
Chambers et al. (1977) Chart review of care given to rural Canadians by NP (*n* = 167 patients) versus MD group (*n* = 1,146 patients)	NP	Primary care visits, hospital days, health service costs	NP-managed patients had 186% increase in primary care visits, hospital visits decreased 35% and hospital days decreased by 5%; NP-managed patients also had an increase in prenatal visits, well-child visits and school exams; costs increased 26% for NPs vs 21% by MD group.
Spitzer (1997) Canadian study comparing NP to family physician care	NP	Mortality, physical functioning capacity, social and emotional functioning	No differences in mortality rates, physical functioning capacity, social and emotional functioning; evidence of acceptance of NP by patients and other health care providers were found.
Russo et al. (1975) Tape-recorded analysis of NPs in evening telephone call management system compared to pediatric house MDs and pediatricians	NP	History taking, disposition, telephone communication skills	NPs averaged 79.6% possible score vs 52.6% for MDs. NPs' evaluation agreed with MD 84% of the time. Study concluded that NPs could effectively share telephone calls with physician backup.
Spitzer et al. (1974) & Sackett et al. (1974) Randomized trial of NP (*n* = 1,058 families) and MD (*n* = 540 families) care in primary care practices in Canada	NP	Clinical activities, diagnosis, procedures, mortality, physical functioning, emotional and social functioning	No difference between MD and NP care for mortality rates and patient physical, emotional, or social functioning; management of care was rated adequate for 69% of NP care vs 66% of MD care.

(continued)

Table 1.7 (continued)

STUDY	APN ROLE	OUTCOME INDICATORS	FINDINGS
Skinner & Kahn (1972) Comparison of care of pediatric NP and residents in primary care facility	NP	Time management, consultation requirements, patient satisfaction	NP spent more time with patients; NP consulted in 79% of patient assessments compared to residents consulting on only 2 occasions; 90% of patients were satisfied.
Duncan, Smith, & Silver (1971) Chart review comparison of care given to 182 pediatric patients in community health clinic by NPs and MDs	NP	Physical examination, diagnosis, treatment	There was total agreement in the findings of the NP and consulting MD in 239 of 278 conditions noted in the 182 children; there was a difference in assessment of 39 (0.7%) conditions and in 37 the difference was not considered significant.
Charney & Kitzman (1971) Comparison of NP-MD team care to newborns ($n = 703$) vs MD care ($n = 517$)	NP	Number of newborn visits, duration of visit, attitudes of parents, costs	There was no difference in total number of visits made between the groups; NP group had twice as many calls and were able to handle 153 of 158 calls independently; NP presence resulted in ↓ MD telephone time by 1/5; parents reported positive satisfaction with NP care.

Table 1.7 (continued)

STUDY	APN ROLE	OUTCOME INDICATORS	FINDINGS
Day et al. (1970) Opinion survey of parents of pediatric patients of NP–MD combined care practice	NP	Services provided, communication, having questions answered, telephone service, home visits, hospital visit care	Parents (94%) expressed satisfaction with NP-MD care; 57% reported that joint care was better than care received from a physician alone; parents were highly satisfied with NP home visits, hospital visits, and care provided to child.
Lewis et al. (1969) Evaluation of NP performance compared to MD using critical-incident technique for care given to medical clinic patients for 86 NP patients and 118 MD patients	NP	Missed appointments, patient satisfaction, frequency of symptoms, change in patient disability level	↑ number of NP patients who had returned to work (40% in NP group vs ↓ in MD group); ↓ in patient symptoms in NP group vs no change in MD group patients; 50% fewer broken appointments for NP vs MD group patients; no differences in severity of patient disease between groups.
Severin & Becker (1964) Comparison of psychiatric CNS consultation in ER compared to MD care	CNS	Formulation of plan of care; consultation required	CNS managed 66% of psychiatric referrals and required only phone consultation in majority of cases to complete a plan of therapy.

Sources for Identifying Outcome Measures and Outcome Instruments

Sources for identifying outcome measures include the literature on outcomes, outcome measurement manuals, regulatory and accrediting agencies, governmental sources, and clinical practice guidelines. A number of data-gathering tools can be used to collect outcomes data, including flowcharts, check sheets, protocols, guideline-based performance measures, critical pathways, and other instruments. A growing number of instruments that have established reliability and validity are available for use in outcome measurement studies. Sources for finding outcome measurement tools include the literature, specialty organizations and institutes, software programs, and Internet sources (Kleinpell, 1997; McDaniel & Nash, 1990; Wogner, 1999).

Other sources of outcome and performance measures include textbooks, journal supplements, software, and Internet sources devoted to maintaining collections of instruments, tests, rating scales, and other tools that can be used for outcomes research. Issues to consider in choosing tools and instruments for outcome measurement studies include instrument purpose and intended study population, length and completion time, degree and type of reliability, and validity testing conducted with the instrument, administration and scoring aspects, and associated fees for use and/or scoring (Frank-Stromberg & Olsen, 1998; Kleinpell & Weiner, 1999). The use of objective documentation tools can also help to evaluate APN work activities and measure performance and outcomes (Kleinpell, 2000; Oermann & Huber, 1999; Whitcomb, Craig, & Welker, 2000; Whitcomb et al., 2002). The chapter by Schwartz et al. in this book further reviews sources of outcome instruments, including Internet resources.

The Future of Outcomes Research in Advanced Practice Nursing

Studies measuring the effects of APN care have found that APNs improve access to care, competently manage care for patients in a variety of health care settings, are accepted by patients, and provide high-quality care. Yet, only a limited number of studies exist, or rather, have been published. Early research on APNs addressed competency aspects and ability to perform in newly defined roles (Sweet, 1986). Additional research on APNs has further explored the effects of APN care on care-related, patient-related, and performance-related outcomes.

Yet, often the overall impact of APN care has been difficult to assess. Many studies group APNs and other midlevel care providers together; other studies, by virtue of their study design, preclude attributing direct causation of an outcome to APN care. The outcome studies on APN care that exist are not enough to describe the true outcomes that result from APN care. A concept analysis of outcomes for APNs highlighted the importance of the measurement of clinically relevant outcomes that reflect the work of the APN (Neis et al., 1999).

The use of nurse-sensitive indicators to develop appropriate measures and outcomes for APNs has also been suggested (Wong, 1998), yet, determining which are most appropriate can be challenging. Identifying domains of APN practice may help in categorizing role functions that are unique to APN practice and that can be examined in terms of their effect on patient outcomes. Beal (2000) examined the practice of nurse practitioners working in a neonatal intensive care unit and identified nine domains of NP practice, including (a) diagnostic/patient monitoring, (b) management of patient health/illness, (c) administering/monitoring therapeutic interventions and regimens, (d) monitoring/ensuring quality of health care practices, (e) organization and work role, (f) helping role, (g) teaching/coaching role, (h) management of rapidly changing situations, and (i) consulting role. The case management role of APNs has also been highlighted (Foss & Koerner, 1997). Evaluating what a particular APN role encompasses in terms of role functions, enables outcomes that are affected by APN care to be more readily identified.

Recent studies have focused solely on comparing APN care to other health care providers. Although it is important to establish that APN care does not differ (or is better) than that of other health care providers, research on the unique contributions and outcomes of APN care is needed. Several synthesis reviews on the impact of APNs on patient outcomes have confirmed that additional studies are needed to demonstrate APN importance to cost and quality outcomes in a variety of populations (Boyle, 1995; Sechrist & Berlin, 1998; Urden, 1999). As the APN role is expanding to a variety of unique practice settings, including inpatient hospital settings, subacute care, urgent care, home care, long-term care, and traditional primary care settings, the impact of the APN in these settings needs to be established.

Recommendations for APN Outcome Studies

The use of practice-level outcome studies has been proposed as a way to practically measure the effect of APN care (Buppert, 2000). As randomized clinical trials are often not feasible in clinical practice settings, the use of practice-level outcome studies can enable measurement of an APN intervention by comparing the patient's improvement with the patient's baseline measurements (Buppert, 2000). Other study designs such as quasi-experimental, qualitative, or descriptive, or the use of case studies can also be employed in assessing APN outcomes. Additionally, APNs and researchers who have conducted outcomes research on the impact of the APN role need to be encouraged to disseminate the results through publications and presentations.

Use of nationally recognized outcome measures and instruments rather than self-developed tools should be incorporated into APN outcomes research. The use of outcome measures that affect health policy (such as costs, access to care, and quality of life) should also be adopted. Additionally, research with the use of randomization and experimental designs that incorporate multiple sites and/or large patient populations are also needed in APN outcomes research. Finally, successful methods and processes used to conduct outcomes research need to be shared to facilitate replication and to disseminate knowledge. The need for outcomes research on the APN role persists. Measuring outcomes of APN care is needed to establish the continued impact of APN care, highlight the effectiveness of APNs, and identify the unique contributions that APNs bring to patient care in the evolving health care arena.

REFERENCES

Ahrens, T., Yancey, V., & Kollef, M. (2003). Improving family communication at the end of life: Implication for length of stay in the intensive care unit and resource use. *American Journal of Critical Care, 12,* 317–323.

Aigner, M. J., Drew, S., & Phipps, J. (2004). A comparative study of nursing home resident outcomes between care provided by nurse practitioners/physicians versus physicians only. *Journal of the American Medical Directors Association, 5,* 16–23.

Albers-Heitner, P., Berghmans, B., Joore, M., Lagro-Janssen, T., Severens, J., Nieman, F., et al. (2008). The effects of involving a nurse practitioner in primary care for adult patients with urinary incontinence: The PromoCon study (Promoting Continence). *BMC Health Services Research, 8,* 84.

Alexander, J. S., Younger, R. E., Cohen, R. M., & Crawford, L. V. (1998). Effectiveness of a nurse-managed program for children with chronic asthma. *Journal of Pediatric Nursing, 3,* 312–317.

Andrus, M. R., & Donaldson, A. R. (2006). Outcomes of a lipid management program in a rural nurse practitioner clinic. *Annals of Pharmacotherapy, 40,* 782.

Aubrey, W. R., & Yoxall, C. W. (2001). Evaluation of the role of the neonatal nurse practitioner in resuscitation of preterm infants at birth. *Archives of Disease in Childhood: Fetal & Neonatal Edition, 85,* 96–99.

Avorn, J., Everitt, D. E., & Baker, M. W. (1991). The neglected medical history and therapeutic choices for abdominal pain: A nationwide study of 799 physicians and nurses. *Archives of Internal Medicine, 151,* 694–698.

Bargardi, A. M. (1999, November). Impact of nurse practitioner-implemented evidence-based clinical pathways on "best practice" in an interventional cardiology program. 72nd Scientific Sessions of the American Heart Association, Abstracts [November 1999 Supplement to *Circulation*].

Barnason, S., Merboth, M., Pozehl, B., & Tietjen, M. J. (1998). Utilizing an outcomes approach to improve pain management by nurses: A pilot study. *Nursing Clinics of North America, 12,* 28–36.

Barnason, S., & Rasmussen, D. (2000). Comparison of clinical practice changes in a rapid recovery program for coronary artery bypass graft patients. *Nursing Clinics of North America, 3,* 395–403.

Batey, M., & Holland, J. (1985). Prescribing practices among nurse practitioners in adult and family health. *American Journal of Public Health, 75,* 258–262.

Beal, J. A. (2000). A nurse practitioner model of practice in the neonatal intensive care unit. *American Journal of Maternal Child Nursing, 25,* 18–24.

Benatar, D., Bondmass, M., Ghitelman, J., & Avitall, B. (2003). Outcomes of chronic heart failure. *Archives of Internal Medicine, 163,* 347–352.

Benkert, R., Buchholz, S., & Poole, M. (2001). Hypertension outcomes in an urban nurse-managed center. *Journal of the American Academy of Nurse Practitioners, 13,* 84–89.

Bergeron, J., Neuman, K., & Kinsey, J. (1999). Do advanced practice nurses and physician assistants benefit small rural hospitals? *Journal of Rural Health, 15,* 219–232.

Bevis, L. C., Berg-Copas, G. M., Thomas, B. W., Vasquez, D. G., Wetta-Hall, R., Brake, D., et al. (2008). Outcomes of tube thoracostomies performed by advanced practice providers vs. trauma surgeons. *American Journal of Critical Care, 17,* 357–363.

Blue, L., Lang, E., McMurray, J., Davie, A. P., McDonagh, T. A., Murdoch, D. R., et al. (2001). Randomized controlled trial of specialist nurse intervention in heart failure. *British Medical Journal, 323,* 715–718.

Bourbonnier, M., & Evans, L. K. (2002). Advanced practice nursing in the care of frail older adults. *Journal of the American Geriatrics Society, 50,* 2062–2076.

Boville, D., Saran, M., Salem, J. K., Clough, L., Jones, R. R., Radwany, S. M., et al. (2007). An innovative role for nurse practitioners in managing chronic disease. *Nursing Economic$, 25,* 359–364.

Boyle, D. (1995). Documentation and outcomes of advanced practice nursing. *Oncology Nursing Forum, 22*(8), 11–16.

Brooten, D., & Naylor M. D. (1995). Nurses' effect on changing patient outcomes. *Image—The Journal of Nursing Scholarship, 27,* 95–99.

Brooten, D., Youngblut, J. M., Brown, L., et al. (2001). A randomized trial of nurse specialist home care for women with high-risk pregnancies: Outcomes and costs. *American Journal of Managed Care, 7,* 793–803.

Brown, J., Brown, M., & Jones F. (1979). Evaluation of a nurse practitioner staffed preventive medicine program in a fee-for-service multispecialty clinic. *Preventive Medicine, 8,* 53–58.

Brown, S. A., & Grimes, D. E. (1995). A meta-analysis of nurse practitioners and nurse midwives in primary care. *Nursing Research, 44,* 332–339.

Bryant, R., & Graham, M. C. (2002). Advanced practice nurses: A study of client satisfaction. *Journal of the American Academy of Nurse Practitioners, 14,* 88–92.

Buchanan, L., & Powers, R. (1997). Establishing an NP-staffed minor emergency area. *Nurse Practitioner, 22*(4), 175–187.

Buppert, C. (1999). *Nurse practitioners business practice and legal guide.* Gaithersburg, MD: Aspen Publishers.

Buppert, C. (2000). Measuring outcomes in primary care practice. *Nurse Practitioner, 25*(1), 88–98.

Burns, S. M., & Earven, S. (2002). Improving outcomes for mechanically ventilated medical intensive care unit patients using advanced practice nurses: A 6-year experience. *Critical Care Nursing Clinics of North America, 14,* 231–243.

Burns, S. M., Earven, S., Fisher, C., Lewis, R., Merrell, P., Schubart, J. R., et al. (2003). Implementation of an institutional program to improve clinical and financial outcomes of mechanically ventilated patients: One-year outcomes and lessons learned. *Critical Care Medicine, 31,* 2752–2763.

Byers, J. F., & Brunell, M. L. (1998). Demonstrating the value of the advanced practice nurse: An evaluation model. *AACN Clinical Issues, 9,* 295–305.

Carzoli, R., Martinez-Cruz, M., Cuevas, L., Murphy, S., & Chiu, T. (1994). Comparison of neonatal practitioners, physician assistants, and residents in the neonatal intensive care unit. *Archives of Pediatric and Adolescent Medicine, 148,* 1271–1276.

Chambers, L., Bruce-Lockhart, P., Black, D., Sampson, E., & Burke, M. (1977). A controlled trial of the impact of the family practice nurse on volume, quality, and cost of rural health services. *Medical Care, 25,* 971–981.

Chang, E., Daly, J., Hawkins, A., McGirr, J., Fielding, K., Hemmings, L., et al. (1999). An evaluation of the nurse practitioner role in a major rural emergency department. *Journal of Advanced Nursing, 30,* 260–268.

Charney, E., & Kitzman, H. (1971). The child-health nurse (pediatric nurse practitioner) in private practice. A controlled trial. *New England Journal of Medicine, 285,* 1353–1358.

Cintron, G., Bigas, C., Linates, E., Aranda, J., & Hernandez, E. (1983). Nurse practitioner role in a congestive heart failure clinic: In-hospital time, costs, and patient satisfaction. *Heart & Lung, 12,* 237–240.

Considine, J., Martin, R., Smit, D., Winter, C., & Jenkins, J. (2006). Emergency nurse practitioner care and emergency department patient flow: Case control study. *Emergency Medicine Australasia, 18,* 385–390.

Cooper, M. A., Lindsay, G. M., Kinn, S., & Swann, I. J. (2002). Evaluating emergency nurse practitioner service: A randomized controlled trial. *Journal of Advanced Nursing, 40,* 721–730.

Corner, J., Halliday, D., Haviland, J., Douglas, H. R., et al. (2003). Exploring nursing outcomes for patients with advanced cancer following intervention by Macmillan specialist palliative care nurses. *Journal of Advanced Nursing, 41*(6), 561–574.

Cowan, M. J., Shapiro, M., Hays, R. D., Afifi, A., Vazirani, S., Ward, C. R., et al. (2006). The effect of a multidisciplinary hospitalist/physician and advanced practice nurse collaboration on hospital costs. *Journal of Nursing Administration, 36,* 79–85.

Cragin, L., & Kennedy, H. P. (2006). Linking obstetric and midwifery practice with optimal outcomes. *Journal of Obstetric, Gynecologic, & Neonatal Nursing, 35*(6), 779–785.

Crosby, F., Ventura, M. R., & Feldman, M. J. (1987). Future research recommendations for establishing NP effectiveness. *Nurse Practitioner, 12,* 75–79.

Crimlisk, J. T., Bernardo, J., Blansfield, J. S., et al. (1997). Endotracheal intubation: A closer look at a preventable condition. *Clinical Nurse Specialist, 11,* 145–150.

Cunningham, R. S. (2004). Advanced practice nursing outcomes: A review of selected empirical literature. *Oncology Nursing Forum, 31,* 219–232.

Curran, C. R., & Roberts, W. D. (2002). Columbia University's competency and evidence-based acute care nurse practitioner program. *Nursing Outlook, 50,* 232–237.

Dahle, K., Smith, J., Ingersol, G., & Wilson, J. (1998). Impact of a nurse practitioner on the cost of managing inpatients with heart failure. *American Journal of Cardiology, 82,* 686–688.

Damato, E. G., Dill, P. Z., Gennaro, S., et al. (1993). The association between CNS direct care time and total time and very low birth weight infant outcomes. *Clinical Nurse Specialist, 7,* 75–79.

Davies, A. R., Doyle, M. A., Lansky, D., Rutt, W., Orsolits-Stevic, M., & Doyle, J. B. (1994). Outcomes assessment in clinical settings: A consensus statement on principles and best practices in project management. *Joint Commission Journal on Quality Improvement, 20,* 6–16.

Day, L., Egli, R., & Silver, H. (1970). Acceptance of pediatric nurse practitioners. *American Journal of Diseases of Children, 119,* 204–208.

De Jong, R. N., Jr. (1981). Use of women's health care specialists in a women's clinic. *Journal of Reproductive Medicine, 26,* 283–288.

Delgado-Passler, P., & McCaffery, R. (2006). The influences of postdischarge management by nurse practitioners on hospital readmission for heart failure. *Journal of the American Academy of Nurse Practitioners, 18,* 154–160.

Dellasega, C., & Zerbe, T. M. (2002). Caregivers of frail rural older adults—effects of an advanced practice nursing intervention. *Journal of Gerontological Nursing, 18,* 40–49.

Dickerson, S. S., Wu, Y. B., & Kennedy, M. C. (2006). A CNS-facilitated ICD support group: A clinical project evaluation. *Clinical Nurse Specialist, 20,* 146–153.

Diesch, P., Soukup, M., Adams, P. C., & Wild, M. (2000). Guided imagery replication study using coronary artery bypass graft patients. *Nursing Clinics of North America, 25,* 417–425.

DiGirol, M., & Parry, W. H. (1983). Consultation to the Pediatric Automated Military Outpatient Systems Specialist (AMOSIST): A comparison of consultation by a pediatric clinical nurse specialist and by a pediatrician. *Military Medicine, 148,* 364–367.

Dobscha, S. K., Gerrity, M. S., & Ward, M. F. (2001). Effectiveness of an intervention to improve primary care provider recognition of depression. *American College of Physicians.* Retrieved June 30, 2008, from http://www.acponline.org

Duncan, B., Smith, A., & Silver, H. (1971). Comparison of the physical assessment of children by pediatric nurse practitioners and pediatricians. *American Journal of Public Health, 61,* 1170–1176.

Edmunds, M. W. (1978). Evaluation of nurse practitioner effectiveness: An overview of the literature. *Evaluation and the Health Professions, 1,* 69–82.

Ettner, S. L., Kotlerman, J., Afifi, A., Vazirani, S., Hays, R. D., Shapiro, M., et al. (2006). An alternative approach to reducing the costs of patient care? A controlled trial of the multi-disciplinary doctor–nurse practitioner (MDNP) model. *Medical Decision Making, 26,* 9–17.

Feldman, J., Ventura, M., & Crosby, F. (1987). Studies of nurse practitioner effectiveness. *Nursing Research, 36,* 303–308.

Forster, A. J., Clark, H. D., Menard, A., et al. (2005). Effect of a nurse team coordinator on outcomes for hospitalized medical patients. *American Journal of Medicine, 118,* 1148–1153.

Foss, N., & Koerner, J. (1997). The advanced practice nurse's role in differentiated practice: Martha's story. *AACN Clinical Issues, 8,* 262–270.

Frank-Stromborg, M., & Olsen, S. J. (2003). *Instruments for clinical healthcare research.* Boston: Jones and Bartlett.

Freij, R., Duffy, T., Hackett, D., Cunningham, D., & Fothergill, J. (1996). Radiographic interpretation by nurse practitioners in a minor injuries unit. *Journal of Accident & Emergency Medicine, 13,* 41–43.

Fulton, J. S., & Baldwin, K. (2004) An annotated bibliography reflecting CNS practice and outcomes. *Clinical Nurse Specialist, 18,* 21–39.

Gawlinski, A., McCloy, K., & Jesurum, J. (2001). Measuring outcomes in cardiovascular APN practice. In R. Kleinpell (Ed.), *Outcome assessment in advanced practice nursing* (pp. 131–188). New York: Springer Publishing Company.

Gracias, V. H., Sicoutris, C. P., Meredith, D. M., Haut, E., et al. (2003). Critical care nurse practitioners improve compliance with clinical practice guidelines in the surgical intensive care unit. *Critical Care Medicine, 31*(12), A93.

Gracias, V. H., Sicoutris, C. P., Stawicki, S. P., et al. (2008). Critical care nurse practitioners improve compliance with clinical practice guidelines in "semiclosed" surgical intensive care unit. *Journal of Nursing Care Quality, 23,* 338–344.

Graveley, E., & Littlefield, J. (1992). A cost-effectiveness analysis of three staffing models for the delivery of low-risk prenatal care. *American Journal of Public Health, 82,* 180–184.

Haddock, K. S. (1994). Collaborative discharge planning: Nursing and social services. *Clinical Nurse Specialist, 8,* 248–252.

Hall, J., Palmer, R. H., Orav, E. J., Hargraves, J. L., Wright, E. A., & Louis, T. A. (1990). Performance quality, gender and professional role: A study of physicians and nonphysicians in 16 ambulatory care practices. *Medical Care, 28,* 489–501.

Hamilton, R., & Hawley, W. (2006). Quality of life outcomes related to anemia management of patients with chronic renal failure. *Clinical Nurse Specialist, 20,* 139–143.

Hankins, G., Shaw, S., Cruess, D., Lawrence, H., & Harris, C. (1996). Patient satisfaction with collaborative practice. *Obstetrics & Gynecology, 88,* 1011–1015.

Hanneman, S. K., Bines, A., & Sajtar, W. S. (1993). The indirect patient care effect of a unit-based clinical nurse specialist on preventable pulmonary complications. *American Journal of Critical Care, 2,* 331–338.

Hill, J., Bird, J., Harmer, R., Wright, V., & Lawton, C. (1994). An evaluation of the effectiveness, safety and acceptability of a nurse practitioner in a rheumatology outpatient clinic. *British Journal of Rheumatology, 33,* 283–288.

Hoffman, L., Tasota, F., Scharfenberg, C., Zullo, T., & Donahoe, M. (2002).Management of ventilator dependent patients: 5-month comparison of an acute care nurse practitioner versus physicians-in-training. *American Journal of Respiratory and Critical Care Medicine, 165,* A388.

Hoffman, L., Tasota, F., Zullo, T. G., Scharfenberg, C., & Donahoe, M. P. (2005).Outcomes of care managed by an acute care nurse practitioner/attending physician team in a subacute medical intensive care unit. *American Journal of Critical Care, 14,* 121–130.

Hoffman, L. A., Miller, T. H., Zullo, T. G., & Donahoe, M. P. (2006). Comparison of 2 models for managing tracheotomized patients in a subacute medical intensive care unit. *Respiratory Care, 51,* 1230–1236.

Hooker, R. S., & McCaig, L. (1996). Emergency department uses of physician assistants and nurse practitioners: A national survey. *American Journal of Emergency Medicine, 14,* 245–249.

Horrocks, S., Anderson, E., & Salisbury, C. (2002). Systematic review of whether nurse practitioners working in primary care can provide equivalent care to doctors. *British Medical Journal, 324,* 819–823.

Hylka, S., & Beschle, J. (1995). Nurse practitioners, cost savings, and improved patient care in the department of surgery. *Nursing Economic$, 13,* 349–354.

Ingersoll, G. L. (2008). Outcomes evaluation and performance improvement: An integrative review of research on advanced practice nursing. In A. B. Hamric, J. A. Spross, & C. M. Hanson (Eds.), *Advanced practice nursing: An integrative approach.* Philadelphia: Saunders Elsevier.

Ingersoll, G. L., McIntosh, E., & Williams, M. (2000). Nurse-sensitive outcomes of advanced practice. *Journal of Advanced Nursing, 32,* 1271–1281.

Irvine, D., Sidani, S., & Hall, L. M. (1998). Linking outcomes to nurses' roles in health care. *Nursing Economic$, 16,* 58–64, 87.

James, M., & Pyrgos, N. (1989). Nurse practitioners in accident and emergency departments. *Archives of Emergency Medicine, 6,* 241–246.

Jennings, B., Staggers, N., & Brosch, L. (1999). A classification scheme for outcome indicators. *Image—The Journal of Nursing Scholarship, 31,* 381–388.

Kane, R. L. (2004). *Understanding health care outcomes research.* Boston: Jones and Bartlett.

Karlowicz, M. G., & McMurray, J. L. (2000). Comparison of neonatal nurse practitioners' and pediatric residents' care of extremely low-birth-weight infants. *Archives of Pediatric and Adolescent Medicine, 154,* 1123–1126.

Kaups, K. L., Parks, S. N., & Morris, C. L. (1998). Intracranial pressure monitor placement by midlevel practitioners. *Journal of Trauma, 45,* 884–886.

Kearnes, D. R. (1994). Impact of a nurse practitioner and physician collaborative practice on older adults admitted to a large urban hospital: Differences in treatment and outcome. *Nurse Practitioner, 19*(8), 32–36.

Kelley, C. G., Daly, B. J., Anthony, M. K., Zauszniewski, J. A., & Stange, K. C. (2002). Nurse practitioners and preventive screening in the hospital. *Clinical Nursing Research, 11,* 433–449.

Kirkwood, B., Pesudovs, K., Loh, R. S., & Coster, D. J. (2005). Implementation and evaluation of an ophthalmic nurse practitioner emergency eye clinic. *Clinical & Experimental Opthalmology, 33,* 593–597.

Kirton, O. C., Folcik, M. A., Ivy, M. E., Calabrese, R., Dobkin, E., Pepe, J., et al. (2007). Midlevel practitioner workforce analysis at a university-affiliated teaching hospital. *Archives of Surgery, 142,* 336–341.

Kleinpell, R. (1997). Whose outcomes: Patients, providers, or payers? *Nursing Clinics of North America, 32,* 513–520.

Kleinpell, R. (2005). Acute care nurse practitioner practice: Results of a 5-year longitudinal study. *American Journal of Critical Care, 14,* 211–219.

Kleinpell, R. (2000). Implementation strategies: Assessing outcomes in the elderly in acute care. *AACN Clinical Issues, 11,* 442–452.

Kleinpell, R., Ely, E. W., & Grabenkort, R. (2008). Nurse practitioners and physician assistants in the ICU: An evidence based review. *Critical Care Medicine, 26,* 2888–2897.

Kleinpell, R., & Gawlinski, A. (2005). Assessing outcomes in advanced practice nursing practice: The use of quality indicators and evidence-based practice. *AACN Clinical Issues, 16,* 43–57.

Kleinpell, R., & Weiner, T. (1999). Measuring advanced practice nursing outcomes. *AACN Clinical Issues, 10,* 356–368.

Krichbaum, K., Pearson, V., Savik, K., & Mueller, C. (2005). Improving resident outcomes with GAPN organization level interventions. *Western Journal of Nursing Research, 27,* 322–337.

Krien, S. L., Klamerus, M. L., Vijan, S., et al. (2004). Case management for patients with poorly controlled diabetes: A randomized trial. *American Journal of Medicine, 116,* 732–739.

Kutzleb, J., & Reiner, D. (2006). The impact of nurse-directed patient education on quality of life and functional capacity in people with heart failure. *Journal of the American Academy of Nurse Practitioners, 18,* 116–123.

Lacko, L. A., Dellasega, C., Salerno, F. A., et al. (2000). The role of the advanced practice nurse in facilitating a clinical research study. *Clinical Nurse Specialist, 14,* 110–115.

Lambing, A. Y., Adams, D. L., Fox, D. H., & Divine, G. (2004). Nurse practitioners' and physicians' care activities and clinical outcomes with an inpatient geriatric population. *Journal of the American Academy of Nurse Practitioners, 26,* 343–352.

Langner, S., & Hutelmyer, C. (1995). Patient satisfaction with outpatient human immunodeficiency virus care as delivered by nurse practitioners and physicians. *Holistic Nursing Practice, 10*(1), 54–60.

Lenz, E. R., Mundinger, M. O., Hopkins, S. C., Lin, S. X., & Smolowitz, J. L. (2002). Diabetes care processes and outcomes in patients treated by nurse practitioners or physicians. *Diabetes Educator, 28,* 590–598.

Lenz, E. R., Mundinger, M. O., Kane, R. L., et al. (2004). Primary care outcomes in patients treated by nurse practitioners or physicians: Two-year follow up. *Medical Care Research and Review, 61,* 332–351.

Lewis, C., Resnik, B., Schmidt, G., & Waxman, D. (1969). Activities, events and outcomes in ambulatory patient care. *New England Journal of Medicine, 280,* 645–649.

Ley, S., J. (2001). Quality care outcomes in cardiac surgery: The role of evidence-based practice. *AACN Clinical Issues, 12,* 606–617.

Lindberg, M., Ahlner, J., Ekström, T., Jonsson, D., & Möller, M. (2002). Asthma nurse practice improves outcomes and reduces costs in primary health care. *Scandinavian Journal of Caring Sciences, 16*(1), 73–78.

Litaker, D., Mion, L. C., Planavsky, L., Kippes, C., Mehta, N., & Frolkis, J. (2003). Physician–nurse practitioner teams in chronic disease management: The impact on costs, clinical effectiveness, and patients' perception of care. *Journal of Interprofessional Care, 17,* 223–237.

Lohr, K. (1988). Outcomes measurement: Concepts and questions. *Inquiry, 25,* 37–50.

Lombness, P. (1994). Difference in length of stay with care managed by clinical nurse specialist or physician assistants. *Clinical Nurse Specialist, 8,* 253–260.

Mackey, T. A., Cole, F. L., & Lindenberg, J. (2005). Quality improvement and changes in diabetic patient outcomes in an academic nurse practitioner primary care practice. *Journal of the American Academy of Nurse Practitioners, 17,* 547–553.

Mahoney, D. F. (1994). Appropriateness of geriatric prescribing decisions made by nurse practitioners and physicians. *Image—The Journal of Nursing Scholarship, 26,* 41–46.

McCabe, P. J. (2005). Spheres of clinical nurse specialist practice influence evidence-based care for patients with atrial fibrillation. *Clinical Nurse Specialist, 19,* 308–317.

McCauley, K. M., Bixby, M., & Naylor, M. D. (2006). Advanced practice nurse strategies to improve outcomes and reduce cost in elders with heart failure. *Disease Management, 9,* 302–310.

McCorkle, R., Dowd, M. F., Pickett, M., et al. (2007). Effects of advanced practice nursing on patient and spouse depressive symptoms, sexual function, and marital interaction after radical prostatectomy. *Urologic Nursing, 27,* 65–77.

McDaniel, C., & Nash, J. (1990). Compendium of instruments measuring patient satisfaction with nursing care. *Quality Review Bulletin, 5,* 182–188.

McGrath, S. (1990). The cost-effectiveness of nurse practitioners. *Nurse Practitioner, 15*(7), 40–42.

Meyer, S. C., & Miers, L. J. (2005). Effect of cardiovascular surgeon and acute care nurse practitioner collaboration on postoperative outcomes. *AACN Clinical Issues, 16,* 149–158.

Miller, S. (1997). Impact of a gerontological nurse practitioner on the nursing home elderly in the acute care setting. *AACN Clinical Issues, 8,* 609–615.

Mitchell-Dicenso, A., Guyatt, G., Marrin, M., Goeree, R., Willan, A., Southwell, D., et al. (1996). A controlled trial of nurse practitioners in neonatal intensive care. *Pediatrics, 98,* 1143–1148.

Monroe, D., Pohl, J., Gardner, H. H., & Bell, R. E. (1982). Prescribing patterns of nurse practitioners. *American Journal of Nursing, 82,* 1538–1542.

Moody, N., Smith, P. L., & Glenn, L. L. (1999). Client characteristics and practice patterns of nurse practitioners and physicians. *Nurse Practitioner, 24*(3), 94–103.

Moore, S., Corner, J., Haviland, J., et al. (2002). Nurse led follow-up and conventional medical follow-up in management of patients with lung cancer: Randomised trial. *British Medical Journal, 325*(7373), 1145.

Morse, K. J., Warshawsky, D., Moore, J. M., & Pecora, D. C. (2006). A new role for the ACNP the rapid response team leader. *Critical Care Nursing Quarterly, 29,* 137–146.

Mundinger, M., Kane, R., Lenz, E., Totten, A., Tsai, W., Cleary, P., Friedewald, W., Siu, A., Shelanski, M., et al. (2000). Primary care outcomes in patients treated by nurse practitioners or physicians. *Journal of the American Medical Association, 283,* 59–68.

Naylor, M. D., Brooten, D., Campbell, R., Jacobsen, B. S., Mezey, M. D., Pauly, M. V., et al. (1999). Comprehensive discharge planning and home follow-up of hospitalized elders: A randomized clinical trial. *Journal of the American Medical Association, 281,* 613–620.

Naylor, M. D., Brooten, D. A., Campbell, R. L., Maislin, G., McCauley, K. M, & Schwartz, J. S. (2004). Transitional care of older adults hospitalized with heart failure: A randomized, controlled trial. *Journal of the American Geriatrics Society, 52,* 675–684.

Neff, D. F., Madigan, E., & Narsavage, G. (2003). APN-directed transitional home care model. *Home Healthcare Nurse, 21,* 543–550.

Neidlinger, S., Scroggins, K., & Kennedy, L. M. (1987). Cost evaluation of discharge planning for hospitalized elderly. *Nursing Economic$, 5,* 225–230.

Newhouse, R. P., Stanik-Hutt, J., Steinwachs, D. M., et al. (2009, in progress). *An assessment of the safety, quality, and effectiveness of care provided by advanced practice nurses.* Unpublished manuscript.

Nies, M., Cook, T., Bach, C., Bushnell, K., Salisbury, M., Sinclair, V., et al. (1999). Concept analysis of outcomes for advanced practice nursing. *Outcomes Management for Nursing Practice, 3,* 83–86.

Ockene, J., Adams, A., Gurley, T., Wheeler, E., & Hebert, J. (1999). Brief physician- and nurse practitioner-delivered counseling for high-risk drinkers. *Archives of Internal Medicine, 159,* 2198–2205.

Oermann, M., & Huber, D. (1999). Patient outcomes—A measure of nursing's value. *American Journal of Nursing, 99*(9), 40–47.

Osevala, M. L. (2005). Advanced-practice nursing in heart-failure management: An integrative review. *Journal of Cardiovascular Management, 16,* 19–23.

Paez, K. A., & Allen, J. K. (2006). Cost-effectiveness of nurse practitioner management of hypercholesterolemia following coronary revascularization. *Journal of the American Academy of Nurse Practitioners, 18,* 436–444.

Paladichuk, A. (1997). Chronic disease management: An outpatient approach. *Critical Care Nurse, 17,* 90–95.

Patton, M., & Schaerf, R. (1995). Thoracotomy critical pathway and clinical outcomes. *Cancer Practice, 3,* 286–294.

Paul, S. (2000). Impact of a nurse-managed heart failure clinic: A pilot study. *American Journal of Critical Care, 9,* 140–146.

Pioro, M. H., Landefeld, C. S., Brennan, P. F., Daly, B., Fortinsky, R. H., Kim, U., et al. (2001). Outcomes-based trial of an inpatient nurse practitioner service for general medical patients. *Journal of Evaluation in Clinical Practice, 7,* 21–33.

Poduri, K. R., Palenski, C., & Gibson, C. J. (1996). Inpatient rehabilitation: Physiatric and nurse practitioner admission assessment of stroke patients and their rehabilitation outcomes. *International Journal of Rehabilitation Research, 19,* 111–121.

Pozen, M. W., Stechmiller, J. A., Harris, W., et al. (1997). A nurse rehabilitator's impact on patients with myocardial infarction. *Medical Care, 15,* 830–837.

Prescott, P., & Driscoll, L. (1979). Nurse practitioner effectiveness: A review of physician-nurse comparison studies. *Evaluation and Health Professions, 2,* 387–418.

Quenot, J. P., Sadoire, S., Devoucoux, F., Doise, J. M., Cailliod, R., Cunin, N., et al. (2007). Effect of a nurse-implemented sedation protocol on the incidence of ventilator-associated pneumonia. *Critical Care Medicine, 35,* 2031–2036.

Rantz, M. J., Popejoy, L., Petroski, G. F., et al. (2001). Randomized clinical trial of a quality improvement intervention in nursing homes. *The Gerontologist, 41,* 525–538.

Reigle, J., Molnar, H. M., Howell, C., & Dumont, C. (2006). Evaluation of in-patient interventional cardiology. *Critical Care Nursing Clinics of North America, 18*(4), 523–529.

Resnick, B. (2006). Outcomes research: You do have the time. *Journal of the American Academy of Nurse Practitioners, 18,* 505–509.

Reveley, S. (1998). The role of the triage nurse practitioner in general medical practice: An analysis of the role. *Journal of Advanced Nursing, 28,* 584–591.

Rhee, K., & Dermyer, A. (1995). Patient satisfaction with a nurse practitioner in a university emergency service. *Annals of Emergency Medicine, 26,* 130–132.

Rideout, K. (2007). Evaluation of a PNP care coordinator model for hospitalized children, adolescents, and young adults with cystic fibrosis. *Pediatric Nursing, 33,* 29–35.

Ritz, L. J., Nissen, M. J., Swenson, K. K., Farrell, J. B., Sperduto, P. W., Sladek, M. L., Lally, R. M., & Schroeder, L. M. (2000). Effects of advanced nursing care on quality of life and cost outcomes of women diagnosed with breast cancer. *Oncology Nursing Forum, 27*(6), 923–932.

Rosenaur, J., Stanford, D., Morgan, W., & Curtin, B. (1984). Prescribing behaviors of primary care nurse practitioners. *American Journal of Public Health, 74,* 10–13.

Rudy, E. B., Davidson, L. J., Daly, B., Clochesy, J. M., Sereika, S., Baldisseri, M., et al. (1998). Care activities and outcomes of patients cared for by acute care nurse practitioners, physician assistants, and resident physicians: A comparison. *American Journal of Critical Care, 7,* 267–281.

Runyan, J. (1975). The Memphis chronic disease program. *Journal of the American Medical Association, 231,* 264–267.

Russell, D., Vorder-Bruegge, M., & Burns, S. M. (2002). Effect of an outcomes-managed approach to care of neuroscience patients by acute care nurse practitioners. *American Journal of Critical Care, 11,* 353–364.

Russell, L. C. (1989). Cost containment of modified radical mastectomy: The impact of the clinical nurse specialist. *Point View, 26,* 18–19.

Russo, R. M. Gururaj, V. J., Bunye, A. S., Kim, Y. H., & Ner, S. (1975) Triage abilities of nurse practitioner vs. pediatrician. *American Journal of Diseases of Children, 129,* 673–675.

Sackett, D., Spitzer, W., Gent, M., & Roberts, R. (1974). The Burlington randomized trial of the nurse practitioner: Health outcomes of patients. *Annals of Internal Medicine, 80,* 137–142.

Safriet, B. (1992). Health care dollars and regulatory sense: The role of advanced practice nursing. *Yale Journal on Regulation, 9,* 417–487.

Sakr, M., Angus, J., Perrin, J., Nixon, C., Nicholl, J., & Wardrope, J. (1999). Care of minor injuries by emergency nurse practitioners of junior doctors: A randomised controlled trial. *Lancet, 354,* 1321–1326.

Salkever, D. S., Skinner, E. A., Steinwachs, D. M., & Katz, H. (1982). Episode-based efficiency comparisons for physician and nurse practitioners. *Medical Care, 20,* 143–153.

Sarkissian, S., & Wennberg, R. (1999). Effects of the acute care nurse practitioner role on epilepsy monitoring outcomes. *Outcomes Management in Nursing Practice, 3,* 161–166.

Schultz, J. M., Liptak, G. S., & Fioravanti, J. (1994). Nurse practitioners' effectiveness in NICU. *Nursing Management, 25,* 50–52.

Scisney-Matlock, M., Makos, G., Saunders, T., et al. (2004). Comparison of quality-of-hypertension care for groups treated by physician versus groups treated by physician–nurse team. *Journal of the American Academy of Nurse Practitioners, 16,* 7–23.

Seale, C., Anderson, E., & Kinnersley, P. (2006). Treatment advice in primary care: A comparative study of nurse practitioners and general practitioners. *Journal of Advanced Nursing, 54,* 534–541.

Sears, J. M., Wickizer, T. M., Franklin, G. M., Cheadle, A. D., & Berkowitz, B. (2007). Nurse practitioners as attending providers for workers with uncomplicated back injuries: Using administrative data to evaluate quality and process of care. *Journal of Occupational Environmental Medicine, 49,* 900–908.

Sears, J. M., Wickizer, T. M., Franklin, G. M., Cheadle, A. D., & Berkowitz, B. (2008). Expanding the role of nurse practitioners: Effects on rural access to care for injured workers. *Journal of Rural Health, 24,* 171–178.

Sechrist, K., & Berlin, L. (1998). Role of the clinical nurse specialist: An integrative review of the literature. *AACN Clinical Issues, 9,* 306–324.

Severin, N., & Becker, R. (1964). Nurses as psychiatric consultants in a general hospital emergency room. *Community Mental Health Journal, 30,* 261–267.

Shebesta, K. F., Cook, B., Rickets, C., et al. (2006). Pediatric trauma nurse practitioners increase bedside nurses' satisfaction with pediatric trauma patient care. *Journal of Trauma Nursing, 13*(2), 66–69.

Sidani, S., Doran, D., Porter, H., LeFort, S., O'Brien-Pallas, L. L., Zahn, C., et al. (2006). Processes of care: Comparison between nurse practitioners and physician residents in acute care. *Canadian Journal of Nursing Leadership, 19,* 69–85.

Simborg, D., Starfield, B., & Horn, S. (1978). Physician and non-physician health practitioners: The characteristics of their practices and their relationships. *American Journal of Public Health, 68,* 44–48.

Sinuff,, T., Cook, D., Giacomini, M., et al. (2007). Facilitating clinician adherence to guidelines in the intensive care unit: A multicenter, qualitative study. *Critical Care Medicine, 35,* 2083–2089.

Skinner, E., & Kahn, L. (1972). A comparison between the pediatric nurse practitioner and the pediatric resident in an out-patient department: A pilot study. *Clinical Pediatrics, 11,* 142–147.

Sole, M. L., Hunkar-Huie, A. M., Schiller, J. S., & Cheatham, M. L. (2001). Comprehensive trauma patient care by nonphysician providers. *AACN Clinical Issues, 2,* 438–446.

Sox, H. (1979). Quality of patient care by nurse practitioners and physician assistants: A ten-year perspective. *Annals of Internal Medicine, 91,* 459–468.

Spisso, J., O'Callaghan, C., McKennan, M., & Holcroft, J. W. (1990). Improved quality of care and reduction of housestaff workload using trauma nurse practitioners. *Journal of Trauma, 30,* 660–665.

Spitzer, R. (1997). The Vanderbilt University experience. *Nursing Management, 28*(3), 38–40.

Spitzer, W., Sackett, D., Sibley, J., Roberts, R., Tech, M., Gent, M., et al. (1974). The Burlington randomized trial of the nurse practitioner. *New England Journal of Medicine, 290,* 251–256.

Stetler, C., Effken, J., Frigon, L., Tiernan, C., & Zwingman-Bagley, C. (1998). Utilization-focused evaluation of acute care nurse practitioner role. *Outcomes Management for Nursing Practice, 2,* 152–160.

Stolee, P., Hillier, L. M., Esbaugh, J., Griffiths, N., & Borrie, M. J. (2006). Examining the nurse practitioner role in long-term care: Evaluation of a pilot project in Canada. *Journal of Gerontological Nursing, 32,* 28–36.

Sullivan-Marx, E., & Maislin, G. (2000). Comparison of nurse practitioner and family physician relative work values. *Image—The Journal of Nursing Scholarship, 32,* 71–76.

Sulzbach-Hoke, L., & Gift, A. (1995). Use of quality management to provide nutrition to intubated patients. *Clinical Nurse Specialist, 9,* 248–251.

Sweet, J. (1986). The cost-effectiveness of nurse practitioners. *Nursing Economic$, 4,* 190–193.

Thompson, R. (1980). Neonatal transport nurses: An analysis of their role in the transport of newborn infants. *Pediatrics, 65,* 887–892.

Thompson, R., Basden, P., & Howell, L. (1982). Evaluation of initial implementation of an organized adult health program employing family nurse practitioners. *Medical Care, 20,* 1109–1127.

Tijhuis, G. J., Zwinderman, A. H., Hazes, J. W., et al. (2002). A randomized comparison of care provided by a clinical nurse specialist, an inpatient team, and a day patient team in rheumatoid arthritis. *Arthritis and Rheumatism, 47,* 525–531.

Urden, L. (1999). Outcome evaluation: An essential component for CNS practice. *Clinical Nurse Specialist, 13,* 39–46.

Topp, R., Tucker, D., & Weber, C. (1998). Effect of a clinical case manager/clinical nurse specialist on patients hospitalized with congestive heart failure. *Nursing Case Management, 3,* 140–145.

Tsay, S. L., Lee, U. C., & Lee, Y. C. (2005). Effects of an adaptation training programme for patients with end-stage renal disease. *Journal of Advanced Nursing, 50,* 39–46.

U.S. Congress, Office of Technology Assessment. (1986). *Nurse practitioners, physician assistants, and certified nurse-midwives: A policy analysis.* Washington, DC: U.S. Government Printing Office.

Vanhook, P. (2000, February). *Presence of nurse practitioner on stroke team reduced morbidity, mortality.* American Heart Association 25th International Stroke Conference Report, Reuters Medical News.

Vazirani, S., Hays, R. D., Shapiro, M. F., & Cowan, M. (2005). Effect of a multidisciplinary intervention on communication and collaboration among physicians and nurses. *American Journal of Critical Care, 14,* 71–77.

Venner, G. H., & Steelbinder, J. S. (1996). Team management of congestive heart failure across the continuum. *Journal of Cardiovascular Nursing, 10,* 71–84.

Weinberg, R., Lijestrand, J., & Moore, S. (1983). Inpatient management by a nurse practitioner: Effectiveness in a rehabilitation setting. *Archives of Physical Medicine Rehabilitation, 64,* 588–590.

Wheeler, E. C. (2000). The CNS's impact on process and outcome of patients with total knee replacement. *Clinical Nurse Specialist, 14,* 159–169.

Whitcomb, R., Craig, R., & Welker, C. (2000). Measuring how acute care nurse practitioners affect outcomes. *Dimensions of Critical Care Nursing, 19,* 34–35.

Whitcomb, R., Wilson, S., Chang-Dawkins, S., Durand, J., Pitcher, D., Lauzon, C., et al. (2002). Advanced practice nursing: Acute care model in progress. *Journal of Nursing Administration, 32,* 123–125.

White, C. L. (1999). Changing pain management practice and impact on patient outcomes. *Clinical Nurse Specialist, 13,* 166–172.

Willoughby, D., & Burroughs, D. (2001). A CNS-managed diabetes foot-care clinic: A descriptive survey of characteristics and foot care behaviors of the patient population. *Clinical Nurse Specialist, 15,* 52–57.

Wojner, A. (1999). *Outcomes management: Application to clinical practice.* New York: W.B. Saunders.

Wong, S. (1998). Outcomes of nursing care: How do we know? *Clinical Nurse Specialist, 12,* 147–151.

Woods, L. (2006). Evaluating the clinical effectiveness of neonatal nurse practitioners: An exploratory study. *Journal of Clinical Nursing, 15,* 35–44.

York, R., Brown, L. P., Samuels, P., Finkler, S. A., et al. (1997). A randomized trial of discharge and nurse specialist follow-up care of high-risk childbearing women. *Nursing Research, 46,* 254–260.

Ziemer, D. C., Goldschmid, M. G., Musey, V. C., Domin, W. S., Thule, P. M., Gallina, D. L., et al. (1996). Diabetes in urban African Americans. III. Management of type II diabetes in a municipal hospital setting. *American Journal of Medicine, 101,* 25–32.

2

Analyzing Economic Outcomes in Advanced Practice Nursing

KEVIN D. FRICK AND PATRICIA W. STONE

The growing proportion of older adults in the U.S. population, various improvements in health care technology, direct-to-consumer advertising for a long list of pharmaceuticals, increasing costs of doing business in other sectors besides health care, and international competitive pressures on wages and benefits have drawn greater attention to the costs of health care over time. The focus on cost is not the only factor raising the importance of studying and factoring-in the cost-effectiveness of health care in the United States. Other relevant factors include (a) the scientific recommendations related to the conduct of cost-effectiveness analyses that have been issued in the United States, (b) a format for formulary submissions offered by the Academy of Managed Care Pharmacy, (c) recognition by parties in the United States of other recommendations around the globe, (d) conferences related to cost-effectiveness sponsored by the National Institute of Nursing Research, and (e) an increasing focus on comparative effectiveness more generally.

Acknowledgment: Drs. Stone and Frick are funded through the Center for Evidence-Based Practice in the Underserved (P30NR010677) to assist nurse researchers in conducting economic evaluation.

In 2006, U.S. health care spending increased 6.7% (greater than the rate of inflation), to a total of $2.1 trillion or 16.0% of the gross domestic product (Catlin, Cowan, Hartman, Heffler, & National Health Expenditure Accounts Team, 2008). This increasing level of expenditure and increasing proportion of the gross domestic product being spent on health care forces policy makers to consider the costs as well as the effectiveness of new treatments, devices, or interventions. Health policy makers increasingly request analyses, including projected economic outcomes prior to the approval of funding for or reimbursement of these new activities. In the current health care environment, advanced practice nurses (APNs) need to be knowledgeable about the interpretation of cost and effectiveness data, particularly when they are combined in a cost-effectiveness study.

The increased demand for economic information has resulted in a number of economic evaluations in the literature specific to nursing (examples include Anderson, Walsh, Louey, Meade, & Fairbrother, 2002; Brooten et al., 2002; Crowther, 2003; Spetz, 2005) and a plethora of cost-effectiveness studies (Neumann, Greenberg, Olchanski, Stone, & Rosen, 2005). In addition to being able to read about the results of studies related to the services provided, APNs and other clinicians are being asked to participate in these analyses or review published reports of economic evidence for appropriateness regarding implementation into practice (examples include Chiu & Newcomer, 2007; Chummun & Tiran, 2008; Lee, Chan, Chen, Gin, & Lau, 2007; Subramanian et al., 2007).

A number of different methods are employed to address economic outcomes of health care. The purposes of this chapter are (a) to present an overview of five different types of economic evaluations an APN may encounter, (b) discuss appropriate outcome measures for each type of analysis, (c) present and critique published examples of each type of economic evaluation, and (d) discuss methodological issues of importance to economic evaluations.

TYPES OF ECONOMIC EVALUATIONS

Five different methods of economic evaluations are commonly used in assessing the economic impact of new health care interventions and technology. Table 2.1 presents a brief overview of these methods (Drummond, Sculpher, Torrance, O'Brien, & Stoddart, 2005). In all of these

Table 2.1

TYPES OF ECONOMIC EVALUATIONS

TYPE OF STUDY	DEFINITION	EFFECT MEASUREMENT
Cost-minimization analysis (CMA)	An analysis that computes the incremental costs of alternatives that achieve the same outcome	Not measured
Cost-consequences analysis (CCA)	An analysis in which incremental costs and effects are computed, without any attempt to aggregate them	Naturally occurring units*
Cost-effectiveness analysis (CEA)	An analysis in which incremental costs and effects are presented in a ratio	Naturally occurring units
Cost-utility analysis (CUA)	A special type of cost-effectiveness analysis, in which quality of life is considered	Quality-adjusted life years
Cost-benefit analysis (CBA)	An analysis in which incremental costs and effects are computed and all benefits and costs are measured in dollars	Dollars

*Examples of naturally occurring units are life-years gained, disability-days saved, or cases avoided.

economic outcome evaluations, alternative strategies are compared and the incremental cost of the competing strategies is computed according to the following formula:

$$\text{Incremental Costs} = C_1 - C_2$$

where C_1 represents the cost of the new intervention and C_2 represents the cost of the comparator (e.g., the next best strategy). There is more variation between methods regarding how effectiveness is measured, although the focus remains on incremental changes in effectiveness (i.e., comparing the outcome of one intervention with that of another).

Cost-Minimization Analysis

In a true cost-minimization analysis (CMA), only the costs are evaluated and the alternatives are assumed or have been found to offer equivalent outcomes. Many of these studies begin as cost-effectiveness studies (discussed in more detail below), in which the investigators expected one intervention to be both more effective and more expensive. As a result, in most published economic evaluations labeled as CMAs, some level of effectiveness of the strategies being compared is measured (examples include Goodman et al., 2007; Patel, Duquaine, & McKinnon, 2007). In each study, clinical outcomes were measured prior to the study being published as a cost-minimization analysis. In the Goodman et al. (2007) study, the authors measured a number of outcomes of a fitness-for-life program and found no statistically significant differences between groups. In the Patel et al. (2007) study, outcomes associated with changes in the dosing of meropenem were found to be similar prior to the study being published as a cost-minimization study.

Cost-Consequence Analysis

A cost-consequence analysis (CCA) is a study in which the costs and the consequences of two or more alternatives are measured, but costs and consequences are listed separately. This methodology is often chosen when there is no obvious summary measure for the outcomes applicable to the interventions being studied. In a CCA, the analyst expects the decision makers to form their own opinions about the relative importance of the findings. To facilitate decision making, the analysts provide an array of consequences applicable to each strategy. Two studies serve as examples of this methodology being used in the nursing literature. Sørensen and Frich (2008) analyzed the consequences of a nurse follow-up intervention for chronic nonmalignant pain patients and described outcomes in terms of the eight SF-36 subscales. Dawes et al. (2007) compared nurse-supported early discharge for women receiving major abdominal or pelvic surgery with those receiving usual care. In addition to studying costs, Dawes et al. examined results from the SF-36, complications, length of hospital stay, readmissions, and satisfaction.

Cost-Effectiveness Analysis

Cost-effectiveness analysis (CEA) also measures incremental costs. In CEA, incremental consequences are measured in a single common natu-

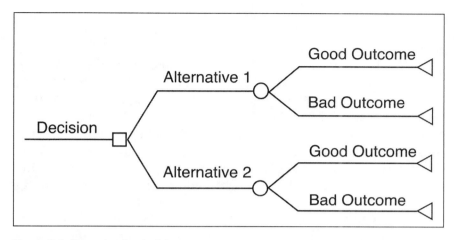

Figure 2.1 Example of a decision tree.

ral unit, such as life-years gained or cases avoided. In addition, costs and effects are summarized in an incremental cost-effectiveness ratio, which is calculated using the following formula:

$$\text{Cost-effectiveness ratio} = (C_1 - C_2)/(E_1 - E_2)$$

where C_1 equals the cost of the new intervention, C_2 equals the cost of the comparator, E_1 equals the effect of the new intervention, and E_2 equals the effect of the comparator. For CEA, analysts often attach the resource utilization data-collection process to a randomized trial, usually powered on something other than the cost-effectiveness result (e.g., Paez & Allen, 2006, examined nurse management of hypercholesterolemia patients), or employ a decision-analytic approach and model the problem through the use of a decision tree (e.g., Honkanen, Mushlin, Lachs, & Schackman, 2005, modeled external hip protectors being used in nursing homes). A sample decision tree is diagrammed in Figure 2.1.

The decision is between choosing alternative 1 or alternative 2. Both alternatives have associated probabilities of good and bad outcomes. In addition, there are the associated costs of each strategy. The use of decision analysis and decision trees is a defined mathematical modeling technique. It is suggested that anyone interested in using this technique seek training opportunities. There are a number of highly readable texts available to the APN wishing to understand this approach better (Drummond et al., 2005; Haddix, Teutsch, & Corso, 2002; Muennig, 2008; Petitti, 2000).

A number of examples of CEA can be found in the recent nursing literature (Ganz, Simmons, & Schnelle, 2005; Honkanen et al., 2005; Paez & Allen, 2006; Rost, Pyne, Dickinson, & LoSasso, 2005). Paez and Allen (2006) provide an excellent example of deriving a cost-effectiveness analysis from a randomized trial. The study included 228 consecutive adults with hypercholesterolemia and chronic heart disease who were hospitalized. The intervention was follow-up care regarding lipid management, including lifestyle modification with services being provided by a nurse practitioner; this was compared with usual care enhanced with a small amount of extra information on lipids. The results were expressed as the extra dollars spent per unit change in low-density lipoprotein cholesterol (LDL-C) at 1 year and per percentage reduction in LDL-C at 1 year. Although this is an acceptable health outcome, it only facilitates comparison with other studies that are focusing on interventions for hypercholesterolemia. In contrast, Ganz, Simmons, and Schnelle used a Markov simulation cohort (i.e., simulating what happens to a cohort of individuals over multiple periods through time) to estimate the cost-effectiveness of having recommended staffing levels. This group used data from the literature, showed the sources very clearly, and expressed their results in dollars per quality-adjusted life year (discussed in more detail below).

The quality-adjusted life year is a common outcome unit at this point in time, as it has been recommended by a number of organizations around the world and facilitates comparisons among different studies. More generally, many economic analysts recommend using a standard outcome measure, such as dollars per life year ($/LY), because it is appropriate to different health care situations. Consequently, results can be compared across a variety of patient populations and settings. Although easy to understand, an outcome measure of $/LY considers only survival, not suboptimal health states and/or quality of life. This is a concern, as quality of life is often considered an important issue to individuals considering different health care treatments. This leads directly into the more detailed discussion of quality-adjusted life years (QALY) and their application which follows.

Cost-Utility Analysis

Cost-utility analysis (CUA) considers the effectiveness of the interventions on both the quantity and the quality of life in a single multidimensional measure, QALY. The QALY is a measure of the quantity of life gained weighted by the quality of that life. Quality of life is measured by a utility, which is a measure of preference for a given health state rated on a scale of 0 (death) to 1 (perfect health). Because dollars spent to gain a QALY are not disease specific, the measure is useful for informing health policy decisions and is recommended for such use by the U.S. Public Health Service's Panel on Cost-Effectiveness in Health and Medicine (Gold, Siegel, Russell, & Weinstein, 1996). However, at a recent meeting of the International Society of Pharmacoeconomics and Outcomes Research (ISPOR), a speaker highlighted that there is variance in the interpretation of what QALYs are actually measuring ("Determinants," 2006) and there is not universal agreement as to what society should be willing to pay to gain a QALY (Hirth, Chernew, Miller, Fendrick, & Weissert, 2000; Ubel, Hirth, Chernew, & Fendrick, 2003), although the figure of $50,000/QALY is still often cited.

One group of researchers considered a nursing intervention to increase adherence to antiretroviral therapy among HIV-infected patients (Freedberg et al., 2006). The design of this study illustrates how data from a randomized clinical trial can be combined with a computer-modeling exercise to conduct the cost-effectiveness analysis. The authors modeled the associated change in virologic suppression as well as changes in cost and quality-adjusted survival. Comparing these results with the costs of the intervention and the therapy, the authors found the intervention to be highly cost-effective, with a ratio of $14,100 per QALY gained compared with standard therapy.

Cost-Benefit Analysis

Cost-benefit analysis (CBA) is a form of economic evaluation in which consequences are measured according to some monetary unit. In CBA, a single dollar figure representing costs minus benefits is calculated. As long as the decision maker agrees with the methods used to place a dollar value on outcomes, this provides the decision maker with a direct indication of whether the value of the benefits is greater than the cost. Simon et al. (2007) determined the net economic benefit of a nurse specialist-led program for patients with depression and diabetes. Their study used a randomized trial design and compared this program with "usual care" intervention. The care provided included psychotherapy and pharmaceutical treatment. A sufficient amount of other health services utilization was saved so that if a day without depression was counted as $10 (the type of assumption necessary for a cost-benefit analysis), the total positive economic benefit per patient was $952. The authors also conducted a statistical analysis to demonstrate that the 95% confidence interval regarding the point estimate of economic net benefit did not include zero.

COMMON ISSUES IN ALL ECONOMIC EVALUATIONS

The basic steps in conducting economic evaluations are illustrated in Figure 2.2. In addition, because this is essentially a new language to many APNs, Table 2.2 defines some of the concepts and common terminology used in these analyses.

Selecting the Type of Economic Evaluation

The first step is to select the appropriate type of analysis to conduct. Considerations should include: (a) the goal of the analysis (e.g., whether to compare only interventions affecting a single disease with a well-defined most important symptom or to compare interventions for different diseases or interventions for a condition with a complex set of symptoms), (b) whether the effectiveness of the interventions is equivalent (and, if so, this suggests a cost-minimization analysis), (c) the effectiveness measures available (e.g., can QALYs be generated), (d) the potential impact of the interventions on either quality or quantity of life (if both, then a cost-utility analysis is most appropriate), (e) the availability of data, (f) the expertise available, and (g) ethical issues.

Framing the Analysis

Once the economic method has been selected, the analysis is framed. This includes selecting the appropriate comparator(s) to analyze. For example, the cost-effectiveness of a new educational program offered

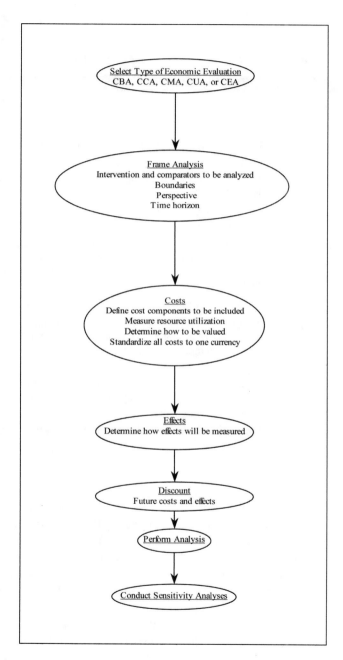

Figure 2.2 Basic steps in economic evaluations.

Table 2.2

COMMON TERMINOLOGY IN ECONOMIC EVALUATIONS

TERM	DEFINITION
Boundaries of the study	The scope of the study
Comparator(s)	The alternative(s) to which the new intervention is compared
Consumer price index (CPI)	A measure of average change in price over time; used to adjust costs that are estimated in different years
Discounting	The process of converting future costs and effects to the present value
Incremental cost-effectiveness ratio	The ratio of the difference of the costs of two alternatives to the difference in effectiveness between the same two alternatives; used in cost-effectiveness and cost-utility analyses
Perspective	The viewpoint from which the analysis is conducted
Sensitivity analysis	Calculations in which a parameter is varied and indicates the degree of influence it has on the analysis; often used when a parameter is uncertain
Probabilistic sensitivity analysis	Calculations in which one or more parameters are varied randomly, using a defined distribution to determine the proportion of times that an intervention is economically favored in comparison with other interventions
Time horizon	The period of time for which the costs and effects are measured

in a hospital setting may be different from an outpatient-focused program or from the absence of teaching altogether. At the least, the comparison of new interventions should be to the current practice, *or* status quo. This also emphasizes the fact that analyses do not compare an intervention with "doing nothing." In addition, often more than one comparator is appropriate to include in the analysis. This is especially true when multiple alternatives have been found to offer similar clinical outcomes *or* potentially there are multiple levels of intensity of the interventions (e.g., increasing home health visits from twice a week to daily).

   Boundaries (i.e., the scope) of the study delimit the costs and effects that are included in the analysis. Many interventions have some spillover effects that must be considered. The question becomes how far to follow such effects to adequately assess the economic impact of the intervention. For example, if the aim of an educational program for mothers of infants admitted to a neonatal intensive care unit is to decrease the mothers' level of anxiety and improve the physiologic outcomes of the infant, then it logically follows that the boundaries would include both the mother and the infant. This intervention may affect the overall parenting skills of the mother, however, and may have additional positive effects on other children in the family. In theory, all these effects are relevant, but in framing the study it is important to draw practical and feasible limits around the analysis.
   In all types of economic evaluations, the *perspective* or viewpoint taken in the analysis also drives the set of costs and benefits included. Studies may be motivated by policy decisions relevant to specific institutions or individuals. In this case, the perspective of primary interest may be that of a managed care organization, hospital, employer, state health department, or other party. An economic evaluation conducted from the perspective of the hospital (i.e., providing a result most relevant to a hospital decision maker) should not consider costs (or savings) associated with family caregiving in the home. If the goal of the analysis is to affect broad resource allocation and health policy issues, however, then the societal perspective is appropriate and recommended (Gold et al., 1996). This perspective incorporates all costs and all health effects regardless of who incurs them. This is advantageous because if a systematic analysis is performed to compare the results of multiple studies and all have used the societal perspective, it makes comparison easier. Gathering data for the societal perspective also allows any other perspective to be calculated as a subset of the societal perspective. A general rule is to take a societal perspective and then, if desired, present the same results from a different perspective.
   The *time horizon* refers to the period of time for which the costs and benefits are measured in the analysis. The time horizon may vary from less than 1 year to the patient's entire life span. The appropriate time horizon to consider will depend on the probable length of effect of the interventions being compared. Once the framing of the analysis is complete, the analyst is ready to estimate costs. The distinction between the time of the intervention and the time horizon for the

analysis must be kept in mind. An intervention that lasts less than 1 year (e.g., nurses providing counseling to adolescents on high-risk behaviors) may have effects that last a lifetime.

Costs

Terminology pertaining to costs of resources has traditionally been divided into "direct" and "indirect" costs (Gold et al., 1996), with other labels like "friction costs" sometimes being applied to the cost of hiring a new employee and sometimes being applied to an entire method of valuing productivity (Brouwer & Koopmanschap, 2005; Gold et al., 1996). However, because economists and accountants do not use the same definitions and sometimes even economists have not been able to agree on a universal set of definitions, the terminology has become complicated. In health economics, direct costs have been defined as changes in resource use directly attributable to the provision of care, whereas indirect costs have referred to costs associated with the loss of productivity from morbidity and/or mortality (Liljas, 1998). Accountants, on the other hand, refer to direct costs as variable costs (e.g., supplies) and indirect costs as overhead costs (e.g., rent) (Anthony & Young, 1994). In light of these past inconsistencies in defining and measuring costs, the APN conducting an economic evaluation should be sure to clarify and clearly communicate how the cost terms are defined. The trend in the CEA literature is to avoid the term "indirect." Given this trend and the potential for confusion, we urge APNs to likewise avoid using this term.

Economists and analysts often use a "two-step" approach to determine the costs attributable to an intervention. The first step in the estimation is determining the amount of resources attributable or consumed. Once the attributable resources have been determined, the "money" valuation or costs of the resources may be estimated. Using a two-step approach increases the clarity and transparency of the analysis and allows readers of the analysis to understand how the costs of attributable resources may be similar or different in their own setting.

The resources and associated costs can be categorized as in Table 2.3, which is an adaptation of a grouping that appeared earlier in the literature (Luce, Manning, Siegel, & Lipscomb, 1996). In CEA, financial health care costs are directly related to the intervention itself and associ-

Table 2.3

COST COMPONENTS TO CONSIDER FOR INCLUSION

COST COMPONENTS

Financial, health care
Intervention
Hospitalization
Outpatient visits
Long-term care
Other health care

Financial, non-health care
Transportation
Social services

Value of time and lost productivity
Patient time receiving care
Family/informal caregiver time

Patient loss of productivity due only to morbidity or mortality*
Other

*Not recommended for inclusion in cost-utility analyses by the U.S. Public Health Service's Panel on Cost-Effectiveness in Health and Medicine (Gold et al., 1996).

ated costs or savings of future health care, which the intervention may impact. For example, financial health care costs associated with a hepatitis B virus (HBV) immunization program should include the costs of obtaining and administering the immunization. In addition, they should include "downstream" costs (as well as savings), such as hospitalizations, outpatient visits, and other treatment costs associated with the diagnosis of HBV itself. Financial costs associated with other related diseases, such as cirrhosis or cancer, should also be included. Similarly, the value of the time a patient spends either seeking care or participating in an intervention constitutes a real use of resources for the individual and society. Thus, relevant patient–time costs may include both the time involved in receiving the treatment and the time spent waiting to receive care.

Consumption of resources other than those associated with the provision of health care also should be considered in economic evaluations conducted from the societal perspective. Financial non-health care costs may include, for example, child care costs for a parent attending a smoking cessation program, increase in a family's food expenditure as a result of a dietary prescription, the cost of transportation to and from a clinic, etc.

Historically, patient time and other non-health care resources have not been consistently included in analyses (Jacobs & Fassbender, 1998; Stone, Chapman, Sandberg, Liljas, & Neumann, 2000). Nonetheless, if an analysis is conducted from the societal perspective, inclusion of such factors is recommended (Gold et al., 1996). In addition, because health care is becoming more community-based, nursing interventions may directly influence these costs. For example, a home visit by an APN case manager may not only increase the ability of the APN to conduct a holistic assessment, but also may save resources related to patient time, transportation, and family caregiving.

Productivity costs are the costs associated with morbidity or mortality. **Morbidity costs** are those associated with lost or impaired ability to work or to engage in leisure activities (e.g., loss of income due to time for recuperation or convalescence after coronary bypass surgery). **Mortality costs** are related to loss of life, and are usually measured according to what the individual would have been capable of earning. Two issues are important to note concerning productivity costs:

- First, the U.S. Public Health Service's Panel on Cost-Effectiveness in Health and Medicine recommended that productivity costs be excluded from CUAs (Gold et al., 1996). The authors expressed concern that including both productivity costs and QALYs would represent a double counting because people may be considering productivity and earning potential when responding to tradeoffs involving health and quality of life. Thus, when QALYs are used, productivity is already included in the denominator of the cost-effectiveness ratio.
- Second, this assumption is controversial and has been debated by experts in the field (Brouwer, Koopmanschap, & Rutten, 1997a, 1997b; Weinstein & Manning, 1997; Weinstein et al., 1997). In light of this controversy, some analysts have presented results both with and without the inclusion of productivity costs (Krahn, Guasparini, Sherman, & Detsky, 1998). APNs conducting CUAs may also wish to present results both with and without the inclu-

sion of productivity costs as well as continue to monitor recommendations made in the United States and elsewhere.

Some interventions (e.g., a successful smoking cessation program) extend life. Costs related to resource consumption in "added life-years" are recommended for inclusion in economic evaluations. Added life-year costs are related to the consumption of health care resources (financial health care costs) and other types of consumption (all other cost categories). Because not all analyses increase life expectancy (e.g., use of cochlear implants or an educational intervention program aimed at decreasing parental anxiety), resource consumption in added life-years is not always applicable. Sometimes, living longer and healthier can cost less annually but more over time (van Baal et al., 2008).

Finally, income transfers such as Social Security payments are redistributions of money and are therefore not real costs to society. Consequently, although these "transfer costs" may be tracked and may be important for analyses from the government's perspective, they should not be included with other societal costs. What should be included in a societal cost analysis are the costs of administering an income transfer program.

When trying to determine which costs to include, the process should begin with an outline of the categories of costs included, using the list in Table 2.3. Once this is complete, a researcher should consider the cost "ingredients" that the intervention impacts under each category (Drummond et al., 2005). After the ingredients are identified, discussions about which costs are most relevant and which are important to measure can take place. Moreover, the perspective of the analysis will drive the decisions about which cost component to include. The treatment of the cost component (e.g., productivity costs captured in quality-of-life adjustments) is determined by the specific economic analytic method chosen.

Once the consumption of resources has been estimated, the resource must be assigned a dollar value. Economists use the term "opportunity costs," which reflects the value of the next-best alternative use of the resources. Determining the actual opportunity cost of a resource is difficult. Following are some general guidelines for assigning a dollar value to a resource.

In many markets, market prices (or charges) equate to costs. This does not apply in health care as often as in other fields. This incongruence is particularly notable for charges associated with hospitalizations, due to institutional "cost shifting." Health care delivery institutions charge a certain amount to patients when sending out bills. Cost shifting is the practice of obtaining higher costs from payers who are willing to pay higher levels of reimbursement or unable to negotiate lower levels of reimbursement. Therefore, for these institutional categories, an adjustment to prices is necessary. However, many customers, such as large insurance organizations, pay only a fraction of these charges. Large payers negotiate payment rates for services rendered based on the cost of the service and allowed profit margins (or excess revenues for not-for-profit institutions). Payers with the least market power (e.g., uninsured individuals) are the only ones who are likely to pay anything near the actual cost. If a hospital were just to break even based on the negotiated rates, then it is clear that the actual amount charged does not represent anything close to the actual cost.

Instead of using charges, a common source of valuation for hospital costs is the hospital's own cost-accounting system. For researchers internal to the institution, these will often be easy to access. These cost-accounting systems are developed by finance departments to help administrative decision making and are based on past accounting studies and algorithms. Although the market price of medical care often does not represent actual costs, the market prices of the goods in the cost-accounting system are expected to represent the relevant cost. If a cost-accounting system is available, the APN can usually determine the specific monetary health care–cost components, such as variable costs (e.g., staffing and supplies) and fixed overhead costs (e.g., rent and percentage of administration costs).

Another alternative is to use hospital cost-to-charge ratios (CCRs), which are calculated by dividing the total costs in a cost center by the total charges for the same resource. CCRs are recognized as a gross adjustment to charges. This type of adjustment is better than using charges alone, but is not preferable to cost-accounting systems when they are available. Published sources also are often used as the source of valuation of the resource (Stone, Chapman, Sandberg, Liljas, & Neumann, 2000). Governmental fee schedules are also often used to represent costs of particular procedures (Armstrong, Malone, & Erder, 2008).

When cost estimations come from various sources, it is important to standardize all costs to the same currency and year. For example, non-U.S. currency figures may be converted into U.S. dollars using the appropriate foreign exchange factor for that year (Federal Reserve Bank of St. Louis, http://www.stls.frb.org/fred/data/exchange.html). A study of stoma therapy nurses demonstrates the concept of exchange rates (Becker, Schulten-Oberbörsch, Beck, & Vestweber, 1999). The concept of purchasing-power parity, which not only accounts for the exchange rate but attempts to yield the capacity to purchase the same quantity of goods, is also commonly used (Urdahl et al., 2003). In addition, because $1 in 1988 does not have the same purchasing power as $1 in the year 2008, the costs from different years must be adjusted into a standard year format by the use of the consumer price index (CPI), for which data are available from the Bureau of Labor Statistics (BLS) Web site (www.bls.gov) and a single year-to-year calculation can be done using the inflation calculator provided at that Web site (http://data.bls.gov/cgi-bin/cpicalc.pl). This inflation calculator is based on general market goods inflation. The BLS also calculates a medical inflation rate. Because the costs of health care are rising more rapidly than costs in most other markets, analysts often use the medical inflation rate to inflate costs that pertain only to health care resources. A recent study of the costs of nurse turnover demonstrates inflation adjustment for calculations that could serve as an input to cost-benefit analyses related to retention efforts (Jones, 2008). Finally, there is discussion as to whether to use the consumer price index or the producer price index for inflation adjustment in general.

Discounting

Once all costs and benefits have been calculated, future costs and benefits are discounted to present value. Discounting reflects the principle that suggests people place greater value on something they have today than on something they will have in the future. Interest rates are an example of this principle. Future costs and benefits are discounted to present value using the following formula:

$$F/(1 + r)^n$$

where F = the future value (usually measured in dollars at today's value), r = the discount rate, and n = the number of years in the future (Stone, 1998). Currently, in the United States, experts recommend using a 3% discount rate, to discount both costs and effects (Gold et al., 1996). However, because prevention interventions are aimed at improving future health, by discounting future benefits the intervention may not seem as beneficial. Therefore, some analysts are uncomfortable discounting future health benefits and only discount costs (Stone et al., 2000). Thus, to increase the comparability of analyses, APNs in the United States should discount both costs and effects at 3% and, if desired, the results without discounting may also be presented (Gold et al., 1996). Moreover, prior to the recommendations being issued by the U.S. Public Health Service's Panel on Cost-Effectiveness in Health and Medicine in 1996, many analysts used a 5% discount rate, so this was suggested as an additional discount rate to use for comparison (Gold et al., 1996).

Analysis

In conducting economic evaluations, data gathered may include resource utilization, value of resources, effectiveness of treatment, and preferences regarding health outcomes. Based on the data gathered, the "base-case" analysis is computed. If the recommendations made by the U.S. Public Health Service's Panel on Cost-Effectiveness in Health and Medicine are followed, this initial analysis is labeled a "reference case" (Gold et al., 1996). A best practice when presenting results (whether they represent the reference case or not) is to include a table listing all parameters, the value assigned to each parameter, and the source of the value.

Sensitivity Analysis

Many of the data points gathered include some assumptions or uncertainty in the parameter. For clarification, the analysis based only on the best point estimates is referred to as the "base case," regardless of whether the recommendations of the Panel are followed. Thus, any cost-effectiveness analysis includes a base case, but not all base case analyses are reference case analyses.

The assumptions that are made in the base case should be clearly stated before the results are presented, to increase the transparency of the analysis. In addition, sensitivity analyses should be conducted to explore the implications of alternative assumptions. Sensitivity analysis is an important element of a sound economic evaluation (Drummond et al., 2005; Gold et al., 1996).

Sensitivity analyses are calculations in which a parameter is varied. These analyses indicate the degree of influence the particular value has on the analysis. The range used for a parameter should be specified along with the point estimate in Table 2.2.

A univariate sensitivity analysis examines the degree to which changing a single assumption changes the outcome of the entire analysis. By varying the value of the variable over a reasonable set of parameters, the investigator is able to determine how that variable may impact the results under different assumptions. The impact on the results has multiple interpretations. One is how the magnitude of the cost-effectiveness ratio changes, in other words, whether the ratio changes from spending $10,000/QALY gained to $30,000/QALY gained. However, a second level of interpretation is whether the decision to implement or not implement a new intervention changes. If a decision maker believes that any program costing less than $50,000 is a candidate for implementation, then the change from $10,000/QALY to $30,000/QALY will not change the decision about whether to consider a new intervention for implementation. Ganz, Simmons, and Schnelle (2005) used a series of univariate sensitivity analyses to explore which parameter led to the greatest change in the incremental cost-effectiveness of raising nurse staffing in skilled nursing facilities from the median level to the recommended level. The authors found that the parameter leading to the largest changes was the probability of admission to acute hospital from the nursing home. They also described the relationship between the incremental cost-effectiveness ratio and other variables.

Although univariate sensitivity analyses are insightful, looking at one source of uncertainty by itself is usually inadequate. The alternative is multivariate sensitivity analysis. A multivariate sensitivity analysis examines multiple sources of uncertainty at one time and may generate a more accurate understanding of the uncertainty of the cost-effectiveness results. This can be done by changing all parameters to their most or least favorable levels—but still working with predetermined levels of the values for each variable. A second approach makes use of the fact that variables can sometimes be expected to change together; in such cases, the analyst might explore how the cost-effectiveness ratio changes as the two variables are varied over their ranges. Finally, an analyst can conduct what is referred to as a probabilistic sensitivity analysis.

In this case, the analyst must define distributions from which the values for parameters may be drawn. A random draw is then taken from each distribution and the results of the analysis are calculated. The results of the first analysis are recorded and the process is repeated—at least thousands and sometimes tens of thousands of times. The analyst must then describe the range of results by describing the distribution of ratios. Honkanen et al. (2007) use this technique to describe the distribution of cost-effectiveness results in a study of hip protector use intended to prevent fractures in a community-dwelling geriatric population. One result this group found was that the incremental cost-effectiveness ratio was less than $50,000/QALY in 68% of repeated random results for women initiating hip protector use at age 75. A decision maker faced with this information would have to determine whether being 68% certain of a favorable economic result is sufficient to move forward with a policy change.

CONCLUSIONS

The checklist in Table 2.4 may be useful when reporting or reading a report of an economic evaluation. This checklist draws on criteria for high-quality cost-effectiveness studies and draws on a number of sets of criteria that have been specified over the past decade (Drummond et al., 2005; Gold et al., 1996; Tarn & Dix Smith, 2005).

With the continuing development of new treatments, technologies, and models of care delivery, health-economics evaluations have become increasingly important. The demand for economic outcome research is growing, as is the number of published analyses. In this chapter, we have introduced various methods used in economic evaluation and have described the concepts and terminology used in these analyses.

The quality of studies has been variable and not necessarily improving. As more studies are conducted and submitted for peer-reviewed publication, editors are not always able to find reviewers with the appropriate expertise, hence, studies that are poorly conducted in general or for which specific elements are poor can make their way into print. APNs who plan to read these analyses need to understand methodology enough to recognize what makes a good study and what makes a study that is barely acceptable or even fails the test of acceptability.

Table 2.4

CEA CHECKLIST FOR JOURNAL REPORT

1. Framework

- Background of the problem
- General framing and design of the problem
- Target population for the intervention
- Other program descriptors
- Description of comparator programs
- Boundaries of the analysis
- Time horizon
- Statement of the perspective of the analysis

2. Data and Methods

- Description of event pathway
- Identification of outcomes of interest in the analysis
- Description of model used
- Modeling assumptions
- Diagram of event pathway/model
- Software used
- Complete information about the sources of effectiveness data, cost data, and preference weights
- Methods for obtaining estimates of effectiveness, costs, and preferences
- Critique of data quality
- Statement of year costs
- Statement of method used to adjust costs for inflation
- Statement of type of currency
- Sources and methods for obtaining expert judgment
- Statement of discount rates

3. Results

- Results of model validation
- Reference case results (discounted and undiscounted): total costs and effectiveness, incremental costs and effectiveness, and incremental cost-effectiveness ratios
- Results of sensitivity analyses
- Other estimates of uncertainty, if available
- Graphical representation of cost-effectiveness results
- Aggregate cost and effectiveness information
- Disaggregated results, as relevant
- Secondary analyses using 5% discount rate
- Other secondary analyses, as relevant

(continued)

(Table 2.4 continued)

4. Discussion

- Summary of reference case results
- Summary of sensitivity analysis assumptions having important ethical implications
- Limitations of the study
- Relevance of the study results for specific policy questions or decisions
- Results of related CEAs
- Distributive implications of the intervention

5. Technical report in appendix or available upon request.

Adapted from Gold et al. (1996).

APNs interested in exploring this type of outcome evaluation are encouraged to seek additional training in these methods.

If APNs participate in and conduct economic evaluations concerning the care they provide, the cost-effectiveness of APN care may be demonstrated. When the analysis uses a standard methodology and the assumptions are transparent, the results are more easily interpreted. If the outcome measure is a standard ratio, such as dollars per QALY gained, the results may furnish a strong argument to health-policy decision makers concerning the funding and continued recognition of APNs as cost-effective health care providers.

REFERENCES

Anderson, P. J., Walsh, J. M., Louey, M. A., Meade, C., & Fairbrother, G. (2002). Comparing first and subsequent suprapubic catheter change: Complications and costs. *Urological Nursing, 22,* 324–325, 328–330.

Anthony, R. N., & Young, D. W. (1994). *Management control in nonprofit organizations* (5th ed.). Boston: Irwin McGraw-Hill.

Armstrong, E. P., Malone, D. C., & Erder, M. H. (2008). A Markov cost-utility analysis of escitalopram and duloxetine for the treatment of major depressive disorder. *Current Medical Research and Opinion, 24,* 1115–1121.

Becker, A., Schulten-Oberbörsch, G., Beck, U., & Vestweber, K. H. (1999). Stoma care nurses: Good value for money? *World Journal of Surgery, 23,* 638–642.

Brooten, D., Naylor, M. D., York, R., Brown, L. P., Munro, B. H., Hollingsworth, A.O., Cohen, S. M., Finkler, S., Deatrick, J., & Youngblut, J. M. (2002). Lessons learned from testing the quality cost model of advanced practice nursing (APN) transitional care. *Journal of Nursing Scholarship, 34,* 369–375.

Brouwer, W. B., & Koopmanschap, M. A. (2005). The friction-cost method: Replacement for nothing and leisure for free? *Pharmacoeconomics, 23,* 105–111.

Brouwer, W. B., Koopmanschap, M. A., & Rutten, F. F. (1997a). Productivity costs measurement through quality of life? A response to the recommendation of the Washington panel. *Health Economics, 6,* 253–259.

Brouwer, W. B., Koopmanschap, M. A., & Rutten, F. F. (1997b). Productivity costs in cost-effectiveness analysis: Numerator or denominator: A further discussion. *Health Economics, 6,* 511–514.

Catlin, A., Cowan, C., Hartman, M., Heffler, S., & National Health Expenditure Accounts Team. (2008). National health spending in 2006: A year of change for prescription drugs. *Health Affairs (Millwood), 27,* 14–29.

Chiu, W. K., & Newcomer, R. (2007). A systematic review of nurse-assisted case management to improve hospital discharge transition outcomes for the elderly. *Professional Case Management, 12,* 330–336.

Chummun, H., & Tiran, D. (2008). Increasing research evidence in practice: A possible role for the consultant nurse. *Journal of Nursing Management, 16,* 327–333.

Crowther, M. (2003). Optimal management of outpatients with heart failure using advanced practice nurses in a hospital-based heart failure center. *Journal of American Academic Nurse Practice, 15,* 260–265.

Dawes, H. A., Docherty, T., Traynor, I., Gilmore, D. H., Jardine, A. G., & Knill-Jones, R. (2007). Specialist nurse supported discharge in gynaecology: A randomised comparison and economic evaluation. *European Journal of Obstetrics, Gynecology, and Reproductive Biology, 130,* 262–270.

Determinants of health economic decisions in actual practice: The role of behavioral economics. (2006). [Summary of the presentation given by Professor Daniel Kahneman at the ISPOR 10th Annual International Meeting First Plenary Session, May 16, 2005, Washington, DC, USA.] *Value in Health, 9*(2), 65–67.

Drummond, M., Sculpher, M. J., Torrance, G. W., O'Brien, B. J., & Stoddart, G. L. (2005). *Methods for the economic evaluation of health care programmes* (3rd ed.). New York: Oxford University Press.

Freedberg, K. A., Hirschhorn, L. R., Schackman, B. R., Wolf, L. L., Martin, L. A., Weinstein, M. C., Goldin, S., Paltiel, A. D., Katz, C., Goldie, S. J., Losina, E. (2006). Cost-effectiveness of an intervention to improve adherence to antiretroviral therapy in HIV-infected patients. *Journal of Acquired Immune Deficiency Syndrome, 43*(Suppl. 1), S113–S118.

Ganz, D. A., Simmons, S. F., & Schnelle, J. F. (2005). Cost-effectiveness of recommended nurse staffing levels for short-stay skilled nursing facility patients. *BMC Health Services Research, 5,* 35.

Gold, M. R., Siegel, J. E., Russell, L. B., & Weinstein, M. C. (1996). *Cost effectiveness in health and medicine.* New York: Oxford University Press.

Goodman, H., Parsons, A., Davison, J., Preedy, M., Peters, E., Shuldham, C., Pepper, J., & Cowie, M. R. (2008). A randomised controlled trial to evaluate a nurse-led programme of support and lifestyle management for patients awaiting cardiac surgery 'Fit for surgery: Fit for life' study. *European Journal of Cardiovascular Nursing, 7,* 189–195. Epub 2007 Dec 21.

Haddix, A. C., Teutsch, S. M., & Corso, P. S. (2002). *Prevention effectiveness: A guide to decision analysis and economic evaluation* (2nd ed.). New York: Oxford University Press.

Hirth, R. A., Chernew, M. E., Miller, E., Fendrick, A. M., & Weissert, W. G. (2000). Willingness to pay for a quality-adjusted life year: In search of a standard. *Medical Decision Making, 20,* 332–342.

Honkanen, L. A., Mushlin, A. I., Lachs, M., & Schackman, B. R. (2007). Can hip protector use cost-effectively prevent fractures in community-dwelling geriatric populations? *Journal of the American Geriatrics Society, 54,* 1658–1665.

Honkanen, L. A., Schackman, B. R., Mushlin, A. I., & Lachs, M. S. (2005). A cost-benefit analysis of external hip protectors in the nursing home setting. *Journal of the American Geriatrics Society, 53,* 190–197.

Jacobs, P., & Fassbender, K. (1998). The measurement of indirect costs in the health economics evaluation literature: A review. *International Journal of Technology Assessment in Health Care, 14,* 799–808.

Jones, C. B. (2008). Revisiting nurse turnover costs: Adjusting for inflation. *Journal of Nursing Administration, 38,* 11–18.

Krahn, M., Guasparini, R., Shennan, M., & Detsky, A. S. (1998). Costs and cost effectiveness of a universal, school-based hepatitis B vaccination program. *American Journal of Public Health, 88,* 1638–1644.

Lee, A., Chan, S., Chen, P. P., Gin, T., & Lau, A. S. (2007). Economic evaluations of acute pain service programs: A systematic review. *Clinical Journal of Pain, 23,* 726–733.

Liljas, B. (1998). How to calculate indirect costs in economic evaluations. *PharmacoEconomics, 13,* 1–7.

Luce, B. R., Manning, W. G., Siegel, J. E., & Lipscomb, J. (1996). Estimating costs in cost-effectiveness analysis. In M. Gold, J. E. Siegel, L. Russell, & M. Weinstein (Eds.), *Cost-effectiveness in health and medicine* (pp. 176–213). New York: Oxford University Press.

Muennig, P. (2008). *Cost-effectiveness analyses in health care: A practical approach* (2nd ed.). San Francisco, CA: Jossey-Bass.

Neumann, P. J., Greenberg, D., Olchanski, N. V., Stone, P. W., & Rosen, A. B. (2005). Growth and quality of the cost-utility literature, 1976-2001. *Value Health, 8*(1), 3–9.

Paez, K. A., & Allen, J. K. (2006). Cost-effectiveness of nurse practitioner management of hypercholesterolemia following coronary revascularization. *Journal of the American Academy of Nurse Practitioners, 18,* 436–444.

Patel, G. W., Duquaine, S. M., & McKinnon, P. S. (2007). Clinical outcomes and cost minimization with an alternative dosing regimen for meropenem in a community hospital. *Pharmacotherapy, 27,* 1637–1643.

Petitti, D. B. (2000). *Meta-analysis, decision analysis, and cost-effectiveness analysis: Methods for quantitative synthesis in medicine* (2nd ed.). New York: Oxford University Press.

Rost, K., Pyne, J. M., Dickinson, L. M., & LoSasso, A. T. (2005). Cost-effectiveness of enhancing primary care depression management on an ongoing basis. *Annals of Family Medicine, 3,* 7–14.

Simon, G. E., Katon, W. J., Lin, E. H., Rutter, C., Manning, W. G., Von Korff, M., et al. (2007). Cost-effectiveness of systematic depression treatment among people with diabetes mellitus. *Archives of General Psychiatry, 64,* 65–72.

Sørensen, J., & Frich, L. (2008). Home visits by specially trained nurses after discharge from multi-disciplinary pain care: A cost consequence analysis based on a randomised controlled trial. *European Journal of Pain, 12,* 164–171.

Spetz, J. (2005) The cost and cost-effectiveness of nursing services in health care. *Nursing Outlook, 53,* 305–309.

Stone, P. W. (1998). Methods for conducting and reporting cost-effectiveness analysis in nursing. *Image—The Journal of Nursing Scholarship, 30,* 229–234.

Stone, P. W., Chapman, R. H., Sandberg, E., Liljas, B., & Neumann, P. I. (2000). Measuring costs in cost-utility analyses: Variations in the literature. *International Journal of Technology Assessment in Health Care, 16,* 111–124.

Subramanian, S., Hoover, S., Gilman, B., Field, T. S., Mutter, R., & Gurwitz, J. H. (2007). Computerized physician order entry with clinical decision support in long-term care facilities: Costs and benefits to stakeholders. *Journal of the American Geriatrics Society, 55,* 1451–1457.

Tarn, T. Y. H., & Dix Smith, M. (2004). Pharmacoeconomic guidelines around the world. *ISPOR Connections, 10*(4), 5–15.

Ubel, P. A., Hirth, R. A., Chernew, M. E., & Fendrick, A. M. (2003). What is the price of life and why doesn't it increase at the rate of inflation? *Archives of Internal Medicine, 163,* 1637–1641.

Urdahl, H., Knapp, M., Edgell, E. T., Ghandi, G., Haro, J. M., & SOHO Study Group (2003). Unit costs in international economic evaluations: Resource costing of the Schizophrenia Outpatient Health Outcomes Study. *Acta Psychiatrica Scandinavica. Supplementum, 416,* 41–47.

van Baal, P. H., Polder, J. J., de Wit, G. A., Hoogenveen, R. T., Feenstra, T. L., Boshuizen, H. C., Engelfriet, P. M., & Brouwer, W. B. (2008). Lifetime medical costs of obesity: Prevention no cure for increasing health expenditure. *PLoS Medicine, 5,* e29.

Weinstein, M. C., & Manning, W. G. (1997) Theoretical issues in cost-effectiveness analysis. *Journal of Health Economics, 16,* 121–128.

Weinstein, M. C., Siegel, J. E., Garber, A. M., Lipscomb, J., Luce, R., Manning, W. G., & Torrance, G. W. (1997). Productivity costs, time costs and health related quality of life: A response to the Erasmus group. *Health Economics, 6,* 505–510.

3

Selecting Advanced Practice Nurse Outcome Measures

SUZANNE M. BURNS

Advanced practice nurses (APNs) are increasingly being asked to demonstrate the effectiveness of their role. In some cases, the inability of the APN to do so results in the dissolution of the role. For many institutions, effectiveness is measured in financial outcomes—or some derivation of financial outcomes, such as patient volume. Unfortunately, many APNs are not in revenue-generating positions and must be creative in demonstrating their effectiveness and "value added" benefit to the institutions in which they practice. The purpose of this chapter is to describe a number of different methods and outcome measures that might be used to evaluate an APN's effectiveness. Examples of actual APN-outcome projects will illustrate the methods and demonstrate the importance of determining appropriate factors for measurement.

SELECTING APN ROLE-SENSITIVE OUTCOME MEASURES

A common approach used to determine APN outcomes is to attempt to link institutional aggregate data such as length of stay (LOS) and cost per case to APN practice. Although these types of measurements are important, and helpful in some cases, they are often not sensitive enough to clearly demonstrate the APN's unique contribution. Rarely does aggregate data show the causal effect of an individual on a patient population; there are simply too many intervening variables that may have contributed to the effect. Thus it is important to consider other, more sensitive indicators. There is also a practical reason for carefully selecting outcome variables: APNs are busy and data collection takes time. The data that the APN collects should be easy to obtain prospectively (in the course of his/her daily role) and should be specific to the APN's role. Data collection should not be extensive but instead limited to selected and role-sensitive indicators. Unfortunately, many APNs are averse to collecting data and believe that having to "prove" their worth is unjustified, since their roles are not revenue-generating. In addition, the APNs may feel that data collection distracts them from their primary roles as clinical experts. But, if the outcome measures are carefully selected, the data will not only help to clarify the APN's value to the institution, but also may be used to focus the role accordingly.

When an APN is hired, the manager, administrator, and physician to whom the APN will report generally have a specific role function in mind (educator, case manager, clinical nurse specialist [CNS], clinical coordinator, nurse practitioner [NP], etc.). Following role negotiation, the APN begins the role focusing on the negotiated objectives. Outcome measures should be specific to the role and should be mutually agreed upon by the APN and the individual who hired the APN. Examples follow.

Acute Care Nurse Practitioner for a Medical Acute Care Floor

If the role is that of acute care nurse practitioner (ACNP) for a medical acute care floor, the collaborating physician may be interested in the number of ACNP-managed patients requiring readmission within a selected time interval. This data is relatively easy to collect and can be obtained from institutional clinical data repositories. The ACNP will need to maintain a secure database of his/her discharged patients in order to query the system on a regular basis (e.g., every 2 months, quarterly, yearly). It may be desirable to compare these to other health care provider data as well.

Unit Educator

Another example is that of an APN hired to be a unit educator. In this case the manager and educator may agree that educational offerings and evidence-based practice (EBP) changes designed and implemented by the educator are the outcome measures of interest. These are relatively easy to document as they are accomplished. Descriptions of these initiatives, including the time required to complete them, will help clarify the complexity of the projects as well as the efficiency and effectiveness of the educator. For some initiatives, the educator may also consider periodic audits to assure adherence with the EBP changes.

Clinical Nurse Specialist

The role of CNS generally encompasses all the domains of advanced practice (e.g., clinical management, education, research, consultation, and change agency). However, it may be that outcome measures may focus on only one or two measures of role effectiveness and that these may change over time. For example, the manager and the CNS may agree that one key objective for the year is to improve medication safety (e.g., reduce medication errors). The CNS in this example might partner with the Quality Assurance (QA) department to track unit medication errors following the implementation of a CNS educational and practice-change initiative. A control chart with an arrow pointing to the initiation of the intervention would clearly demonstrate the effect the APN had on the outcome. See Sidebar 3.1 for an explanation of control charts (Wheeler, 2000) and Figure 3.1 for a medication error example. In this case, the APN doesn't actually need to collect data, but instead partners with the QA contact to assure that the intervention date is marked accurately on the control chart. Very few examples like this one would be needed to demonstrate the APN's "worth" to the institution. More important, the APN can use the data to readjust or change the intervention if necessary.

The CNS may also monitor the effect of a change initiative on practice and patient outcomes. Perhaps the initiative is one designed to incorporate prone positioning into the care management protocol for patients with acute respiratory distress syndrome (ARDS). A prospective audit by the CNS following implementation of the educational and competency-based initiative would be relatively easy to accomplish

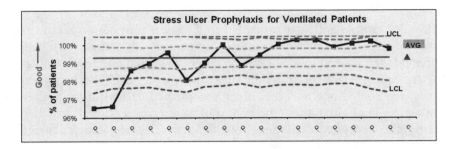

Figure 3.1 Control chart with upper and lower control limits. In this example, the percentage of patients receiving appropriate stress ulcer prophylaxis is being monitored over time. The benchmark for the lower control limit has been derived from regulatory agency benchmark goals of 90%. As demonstrated in the chart, this critical care unit easily meets the benchmark, with an average goal attainment over time of greater than 96%. *Note:* The broken dotted lines represent the corresponding percentage. The "undulations" reflect the differences in the total patients for the sample (i.e., the denominator).

while the CNS is on the unit. Elements to track would be protocol adherence (i.e., Was it implemented?), accuracy (Was it done correctly?), and what was the patient's response (e.g., PaO_2 following prone positioning). Little data collection would be necessary, since the maneuver is generally used infrequently. The reason such an initiative is a reasonable one to use as a CNS outcome is because the procedure is potentially risky and is almost entirely nurse managed. The CNS's effectiveness in safely implementing such a protocol is essential, as it speaks to integration of all the CNS-role components and demonstrates effective leadership and follow-through. In addition, the CNS can use the data to quickly adapt and adjust the protocol as needed. This "real time" monitoring, with short cycles of intervention, evaluation, and correction, assures quality.

Using Aggregate Data

Aggregate data is defined as data collected and reported by organizations and/or departments (e.g., QA, clinical data repositories) as a sum or total over a given time period (e.g., monthly or quarterly) (The Joint Commission, n.d.). The data is helpful and attractive to organizations because it can be translated into financial savings (or in most cases estimates of financial savings). Despite the common use of such outcome

Sidebar 3.1

Control Charts

Most data used to monitor the effect of system interventions in health care are displayed as numerical comparisons (lists or tables of data, etc.). Unfortunately, these approaches have serious drawbacks. The comparisons made with lists of numbers are often narrowly focused, weak, and difficult to interpret because they rarely help us understand the context (e.g., how stable the historical data has been). Tables, on the other hand, often present too much data and are hard to interpret. Graphs provide a solution to these problems because they include previous data by which to compare the effect of the intervention. Essentially, the context for interpreting the current value is integrated into the chart. Additionally, the charts are easier to understand because the data are represented visually rather than numerically.

Control charts (Figure 3.1) start with a time series graph, but control limits and a central line are added to visually delineate the variability of the measure-of-interest. By having control limits, the tendency to inappropriately intervene (called "tampering"), which is costly and time- and effort-intensive, may be avoided. Generally, three consecutive points above the upper or lower control limit are considered significant (e.g., where action should be taken). This approach may help prevent the often counterproductive response of many to "random variation" in the system. Refer to Wheeler (2000) for a more in-depth discussion of control charts.

Time series (or running record graphs) are especially helpful to trend the effect of an intervention over time (see Figure 3.2).

data, it is rarely possible to attribute such data to any one source. Thus, monitoring outcomes specific to the APN role is very difficult unless carefully considered and presented. For example, if the APN begins an educational initiative aimed at decreasing ventilator-associated pneumonia (VAP) in a medical intensive care unit (MICU) population, it is important to first determine if the institutional data may be used to track the outcome. In some cases this would be possible, and all that would be necessary is that the APN intervention be marked so that a control chart might be developed to demonstrate effect over time. However, this example using aggregate data can also be illustrative of how such institutional data is fraught with problems. Unless all other interventions that may potentially affect the outcome are controlled (meaning

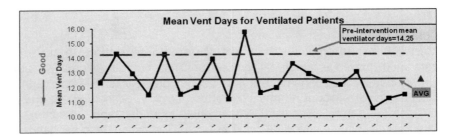

Figure 3.2 Time series graph. This graph represents the mean ventilator days for all patients who require long-term mechanical ventilation in five adult critical care units. The data compares the historical data (mean ventilator days = 14.25) to the current data over time resulting from a process intervention (mean of 12.53 days). Tighter control is noted with time.

they are stable and unchanging during the study period), the outcomes will not be attributed to the APN practice initiative. Instead, the outcomes may be attributed to an attending physician's practice, introduction of a continuous subglottic suctioning endotracheal tube in patients admitted through the emergency department (ED), a hospital-wide "increased awareness campaign," or a new sinusitis prophylaxis regime.

For the APN to clearly demonstrate his/her effectiveness in successfully initiating a practice change that positively affects VAP rates, other data may be required. In this case, the APN's educational initiative was to teach every bedside caregiver to maintain the head of the bed in a 30-degree "head up" position. An audit prior to the intervention of head-of-bed elevation in the units, and on different shifts, demonstrated that adherence was very low (< 20%). This data served as a baseline for comparison following the intervention. At intervals of 1 and 3 months, adherence was again audited and found to be improved (> 70%). Being able to identify that the VAP intervention was occurring allowed for greater assurance that the APN initiative might be linked to the VAP rate improvement. Control charts may be used to mark the beginning of the initiation and subsequent "reteaching" episodes as they relate to the VAP rate over time. The financial results of a successful initiative such as this one are easily calculated and the APN may be recognized as having contributed to the positive results.

The selection of outcome variables to monitor APN effectiveness must be specific to APN role elements. It is important that APNs recognize that data need not be cumbersome to collect; in fact, if it is, the monitoring is likely to be abandoned. Nor does the APN need to collect data on everything he/she does. While the use of aggregate data may be helpful in some cases, the effect of the APN on the variable-of-interest is likely to be profoundly diluted and impossible to attribute to the APN. Some specific categories of outcome measures and the attendant associated problems with each are discussed below.

CATEGORIES OF APN OUTCOME DATA

A variety of indicators may be used to demonstrate the effectiveness of an APN. The strengths and weaknesses of the indicators are described.

Satisfaction (Patient, Family, Caregivers, Physician)

Satisfaction is a variable that speaks directly to the institution's "market share" of customers. If customer satisfaction is not good, the customer will not return. In addition, the customer's negative advertisement of the hospital will have far-reaching implications for the institution. For every disgruntled customer, 23 potential customers may be negatively influenced. Few hospitals exist today that are arrogant enough to ignore satisfaction as an outcome measure. However, as we know, satisfaction is not always synonymous with quality. Regardless, it is an important variable to monitor. The satisfaction of other staff and physicians with the APN practice may also be of interest as an outcome measure.

Most institutions routinely measure patient satisfaction in a global manner. Like other aggregate data, it is hard to specifically attribute the outcomes to APN practice. For example, in many cases the satisfaction instrument will not distinguish the APN from the bedside nurse or the physician. Further complicating the matter, many institutions collect only data related to service line (e.g., medicine or surgery). Thus, for satisfaction to be linked to APN practice, a separate survey may be necessary. However, even this may be a stumbling block. In some institutions, patient satisfaction surveys are closely controlled and may only be distributed via the institutional mechanism in place. There are good reasons for this—the institution doesn't want the patients and families "bothered" with numerous forms and questionnaires. Further, more specific and detailed questions are difficult to design, take the patient additional time to complete, and often require interpretation. If satisfaction is a desired APN outcome measure, it is necessary to determine whether the existing institutional survey is sensitive enough. If not, the APN may need to design his/her own survey. As noted, this may be unduly complicated since institutional requirements may be in place that limit distribution of such surveys.

Surveys of staff and physician satisfaction may also be an effective and useful measure of APN practice. The satisfaction of caregivers is important because their dissatisfaction can affect recruitment, retention, quality of care, and other financial outcomes. Institutional costs of nursing turnover are cited to be from $22,000 to over $64,000 (U.S.) per nurse (Jones & Gates, 2007). Additionally, frequent turnover makes the assurance of quality care difficult. Training costs alone (in time and money) are likely to be high even to assure "safe" care delivery following orientation. In this time of "nursing shortages," retention is essential and nurses' satisfaction with their work environment, professional development opportunities, and ability to "make a contribution in a collaborative manner" are important variables to consider. The APN may well have an important part to play in satisfaction as it relates to one or more of these variables. Satisfaction surveys related to these and other specific aspects of APN practice may be useful and relatively easy to accomplish via mechanisms such as the unit or service-line intranet.

Physician satisfaction is another variable that may be measured. Physicians generate revenue and the APNs with whom they work contribute to the efficiency and effectiveness of the physicians' practice. In these cases, physician satisfaction with the collaborative relationship and results of same are important to follow.

Clinical Outcomes Measures

APN-sensitive clinical outcomes may be difficult to identify because many factors may potentially affect them. It is important to remember that clinical outcome measures need not encompass everything the APN practice may affect, but rather those that are the most easily and clearly attributed to the APN practice. For example, consider the NP charged with managing the care of a neurosurgical patient population. Because in this case the NP's role is focused on managing the medical aspects of care of the patients, selected aspects of care may yield sensitive indicators of effectiveness. Examples include such indicators as urinary tract infection (because the NP is responsible for ordering catheter removal), decubitus ulcer formation (secondary to initiation of mobilization), and selected discharge outcomes.

A common error made by APNs such as case managers or outcomes managers who manage large groups of patients is to collect a large data set in the hope that it will show something. This approach, known as "fishing in the data," is unnecessary and a poor use of the APN's time. A general rule, as with any research study, is that the question should be clear and the variables-of-interest measurable. For example, perhaps the APN's role is focused on improving outcomes of patients who require prolonged mechanical ventilation. It is important that the APN have benchmark data available on ventilator duration so that a comparison may be made. LOS, though sometimes related to ventilator duration, may not be directly affected by the APN, since the clinician's role may not extend to the unit to which the patient is transferred following successful weaning. *Duration of ventilation*, in contrast, *is* attributable, because the APN is the one charged with assuring proper application of and adherence to a weaning protocol. In this example, the data is relatively easy to collect because it is congruent with the role of the APN and can be easily collected in the course of a practice day. As with any outcome measure, it is essential that monitoring be done long enough that the effect can be evaluated.

Efficiency (Time-Saving) Outcomes

Time and efficiency are appropriate outcome measures for APNs and can be measured in a number of different ways. Again, the appropriateness of the measures depends on the specific role of the APN. For example, if the role of the APN is to coordinate care of transplant patients, the APN might keep a log of telephone conversations with patients and categorize them into different content areas. Representative categories, such as medication advice, updates on lab and other tests, consultations about when to come in to the hospital or clinic, or other topics, might be selected. The conversations can be monitored in time increments. Once summarized, the time increments may represent at least a portion of the physician's time that is "freed up" by the nurse, potentially allowing for more patients to be seen by the physician. It must be recognized, however, that the time increments must all have value to the physician or administrator paying for the APN or be acknowledged as important additions to the practice. By monitoring these data, then, aggregate data related to patient volume (in this case, the APN's contribution to freeing physician time) may be more accurately interpreted. In addition, this kind of "availability" of the APN to patients and families is very attractive to worried patients and families. The element may also be measured in a satisfaction survey.

Other time-related measures may demonstrate the APN's effectiveness as well. An example might be an initiative that emerges because ED patients are not being seen in a timely manner and satisfaction has suffered. APNs are frequently charged with system initiatives like this one, but often do not measure the effects of the initiatives. In this case, it would be appropriate to measure satisfaction and waiting times resulting from the initiative. Though in any system initiative there are numerous people who also play a role in making the approach successful, the APN heading the project could use the results as an indication of his/her effectiveness.

Time is money, and the translation of time to money (i.e., cost savings) is relatively easy to do. This type of measure is underused by APNs, who frequently play a very important role in improving the quality and efficiency of care initiatives.

Financial Outcomes

While virtually any outcome measure can be translated into financial outcomes, some financial data is especially of interest to institutions. An example is the use of cost and profit data. As noted earlier, the data is difficult to ascribe to any one APN; however, it can be used to trend the effect of an intervention coordinated or spearheaded by the APN. An example is an initiative such as the "outcomes manager" (OM) role for patients who require long-term mechanical ventilation. In this case, the OM is charged with managing and coordinating selected elements of care of patients assigned to a multidisciplinary clinical pathway. All key stakeholders are recognized as important to the initiative; however, improvements in the variables-of-interest (generally using retrospective/prospective data comparisons) strongly speak to the effectiveness of the APN in managing the program of care. An example of this is described in more detail later in this chapter.

Aggregate Data and/or Hospital Benchmark Data

Aggregate data (described previously), also referred to as hospital bench-mark data, is often used to compare an institution's outcomes to those of other like-sized facilities. Given the volume of data available in institutional data banks, it is easy to understand why administrators and clinicians alike attempt to assign causality to this type of aggregate outcomes data. The assumption that the data represents the effect of specific interventions or care is often unwarranted. This is especially a problem when an attempt is made to infer the reasons for the outcomes and impose solutions. Those upon whom the solutions are to be imposed comment that the data isn't representative of their patients, that they are "sicker" or "different," and that the data is not sensitive enough to stratify appropriately. In fact, the approach often engenders irritation, frustration, and lack of buy-in for the initiative. For example, say the APN has been charged with a hospital-wide initiative on wound care. The APN learns that decubitus ulcer rates can be retrieved from the institutional data banks by service center. Unfortunately, when the APN tries to separate the data by specific units, she/he learns that the data is not available in that form. In fact, the data does not distinguish which patients had preexisting ulcers (and where they originated) or where the majority of the care was delivered when the ulcer developed, since the "service line" designation is by discharge unit, not the unit in which the decubitus developed. Thus, the data may be helpful in looking at overall hospital trends, but will be less useful if a targeted intervention is to be developed. In this case, unless the APN can "drill down" and find the answers, the intervention might be applied to all the units even though it may only be warranted in one.

The use of aggregate data may be helpful in following trends, but requires an in-depth understanding of the variable-of-interest to assure accurate interpretation. An example is the use of LOS data. Take, for example, LOS data related to patients with tracheostomies. If one institution is able to transfer patients to discharge facilities with the tracheosto-mies in place (and requiring mechanical ventilation), the data on LOS may be inaccurately compared to an institution where similar transfer facilities do not exist. If this fact is not understood, erroneous compari-sons between the two hospitals may be made. Instead, a more sensitive indicator of quality for these patients may be weaning and reintubation rates and ventilator duration.

Profit-per-case and cost-per-case may also be misleading, since the factors affecting the numbers may have little to do with the intervention-of-interest. Take, for example, the ventilator-weaning initiative mentioned earlier. Cost of care may be higher in patients transferred to a MICU from a cardiovascular critical care unit than for patients who originate in the MICU. This may inaccurately assign cost-per-case to the MICU, since all costs are attributed to the discharge unit (in this case, the MICU) versus the unit in which the larger proportion of the costs was accrued. Thus, if these financial measures are used to chart progress, they may easily be misinterpreted unless appropriate "drill down" is accomplished.

Institutional aggregate data are useful in some cases; however, a thorough understanding of the data is necessary if the outcomes are to be attributable to APN practice.

CASE EXAMPLES: DIFFERENT APN ROLES AND OUTCOME MEASURES

As described previously, the selection of outcomes data to demonstrate role effectiveness requires, of necessity, that the data be reflective of the APN's practice. A few categories of outcome criteria have been discussed in this chapter and others are discussed in other chapters in this book. The following case examples of APN practices and the specific outcome data they use to evaluate their role effectiveness will illustrate how some of those variables might be used.

Cardiac Cath Lab ACNPs

A cardiology department hired ACNPs to manage patients admitted for cardiac catheterization. This was done because cardiology fellowships had decreased substantially, yet interventional procedures such as cardiac catheterization had increased. In the past, the cardiology fellows did all pre-cath workups, ordered all necessary labs and other diagnostic evaluations, and managed the patients who required overnight stays in the hospital following catheterization. To meet the needs of the cardiology department, the hospital administration, in conjunction with the cardiologists, decided to hire ACNPs to fill the void. The ACNPs performed all the functions previously performed by the fellows, leaving the attending physicians and fellows free to perform the catheterizations.

Though the ACNPs were receiving positive feedback from floor nurses, physicians, and patients, they had not formally considered how to demonstrate their "value added" and were asked to do so by the administrator who was paying their salary. The ACNPs considered why they had been hired and designed outcome measures that would represent their effectiveness in the role. The variables selected included (a) catheter selection (previously a problem because catheters were selected based on physician preference rather than on established cardiology guidelines), (b) time to sheath removal, (c) response time to calls from floor nurses, (d) patient flow (preadmission-to-discharge times), (e) patient teaching and follow-up, and (f) physician satisfaction. Though the ACNPs would have liked to obtain data on patient satisfaction, as noted earlier, this was not possible given the institutional requirement that all patient-satisfaction measurement occur via the larger, hospital-wide mechanism. In all measures, the ACNPs were able to demonstrate very positive results.

Congestive Heart Failure ACNP

In a role collaborating with a cardiologist, the ACNP manages congestive heart failure (CHF) patients in the cardiology clinic. Prior to the ACNP's practice in the clinic, clinic patients would learn of test results upon returning to the clinic or would call the secretary or doctor to learn the results. The ACNP quickly identified that this practice was not optimal and assumed responsibility for this component of the practice, as well as management of the patients during clinic visits. She subsequently began to maintain a log of phone consultations, both by time allotment and by category (medication adjustment, information, symptoms, etc.). Patient and family satisfaction have increased (as evidenced by unsolicited comments and letters) and the physician has noted that his efficiency has been enhanced. The NP is able to translate the time log into patient interactions. The combination of increased physician efficiency and patient satisfaction in combination with a decreased readmission rate since the NP began her practice is convincing evidence that she is effective in her role.

Pulmonary Outcomes Manager

This role began in 1995, following the completion of a research study designed to test an outcomes-managed approach to the care of patients who required prolonged mechanical ventilation in a MICU. At the heart of the initiative was a multidisciplinary clinical pathway managed and monitored by those pulmonary APNs called "Outcomes Managers" (OMs). The outcome variables for the study included ventilator duration, LOS, mortality, and outcome status (stratified as "weaned," "partial ventilatory support," "full support," "death," and "withdrawal"), in addition to cost outcomes for patients with and without a tracheostomy. The results of the study demonstrated a trend toward better outcomes in all categories and significant cost savings in the patients managed via the approach (Burns et al., 1998). The program was extended to all adult critical care units and data were prospectively collected by the APNs and shared quarterly with the adult critical care units. The outcomes of the program were positive and sustained over time (Burns et al., 2003). These measures have been accepted institutionally as representative of the team approach led by the APNs.

Surgical Service Coordinators

Two clinicians began their roles as APNs, but adapted the roles to encompass additional role components reflective of NP practice following the completion of an ACNP program. Their roles are designed to coordinate care of surgical patients in the surgical service line by working with specific surgeons. Since the surgeons take care of different types of patients, their patient populations differ somewhat. Regardless, methods they have selected to monitor their effectiveness include a combination of aggregate institutional data and prospective data. Their prospective data collection includes the number and types of follow-up consultations they perform (phone, clinic visit, in-hospital consultation with ward nurses or other health caregivers, etc.), complications, time-to-interventions (such as initiation of antibiotics or pain relief), staff education and satisfaction of physicians, nurses, and social workers. Since one of the APNs manages a number of very complex patients who continue to have many needs following discharge, some of the episodes of "time out of hospital" are also used to demonstrate her effectiveness. The nurses have also shown that ED visits following discharge have decreased in comparison to when the surgical housestaff managed the patients (prior to institution of the coordinator roles). While these clinicians do monitor more outcome measures than most, the majority of the data is relatively easy for them to collect during their workday.

Lung Transplant Coordinators

These clinicians are intimately involved in the care of lung transplant patients before and following surgery. Their outcome measures include length of time to evaluation of the recipients (they compare this to data attained prior to role initiation and also to the team goals), readmissions before and following transplant, and hospital LOS. As with other roles described previously, these clinicians work as part of a large multidisciplinary team. Thus, the results of outcome measures are attributable to the team and not solely to the APNs. Regardless, their contributions are visible and, to date, their outcomes have been viewed very favorably.

Neuroscience Outcomes Managers

Two ACNPs were asked to serve as OMs for the neurological intensive care unit and a neurosurgery floor. The request came from the administrators of the neuroscience service line, who were concerned that institutional data on cost, volume, and LOS were not comparing favorably to other hospitals in the consortium. Data important to the administrators included the institutional aggregate data on LOS, cost, and profit. The ACNPs recognized that multiple care elements were likely responsible and to that end determined that retrospective data collection on selected factors prior to initiation of their role was necessary for comparison. A variety of nurse-sensitive clinical variables, such as time-to-mobility, Foley catheter removal, time-to-stabilization-of-Dilantin-levels, and patient teaching, were selected for both retrospective and prospective data sets. The intervention was the active care management of the ACNPs who managed these and other care elements. The initial goal, to complete a 6-month pilot interval of OM-managed care in order to evaluate trends, yielded extremely favorable results, and a commitment was made by the neuroscience service line to continue the mode of care. Analysis of the ACNP OM project 1 year following implementation demonstrated increased nurse, physician, and patient satisfaction, a statistically significant improvement in the majority of clinical variables-of-interest monitored, and a $2 million total cost savings (Russell et al., 2002)! The results continue to be extremely positive and have resulted in the hiring of additional ACNPs for the neuroscience service line (Yeager et al., 2006).

SUMMARY AND CONCLUSIONS

The effectiveness of APNs has been called into question many times in the past. Often, when cost shortfalls are realized, constraints are placed on practicing clinicians. APNs, whose practice in the past has not easily been linked to outcomes, are often targeted. While these solutions may "save money" in the short term, the effect on quality, and ultimately finances, may be significant. APNs are essential to the quality system initiatives that occur in hospitals. Their work is important, but is too often not recognized because it is "invisible." Using carefully selected data to demonstrate the APN's effect on some of these system initiatives is possible and important if APNs are to demonstrate their "value added" contributions. Though, as noted, system outcomes are hard to ascribe to any one individual, the contributions of APNs are more likely to be acknowledged if data are available.

This chapter provides some examples of outcome measures that may be selected and used to accurately demonstrate the impact of APN practice. It is essential that APNs recognize that the measures should be selected carefully and be clearly linked to the APN role. Aggregate data are perhaps the least sensitive for demonstrating the effectiveness of individuals, but may be used to demonstrate trends in system approaches led by the APN. While financial data is an appropriate indicator of APN "value added" in some cases, it may be less so in others, especially if the role is not specifically linked to direct patient management.

APNs are essential to the provision of quality patient care. They are responsible not only for a wide variety of evidence-based practice changes and system initiatives, but also for the direct provision of evidence-based care. APN practice outcomes can and should be monitored to more strongly demonstrate the APN's positive contributions to health care.

REFERENCES

Burns, S. M., Earven, D., Fisher, C., Lewis, R., Merrel, P., Schubart, J., et al. (2003). Implementation of an institutional program to improve clinical and financial outcomes of mechanically ventilated patients: One-year outcomes and lessons learned. *Critical Care Medicine, 31,* 2752–2763.

Burns, S. M., Marshall, M., Burns, J. E., Ryan, B., Wilmoth, D., Carpenter, R., et al. (1998). Design, testing and results of an outcomes managed approach to patients requiring prolonged mechanical ventilation. *American Journal of Critical Care, 7,* 45–57.

The Joint Commission. (n.d.). *Aggregate data* [definition]. Retreived June 22, 2008, from The Joint Commission Web site, Sentinel Event Glossary of Terms: http://www.jointcommission.org/SentinelEvents/se_glossary.htm

Jones, C. B., & Gates, M. (2007). The costs and benefits of nurse turnover: A business case for nurse retention. *OJIN: The Online Journal of Issues in Nursing, 12*(3), Manuscript 4. Retrieved from www.nursingworld.org/MainMenuCategories/ANAMarket place/ANAPeriodicals/OJIN/TableofContents/Volume122007/No3Sept07/Nurse Retention.aspx

Russell, D., VorderBruegge, M., & Burns, S. M. (2002). Effect of an outcomes-managed approach to care of neuroscience patients by acute care nurse practitioners. *American Journal of Critical Care, 11,* 353–364.

Wheeler, D. J. (2000). *Understanding variation: The key to managing chaos* (2nd ed.). Knoxville, TN: SPS Press.

Yeager, S., Shaw, D., Casavant, J., & Burns, S. M. (2006). An acute care nurse practitioner model of care for neurosurgical patients. *Critical Care Nurse, 26,* 57–64.

4

General Design and Implementation Challenges in Outcomes Assessment

ANN F. MINNICK

The conduct of outcomes assessment studies is expensive in terms of human resources that might be applied to any number of other important activities. The results of outcomes assessment studies are needed to determine public policies and institutional efforts. Both of these facts make it imperative that outcomes assessment studies be designed to avoid common design flaws and make parsimonious use of resources during their execution. Simply put, you need to avoid wasting your time and someone else's money while producing valuable information.

This chapter is based on the assumption that few practitioners want to simply describe a single outcome but rather are trying to devise assessments of patient outcomes that will help them improve care. This chapter discusses solutions to the four most common design problems and four implementation challenges. Recognition of these basic problems and challenges will lead to the discovery of other issues that can be threats to the execution of outcomes assessment studies. Although the list of potential solutions is not exhaustive, it is designed to arm the person embarking on such studies with a basic set of effective responses.

SOLVING DESIGN PROBLEMS

Four common design problems in outcomes research are (a) ensuring that the study design can meet the study's purpose, (b) selecting outcomes, (c) maximizing the ability to link cause and effect, and (d) selecting a design that is amenable to resolving analytic quandaries.

Linking Purpose and Design

Common Problems

The first and perhaps most important step is to determine what question(s) the outcomes assessment project seeks to answer. Many novice researchers have found themselves embarked on a design only to discover that they never determined specific questions they sought to answer. This occurs most often when clinicians note that some naturally occurring event, such as a change in practice at one site, will result in what seems like experimental and control groups. They then begin to track outcomes, but, because specific questions were never posed, find that they neglected to collect data on some important variable or that the pre-/postintervention design they used cannot really capture the additional ongoing changes in other aspects of practice at the sites.

Another problem in linking purpose and design is the failure to plan a study that could have answered, with only a few design changes, many more questions that are of interest to the larger world of institutional and public policy making. Many practitioners can verbally explain the larger issues for which outcomes assessments are needed, but they design studies that do not help inform the important debates over outcomes and how best to achieve them. At a minimum, any outcomes assessment usually needs to include some exploration of patients' physical and psychosocial outcomes as well as some elements of service costs.

Solutions

There are a number of steps persons planning to embark on outcomes assessments can take to avoid these two problems:

1. Write the questions your outcomes assessment study seeks to answer.

Answer the question: How will answering these questions lead to actions that will improve outcomes for patients, the practice/institution, and the public?

2. For each question, identify who cares about the answer and write the level at which each person/agent functions in terms of making decisions that might influence changes your study might suggest. For example: Is it a professional nurse practitioner group, the practice manager for your group, or a state agency? Or could it be all of them if the design were changed? You will need resources for your study, even if your plans encompass only an assessment of outcomes within your own practice. These people/agencies could be sources of support. The first rule of sales (and gaining support for any type of study *is* marketing) is to meet the customer's needs. Be sure your study does so.

3. If in Step 2 you could not identify more than one audience of interest, reconsider the questions. Outcomes assessment studies are too expensive to be one-trick ponies. If you identify someone who has resources, but whom you believe will not be supportive, consider how at least one question of interest to him/her can be included and properly designed to be answered as *part* of the study. Note that in providing an answer for what the individual or institution may *think* is the most important aspect of an outcomes assessment, you will have the opportunity to bring these other questions (and findings!) to their attention.

4. Verify through your review of the literature and consultation with persons at each of the specified levels that these are the most important questions. "Important" means those questions that arise because there are great gaps in understanding and for which solutions are most urgently needed.

5. Seek consultation to ensure that it is possible to design an assessment that produces data that can answer the questions.

Selecting Outcomes

Problems

Once the first five solution steps are taken, it becomes easier to address the problem of defining outcomes for the outcomes assessment. Taking these steps helps guarantee that the outcomes selected have one of the three attributes needed in any outcome worth the investment: *salience*. Salience is defined as the quality of being related to the phenomenon of interest. The other two qualities, *objectivity* and *common currency*, remain to be addressed.

Objectivity is the ability of an outcome to be measured without bias. For an outcome to be said to be based in reality, it must be one that has the quality of being true to life. One example of a bias problem is illustrated by a seemingly simple outcome: rehospitalization within 60 days after treatment. In one study, we had to grapple with the bias inherent in defining rehospitalization as having occurred only if it happened at the single hospital where most nurse practitioners had privileges. There was the chance that some patients were being rehospitalized at several other hospitals at which a few of the nurse practitioners also had privileges.

Another example of this problem involves physical restraint use as an outcome. Once the physical restraint is defined, it should be fairly easy to determine if someone is restrained. The issue arises in counting restrained persons. If patients are transported to a unit in restraints, should they be counted against the receiving unit in a project seeking to assess the outcomes of a restraint-reduction program? If not, how long should the unit be given to use restraint alternatives before they are counted? Should there be another outcome such as "duration of restraint use for patients admitted in restraint"? How much detail is necessary?

Reality can be defined as the extent to which the outcome definition has some fidelity to nature, that is, is true to life. Depression, quality of life, and spiritual health are examples of outcomes for which there are readily acknowledged problems in capturing the reality of the situation. Other outcomes, although seemingly immune to this problem because they are behaviorally based, are just as vulnerable. Consider the outcome "ambulation sufficient to accomplish five activities of daily living." If the outcome is operationalized as the ability to do this in a setting assumed to be a one-story home, but many patients live in multistory dwellings, there is little that is true to life about the study because many people need to be able to not just ambulate but also climb. Resources to consult in the definition and measurement of common outcomes are listed at the end of this chapter. The books listed highlight the advantages, disadvantages, and design issues associated with each approach.

A final problem revolves around what outcomes researchers often assume is "common currency" in defining outcomes. For example, if death is an outcome and the performance of numerous hospitals is being measured in the outcomes assessment, the death rates will be very different in the hospital that includes its hospice unit in the report versus those that do not have such a unit. A hospital may include deaths in the emergency room and another may not. If a hospital is the public receiving facility for the pronouncement of death in police and fire cases, should these deaths be included in the operationalization of the definition of death? Responsible persons at each hospital often believe everyone at other hospitals uses the same definitions for outcomes when in fact there is no common currency.

Solutions

Solutions obviously lie in rigorous definitions:

1. Each time an outcome is mentioned in the study questions, underline it. Within the context of each question, define the outcome in terms that can be objectively applied within the context of the study. It is important that you do this with each question independently. You may find that the outcome you are referring to as "mobility" in question 1 may be very different by question 4. To define is to choose outcomes.
2. Discuss your definitions at sites where you plan to conduct the assessment, to determine if data are currently amassed using this definition. Ask the responsible parties to describe any special situations they may have that could influence their outcomes, even when their definition is the one you propose. Be prepared to give examples of situations. Remember, most people do not believe their situation is the exception.
3. Simultaneous with Step 2, complete a review to determine what definitions were used in the most important outcomes studies published to date. Although you may choose to define an outcome in a new way and may in reality be developing a new outcome of interest, an outcomes assessment is strengthened if there can be some comparison with findings from previous stud-

ies. For example, in a study of physical restraints, we measured prevalence and incidence, although earlier studies had relied almost exclusively on the latter. We were thus able to ascertain that the lower usage we documented was in fact a decline based on comparisons with earlier reports as well as demonstrate that there were very great differences between incidence and prevalence. Consult the Agency for Health Care Policy and Research Web sites listed at the end of the chapter to learn how outcomes of interest to your project have been defined and measured.

Tracing Cause and Effect

As students of traditional research know, a well-executed, double-blind, randomized pretest-posttest design is effective when one seeks to establish that a particular intervention produces measurable effect(s). In the world of outcomes assessment, this approach is usually not an option because of real-life issues. For example, it is often not possible to randomize patients or to blind providers to treatment. Seven challenges are common to the researcher's ability to make conclusions about causation and identify interventions that might result in outcomes improvement. These seven challenges are:

1. Patient autonomy. The patient may be following the treatment advised, on a continuum ranging from "entirely" to "not at all." The patient may be following one aspect of the treatment entirely and another not at all. The patient may follow a treatment plan one day and not at all the next.
2. Multiplicity of health problems in a single individual. Almost no patient presents with a single health challenge. Multiple system failures are common and the simultaneous presence of physical and mental disorders has been well documented. This makes assessment of a single outcome related to a particular disorder difficult.
3. Nonclinical characteristics. Income, education, insurance coverage, geographical location, exposure to violence, and numerous other variables can influence outcomes.
4. Multiplicity of health providers. This includes known as well as unknown providers using many different types of treatments. Some of these treatments may have been obtained from ethnic healers. Some medications may have been obtained illegally.

Other providers might be recognized in foreign countries and their advice obtained by the autonomous patient through the Internet. Even if the providers are known, their skill in providing a specific treatment may vary. Depending on the schedule, the patient may have received each treatment in a repetitive series from different providers.

5. Unknown time delay between intervention and expected outcome. The classic example of this challenge is the difficulty in determining the outcomes of providers' health-promotion activities because many years (and many intervening messages and experiences) will often pass before a condition manifests itself.

6. Lack of baseline measurements. Patients often change providers and accumulating good baseline measures of health status, quality of life, and other variables are expensive to collect de novo. Even if there is support for de novo measures, it is often impossible to collect a full record that captures the rich and complex changes in human life that may influence response to treatment.

7. The complexity of nonpatient, nonindividual provider variables. These variables include labor (staffing quantity and quality) and capital inputs (e.g., equipment) as well as conditions of employment and leadership. In studies of whether or not a particular practice influences outcomes, these types of variables rather than the practice itself may be paramount in the actual execution of the practice. For example, staff may have the same beliefs and knowledge about ways to avoid extubation accidents, but a shortage of supplies or staff may make the execution of these steps impossible. Merely assessing extubations by practice group or before and after an educational session with the staff will not assist in tracing why an outcome is occurring.

Solutions

All of the solutions depend on the outcomes assessor having a broad knowledge of patients, providers, and system variables. Consultants for each of these areas during the design phase can be worthwhile to ensure that the potential effects of these variables are at least considered.

Through interviews with providers and patients as well as review of clinical documents, such as medical records, determine what the potential is that aspects 1 through 4 may influence the outcomes assessment. During this process, attempt to determine if these aspects are evenly distributed across cases or if only select groups are influenced by this variable. For example, many patients at one clinic site may visit a traditional healer down the street and patients at another site might not. As with the issue of defining outcomes, patients and providers will not necessarily think that their situations are unique. During the project-planning phase, you will need to ask questions that will provoke a wide-ranging discussion, such as "Tell me about some of the things you do for your arthritis besides coming to the clinic."

Plan on multiple measurement over time. Multiple measures over time will help to ascertain any change/attenuation of effect on outcomes. This is especially important if the outcomes assessment is part of an intervention effort. Outcome may at first seem to be favorably influenced, but there may be rapid attenuation. Conversely, it may take an unknown period of time for full effects to be realized.

After reviewing the availability of baseline data, recognize that significant outcomes assessment resources may need to be assigned to build a database. The project budget needs to reflect this expense. Make it a priority to explore how to maintain the elements of these data after the assessment project is complete. Experience has shown that once providers and institutions have access to such a database, they are willing to devote the resources necessary for its maintenance because a well-designed database can be used for many outcomes assessment projects and to meet accreditation data demands.

Use a framework such as the one in Figure 4.1 to ascertain that you have assessed the system variables that are most likely to influence outcomes. Many times the key to improving outcomes is to attempt to modify system—rather than individual provider or patient—variables. For example, in the last century anesthesia outcomes were improved significantly when the tubing connection ends of various gases provided during surgery were made compatible only with the appropriate delivery device.

Analytic Issues

Problems

As can be deduced from the discussion of the many variables that need to be accounted for in an outcomes assessment project, multivariate

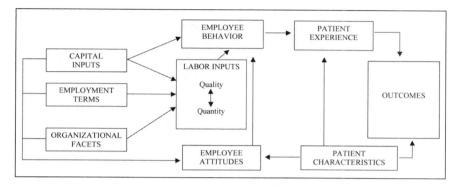

Figure 4.1 A framework of variables influencing patient outcomes.
Source: Developed by A. Minnick and M. J. Roberts (1991).

analysis becomes a necessity. Any outcome may be affected by what Ferketich and Verran (1992) have referred to as attribute variables, contextual variables, and specific treatment effects. The problem with such an approach is that one usually does not know at the beginning of a project if the variables of interest are orthogonal to one another (an assumption of many statistical techniques). This problem is known as collinearity. Another problem is the definition and treatment of attribute and contextual variables. More analytic problems occur when an outcome is rare or at best infrequent. Finally, there is the problem that data of interest are drawn from different levels. For example, an outcome may be drawn from individual patient records, but variables such as staffing may be unit based with others drawn from an institutional level. Special techniques are needed for the analysis.

Solutions

Few practitioners are equipped to deal with these problems. The following steps are advisable for practitioners who have not developed advanced statistical and design expertise:

1. Recognize what one does not know and consult experts during the design phase. The timing is essential because many of the solutions to these problems are rooted in selecting the proper design. For example, in the case of rare outcomes, a case-control approach may be advised.

2. The practitioner should, however, be knowledgeable enough to recognize the possibility that all three problems exist and to ask a statistician how the problems can be addressed. In asking the statistician for advice, inquire about the advantages and disadvantages of each proposed solution.

ADDRESSING IMPLEMENTATION CHALLENGES

Analytic Issues

Having considered the complexity of the design issues described above, thoughtful practitioners may be tempted to run from the very idea of launching a systematic outcomes assessment. This section is devoted to providing "doable" solutions for the four major implementation challenges: (a) assembling a competent, productive team, (b) securing the resources to complete the project, (c) obtaining institutional cooperation, and (d) enlisting the cooperation of providers and patients.

Solutions

The solutions are based on the belief that the process of getting this type of project done is no different than the steps one would take in any type of project, from remodeling one's home to opening a new clinic. You would not attempt to do either of these projects alone, nor would you attempt to go forward without adequate resources.

1. Assemble a team of people who are as interested in the idea as you are. If no one is interested, begin building interest one person at a time. Put yourself in that person's position. What responsibilities or needs would this type of project help that person address? Use these points in talking with them. Try to include formal resource allocators as well as informal opinion makers in this effort.

2. Consider all sources of support, including those outside of your institution. Your well-designed project and its findings could serve as a model for others. Foundations as well as federal agencies are interested in models and in projects that are large enough to produce generalizable findings about the outcomes.

Once you have ascertained why your institution or an outside agency should be interested, prepare a (no more than) three-page discussion paper that explains the need for the project, the answers it will produce, and why they will be valuable to the funder. Include an estimate of the general costs. This is a major marketing tool. People who are asked for resources need to know what they are buying, why they need it, and what it is going to cost.

3. Build alliances with the database, statistical, and design experts whose help you will be able to afford once Step 2 is accomplished. You will need to begin building these alliances prior to approaching resource holders to get a general idea of costs and to amass the technical expertise that will make the proposal a solid one.

4. Consider banding together with like-minded providers, institutions, professional associations, or health care systems. This cooperation can drive down costs by spreading the fixed expenses (e.g., statistical help) over a greater number of supporters. It also is a wonderful way to gather data on rare events and to develop a database that allows for exploration of multiple factor influences on outcomes. For example, if you are in Nebraska you may not have sufficient population to explore the effect of varied ethnicity on patient outcomes. A project that includes sites in Illinois, New York, or California would make this possible.

As noted in the beginning of this chapter, outcomes assessments are important sources of information upon which public policies and private actions are based. Given this fact and the expense of these assessments, outcomes assessment can truly be said to be one of those activities in which "if it is worth doing, it is worth doing well." A poor outcomes assessment can be worse than none at all. With an awareness of the design pitfalls and access to solutions and experts, practitioners can help ensure that outcomes assessments truly are worth the investment.

REFERENCE

Ferketich, S. L., & Verran, J. A. (1991). *Analysis issues in outcomes research.* Paper presented at Patient Outcomes Research: Examining the Effectiveness of Nursing

Practice conference sponsored by the National Center for Nursing Research (currently the National Institute of Nursing Research), September 11–13, 1991, Rockville, MD. Retrieved June 16, 2007, from http://www.ninr.nih.gov/NR/rdonlyres/B3322AAC-2C54-4309-BE83-E09AAD41D1AB/4743/AnalysisIssuesinOutcomes Research.pdf.

RESOURCES—BOOKS AND WEB SITES

AHRQ, the Agency for Healthcare Research and Quality (http://www.ahrq.gov/), is "the nation's lead Federal agency for research on health care quality, costs, outcomes, and patient safety" and is a key source for information about national outcomes assessment efforts.

CAHPS, the AHCPR's Consumer Assessment of Healthcare Providers and Systems program (https://www.cahps.ahrq.gov/default.asp), is "a public–private initiative to develop standardized surveys of patients' experiences with ambulatory and facility-level care." The CAHPS Web site provides free information and AHRQ tools to measure consumers' assessment of their health care experiences. Survey tools can be downloaded and technical advice is available.

Frank-Stromborg, M., & Olsen, S. J. (Eds.). (2004). *Instruments for clinical health care research* (3rd ed.). Sudbury, MA: Jones and Bartlett.

Kane, R. L. (Ed.). (2006). *Understanding health care outcomes research* (2nd ed.). Sudbury, MA: Jones and Bartlett. [Although aimed at researchers, this classic work points out many issues that could influence outcomes assessments.]

McDowell, I., & Newell, C. (2006). *Measuring health. A guide to rating scales and questionnaires* (3rd ed.). New York: Oxford University Press.

Medical Care Research and Review. (2007). [In April 2007, this journal sponsored a special supplement (Vol. 64, No. 2 Suppl.) on Performance Measurement and Outcomes of Nursing Care. The Contents for this supplement, with downloadable PDFs of separate articles, is available online: http://mcr.sagepub.com/content/vol64/2_suppl/]

Muennig, P. (2002). *Designing and conducting cost-effectiveness analyses in medicine and health care.* San Francisco: Jossey-Bass. [Although assessing cost-effectiveness as an outcome requires specialized skills, this book is a good basic primer toward understanding this complex outcome.]

5

Locating Instruments and Measures for APN Outcome Assessments

MARILYN WOLF SCHWARTZ, ROGER GREEN,
AND JAN BUFFO DEMPSEY

Advanced practice nurses (APNs) and researchers need to know how to find surveys, questionnaires, and other measurement instruments to determine whether a treatment is effective. In the evidence-based health care era, APNs as well as researchers need to study, measure, and report significant changes in interventions. When APNs report evidence-based findings in the literature, they are improving the quality of health care and contributing to the professions. This chapter is intended to help APNs find the instruments that measure the impact of APN care and APN interventions.

The authors present major resources that librarians and clinicians can use to find instruments. The terms "instruments," "questionnaires," "surveys," and "tools" are used interchangeably. "Instrument" is the preferred term, however, because that is what the database Cumulative Index to Nursing and Allied Health (CINAHL) uses in indexing the search terms for instruments and tools in the literature.

In this chapter, readers will find:

1. Books: The books described herein are standard reference texts regarded as the first sources to check in finding instruments.

2. Bibliographic databases: These are defined in the order of importance to nursing applications. Examples of search strategies are shown for CINAHL and for another database called Health and Psychosocial Instruments (HaPI). Only *CINAHL* and *HaPI* searches were processed, because of their relevance to advanced practice nursing. The reader may then apply some of the same techniques to searching other databases. It is important to consult a medical librarian, when available, to process searches, especially when doing an evidence-based study or when publishing or presenting papers. Using the controlled vocabulary or thesauri for retrieval in databases is important and medical librarians are adept at using them effectively.

3. Internet resources: Those listed include the Web sites of professional organizations and government agencies as well as library guides to tools. The Internet resources listed are by no means exhaustive, but considered selective.

STANDARD BOOKS

In this age of technology, standard textbooks are not the most popular sources of information. However, following are some tried-and-true measurement tools in book form. Note additional books listed in the Suggested Reading lists at the end of this chapter, many of which are more specific to nursing and medicine. The books to consult are too numerous to describe individually. Many nursing and medical libraries own the books listed here. Of course, most books may be purchased from online book vendors such as Amazon. Where Web sites are given, all sites were active as of June 19, 2008.

Mental Measurements Yearbooks

Mental Measurements Yearbooks (MMYB) is published by the Buros Institute of Mental Measurements. According to the Web site http:// www.unl.edu/buros, this group has been around for 70 years and employs experts in the field. This standard reference text is available in most university and public libraries on reference shelves. It is updated every 2 years and may be accessed online through many library online database menus. It has been published since 1938. The book lists tests in alphabetical order with descriptive information on purpose, intended population, acronyms, authors, scores, time, prices, publishers, and cross-references. Each volume provides information on reliability and validity and includes reviews of test and test materials. Many libraries also have access to this book online. Buros also publishes *Test Reviews Online*. There is also a link to test reviews through http://buros.unl.edu/buros/jsp/search.jsp. This Buros site contains only reviews for tests, which the user may decide whether or not to purchase.

Tests in Print

Tests in Print (TIP) is also published by the Buros Institute of Mental Measurement. TIP lists target audience, length, score(s), and cost and is a companion to the MMYB. The TIP and the MMYB are the main resources for finding information on published tests.

Tests: A Comprehensive Reference for Assessments in Psychology, Education, and Business

Tests: A Comprehensive Reference for Assessments in Psychology, Education, and Business, currently edited by Taddy Maddox, has been published by PRO-ED, Inc., from 1983 to the present, with a 2008 edition. Descriptions are brief and contain information on test population, purpose, format, scoring, and cost. It does not include reviews or evaluations of tests.

Test Critiques

Test Critiques has been published since 1984 by Test Corporation of America, Kansas City, Missouri. This multivolume set is a companion to *Tests* and includes reliability and validity information. For a complete description of *Test Critiques*, see the American Psychological Association's Web site: http://www.apa.org/science/testing.html. This resource publishes in-depth reviews of frequently used psychological, education, and business tests. Provides descriptions, practical applications, technical aspects, and critiques of tests. Each volume has a cumulative index.

Directory of Unpublished Experimental Mental Measures

The *Directory of Unpublished Experimental Mental Measures*, edited by B. A. Goldman and D. F. Mitchell, has been published by the American

Psychological Association since 1970 (latest volume published 2007). This directory includes information on recently developed noncommercial experimental tests in 24 categories. The entries cover 36 relevant professional journals published in the United States. Measures described in dissertations are not included. Volumes do not include reviews and do not have title indexes. Check the category index. Some of the categories of measurement are achievement, adjustment, aptitude, attitude, behavior, communication, concept meaning, development, motivation, perception, personality, problem solving and reasoning, trait measurement, values, and vocational interest and evaluation.

Please note many additional books listed in the Suggested Reading lists at the end of this chapter. McDowell's book (2006), in particular, with its guide to rating scales and questionnaires, is an excellent source for finding health-related instruments. University libraries usually carry the books listed and some are in reference sections. Remember that most university libraries now have their catalogs available online, so that if a library itself has a collection of tests or instruments, the information on those tests may be found through the catalogs. Library staff may request interlibrary loans for books not in their own collection. Reference librarians and acquisition librarians usually welcome requests for purchase of instrument resource books that are not owned by the library.

BIBLIOGRAPHIC DATABASES

Searching bibliographic databases retrieves references to articles about instruments, but such articles do not always include copies of the instruments in question. However, remember that searching databases may provide references to articles that occasionally do include the instruments described. Full-text journal articles found online in databases may or may not include copies of instruments. In the Internet Resources section of this chapter is a description of how to find dissertations, which usually include instruments used in doctoral work.

Levels of Evidence

The MEDLINE and Cochrane databases contain references to the highest quality journals or peer-reviewed literature, as do the CINAHL, Psyc-

INFO, and Educational Resources Information Center (ERIC) databases. Database producers, especially MEDLINE, publish statements of criteria required for journals to be indexed on their Web sites. APNs reviewing the instruments and articles describing the tools need to critically appraise the literature to make sure the evidence created in using the instruments is sound.

The next two sections (on CINAHL and HaPI) briefly describe important databases, give examples of questions that need to be studied, and suggest how to find the relevant measurement tools. The first two examples deal with the concept of pain. Pain is one of the most common symptoms to measure because The Joint Commission and Institute of Medicine state that pain is an indicator for measuring the quality of care, and pain is measurable. The third question deals with posttraumatic stress disorder (PTSD), which is a major concern in these times. The databases are discussed in an order that gives priority to the best chances for relevant retrieval in nursing.

Cumulative Index to Nursing and Allied Health

CINAHL is available from the EBSCO Publishing database vendor and journal subscription agency. For access information, go to http://www.ebscohost.com/CINAHL. It is a starting point for finding any instrument because instruments may be searched directly in the instrumentation field of the bibliographic record. Once you log into CINAHL, search directly on the "Instrumentation" field from the "Indexes" on the main screen. If you search the "Publication Type" field and choose "Research Instrument," you may actually find the full text of an instrument. This database is not free to the public; users must request codes from institutional libraries, ask a librarian, or pay for a service to perform searches.

Below are examples of common questions and brief descriptions of strategies for searching for articles on instruments in EBSCO's CINAHL database.

SEARCH EXAMPLES

Question: A copy of the Visual Analog Pain Scale is needed. This is a search for a specifically named scale. Following is a step-by-step description of a basic strategy for finding articles that may report use of the Visual Analog Pain Scale. (This is an example of how to search for a specific scale; the next example will show how to find *any* instrument with the term "pain" in it.)

Strategy

- Login by using institutional codes or by going to a library.
- Click the "Indexes" (upper right, below "Choose Databases" tab).
- In **Browse an Index**: select "Instrumentation" from the drop-down menu.
- Next to **Browse for**: type in "Visual Analog Pain Scale (VAPS)."
- Click "**Browse**" button.
- Choose the scales of interest by clicking the boxes to the left of the terms. The "OR" is the Boolean logical connector meaning "any of the scales will be retrieved." Select one or more of the following terms and add to search using OR:
  - VISUAL ANALOG PAIN SCALE
  - VISUAL ANALOG PAIN SCALE (VAPS)
  - VISUAL ANALOG SCALE
  - VISUAL ANALOG SCALE (BOND AND LADER)
- Click **Add** button to put scales in the search box.
- The search box has the word **Find** on the left.
- Click the **Search** button.
- References will appear when scrolling down.
- Click on underlined title(s) of interest to see complete reference(s).
- Scroll down on complete record to see where "Instrumentation" appears on the left.
- Note the list of instruments that includes VAPS.
- Remember that as technology changes for the vendors, screens may change. Call the Technical Support number or email the vendor to learn how to search the indexes or (as some vendors call them) fields.

Some of the articles may have the instrument(s) printed in them. With an EBSCO subscription to CINAHL, full-text articles may be retrieved.

Question: Suppose a nurse needs to see what pain scales might be used for various diabetic problems. The APN does not have a particular pain scale in mind, but wants any pain instrument used in measuring diabetic problems and interventions.

Strategy

- Login by using institutional codes or by going to a library.
- Next to the **Find** box, type in "pain."
- In "Select a Field" box, select "Instrumentation" from drop-down menu. In box under "pain," type in "diabet*."
- Next to where "diabet*" is typed, open the drop-down menu, select a field, and choose "MW Word in Heading." MW Word in Heading means that *diabetes* or *diabetic* must be the main focus of the article to be retrieved.
- The AND between the two lines of terms is the Boolean logical connector meaning both that the term *pain* has to be in the "Instrumentation" field and that the term *diabetes* (or a derivative thereof) must be the main focus of the article.
- Click **Search** button.
- References will appear when scrolling down.
- Click on underlined title of interest.
- Scroll down on complete record to see where "Instrumentation" appears on the left.
- Note the list of instruments, which will have one or more instruments with the word *pain* related to diabetes/diabetic studies.
- Again, remember that as technology changes for the vendors, screens may change. Call the Technical Support number or email the vendor to learn how to search the indexes or (as some vendors call them) fields.

Note that the truncation or wild-card symbol is an asterisk (*) and retrieves references on diabetes or diabetic(s).

Question: What is available to diagnose posttraumatic stress disorder/syndrome? Again, the APN may not need a specifically named instrument, but needs to see what might be available in general.

Strategy

- Login to EBSCO's CINAHL by using institutional codes or by going to a library.
- Click the "Indexes" (upper right, below "Choose Databases" tab)
- In **Browse an Index:** select "Instrumentation" from the drop-down menu.
- Next to **Browse for:** type in "Posttraumatic Stress."
- Click "**Browse**" button.
- Choose the scales of interest by clicking the boxes to the left of the terms. The "OR" is the Boolean logical connector meaning "any of the scales will be retrieved." Select one or more of the following terms and add to search using OR:
  - POSTTRAUMATIC STRESS (PTS) SCALE
  - POSTTRAUMATIC STRESS (PTS)-RELATED SYMP
  - POSTTRAUMATIC STRESS CHECKLIST (PCL)
  - POSTTRAUMATIC STRESS-CHECKLIST-CIVILIAN
- Click **Add** button to put scales in the search box with **Find** on the left.
- Click the **Search** button.
- References will appear when scrolling down.
- Click on underlined title of interest.
- Scroll down on complete record to see where "Instrumentation" appears on the left.
- Note the list of instruments of which any of the POSTTRAUMATIC STRESS instruments may be mentioned.
- Again, remember that as technology changes for the vendors, screens may change. Call the Technical Support number or email the vendor to learn how to search the indexes or fields, as some vendors call them.

Health and Psychosocial Instruments

The HaPI database is produced by Behavioral Measurement Database Service (BMDS), Pittsburgh, PA 15232-0787. This database lists evaluation and measurement tools, questionnaires, and test instruments. HaPI is available through the database vendor Ovid, a division of Wolters Kluwer Publishing. Go to http://www.ovid.com/site/index.jsp for access information. Ovid databases are available through many medical libraries and some major university libraries. Contact the HaPI publisher for direct access and to find other database vendors who provide access.

The HaPI database does not provide copies of instruments. However, this database shows information on how to obtain the tool/instrument and often gives the address and phone number. This database is bibliographic, meaning that it retrieves references to articles about the instrument. Each reference is indicated as a secondary source, then below the citation the primary source tells where the instrument was originally described, and usually where to call or write to get a copy. This database is not free to the public; users must request codes from institutional libraries, consult a librarian, or pay for a service to process searches.

Using the same examples of pain scales or posttraumatic stress as given earlier, the following is a step-by-step example of handling the same question using the Ovid vendor to search.

Strategy

- Login to Ovid.
- Under **Basic Search**, type in "visual analog pain scale" or a more general term "visual pain," "posttraumatic stress," or the type of instrument in which you are interested.
- Click **Search** button.
- Scroll down to display and click.
- Choose references that are relevant and click "Complete Reference" on the right of the citation.
- The article source shows a reference to an article about the instrument typed in.
- Note the "Primary Source," which is a reference to the original work describing the instrument. This often shows where to write or call to get a copy of the instrument. Note that you may limit retrievals in different ways and that "Primary Source" is one of the limiters.

MEDLINE/PubMed

PubMed.gov is the gateway to the National Library of Medicine's databases, which includes MEDLINE (Medical Literature Analysis & Retrieval System Online). APNs may search this database for references to articles on a specific instrument. The references often discuss the reliability and validity of the instrument. Occasionally, an article reproduces a copy of the instrument discussed. In MEDLINE, email addresses are provided with the authors' names, making it easier to find an author to write for further information about an instrument that may have been discussed in the article. The limiters available for searching include the publication types, including questionnaires.

This database is free to the public at http://pubmed.gov. Check with local medical resource libraries and librarians for instruction on using PubMed. Note that this database has brief tutorials at http://www.nlm.nih.gov/bsd/disted/pubmed.html (retrieved June 18, 2008) as well as a detailed tutorial that may take several hours to complete. The time invested in looking at the tutorials usually pays off in terms of saving time in using the database.

Cochrane Databases

The Cochrane databases are products of the Cochrane Collaboration, an international and independent not-for-profit organization dedicated to making up-to-date, accurate information about the effects of health care readily available worldwide. These databases are excellent resources for finding the highest-level evidence-based studies that may describe instruments. These databases are usually available through libraries or through institutions such as hospitals or drug companies. Ovid and EBSCO are two vendors providing access to many of the Cochrane databases, including:

- Cochrane Database of Systematic Reviews
- Cochrane Database of Abstracts of Reviews of Effects
- Cochrane Central Register of Controlled Trials
- Cochrane Methodology Register
- Health Technology Assessment
- ACP Journal Club

The main Web site of the Cochrane Collaboration, http://www.cochrane.org (retrieved July 6, 2008), gives free access to a few references to reviews. Another Web site that has free information from the Cochrane Database of Systematic Reviews is http://www.mrw.interscience.wiley.com/cochrane/cochrane_clsysrev_articles_fs.html (retrieved July 6,

2008). You can also try a Google search at http://www.google.com or a Google Scholar search at http://scholar.google.com on the search term "Cochrane Databases" to read more. Use the "Advanced Search" button on Google to narrow your search, because basic searches often retrieve thousands of entries. Many university library sites have information on the Cochrane databases and how to search them.

When searching the Cochrane databases on Ovid or EBSCO, limit topics by using the terms "instrument(s)," "questionnaire(s)," "scale(s)," or "survey(s)." Use the truncation symbol of a dollar sign ($) at the ends of root words for Ovid; and the asterisk (*) for EBSCO to retrieve various spellings. For example, type in "instrument$" or "instrument*" to retrieve data about instrument, instruments, or instrumentation.

Education Resources Information Center

The ERIC database is produced by the Institute of Education (IES) of the U.S. Department of Education, Washington, DC. This database lists evaluation and measurement tools, questionnaires, and test instruments. ERIC's Clearinghouse on Assessment and Evaluation (AE) has a Test Locator (http://ericae.net/testcol.html) that includes free tests. This site also has a link to Buros Institute of Mental Measurements at http://buros.unl.edu/buros/jsp/search.jsp, which allows shopping and purchase of tests. *Test Reviews Online* is also on this link.

APNs often participate in educating patient or staff in treatments or procedures. The challenge in the educational process is to show that what was presented caused a change in knowledge and practice. Even though the ERIC database contains a limited number of health or medical literature references, it does provide references to general educational concepts that may be applied to measure the impact of educational interventions. This database is free to the public at http://www.eric.ed.gov/ (retrieved June 18, 2008).

PsycINFO

PsycINFO is produced by the American Psychological Association and contains references to articles about various psychological instruments. Many database vendors offer PsycINFO, including Ovid, EBSCO, and Dialog/Knight-Ridder, and each has its own search engine.

Depending upon what the APN is studying, the PsycINFO database may include references to articles relevant to measuring psychological changes. This database covers professional and academic literature in psychology and related disciplines, including medicine and nursing. PsycINFO is international in scope and includes abstracts for citations in over 2,150 journals, dissertations, books, and book chapters. Some university libraries allow access to this database for users in the library or for students and staff remotely. Some libraries may require you to access the database via a professional librarian.

The strategy for using PsycINFO is different from that used with CINAHL or HaPI. A search hint in using PsycINFO is to use the "Measurement" heading in the database's thesaurus to find related topics that may be of use. In PsycINFO, retrieval may be limited to "tests & measures," using the limit button on Ovid. Retrieval will be for article references, though it is possible that an actual instrument may be reproduced in the article occasionally. Rely on PsycINFO to find articles on validity or reliability of particular measures. Articles may be found on various measures used for a particular health or psychological issue. The American Psychological Association Web site listed in the Internet Resources reading list is an excellent source for finding the actual instruments.

Dissertation Abstracts International

Dissertation Abstracts International (DAI) is the index of doctoral dissertations and master's theses written at most North American graduate schools. The CINAHL database also contains dissertations. The dissertations may be searched and ordered through UMI/ProQuest company. Go to the following Web site to order a dissertation online: http://www.proquest.com/products_umi/dissertations/disexpress.shtml (retrieved June 18, 2008). This site's name is Dissertations Express. In 2008, the average cost for a dissertation was $41.00 plus shipping. On this database, the user may order a dissertation as an individual for the stated fee or, if your library/institution subscribes to this database, the library service may request it for you.

If a dissertation is not available through Dissertations Express, check with a local medical librarian to request an interlibrary loan from the institution that required and published the dissertation.

Dialog/Knight-Ridder

Previously known as Dialog, Knight-Ridder is a vendor that sells access to hundreds of databases that most universities and many hospitals use to conduct searches for library patrons: http://support.dialog.com/publications/dbcat/dbcat_2008.pdf (retrieved June 11, 2008). This 128-page catalog of databases lists all databases to which libraries and librarians have access. The catalog may be viewed by the general public.

INTERNET RESOURCES AND ONLINE LIBRARY RESOURCES

Please note the Internet Resources and University Library Web Sites reading lists at the end of this chapter to find links to library Web sites that have guides to finding instruments. This list is not exhaustive, but does feature quality sites. Use Google to find other Web sites that may be helpful.

Google and Google Scholar

Google (http://www.google.com) may be used as a starting point or as a last resort. In using Google, try to use the "advanced search" if the basic search does not retrieve information needed. Use Google Scholar (http://scholar.google.com) for articles about an instrument. A Google search on the Visual Analog Pain Scale takes you to http://www.ndhcri.org/pain/Tools/Visual_Analog_Pain_Scale.pdf (retrieved June 11, 2008). This is only one of many pain scales that are visual.

University Library Web Sites

Note sites in the University Library Web Sites reading list. Some of the university sites have charts and tables describing databases and step-by-step methods for finding instruments. Many of these Web sites include most of the information in this chapter.

Professional Association Sites

The American Nurses Association publishes books and pamphlets that may help in finding instruments. Note the URL site for one such publication: http://nursingworld.org/books/pdescr.cfm?cnum=11#MI20 (retrieved July 6, 2008). Other specialized advanced practice nursing sites may provide clues to instrument information. For example, check the sites for the American Academy of Nurse Practitioners, the American Academy of Clinical Nurse Anesthetists, the National League of Nursing, American Nephrology Nurses, Emergency Nurses Associations, and others. If an APN is part of a specialized professional association, encourage the Web site manager to include dissertations or articles of members who may have used or developed instruments.

The Sigma Theta Tau International Honor Society of Nursing Virginia Henderson Library may be another source of information for instruments. The Web site describing their evidence-based practice publication is at http://www.nursinglibrary.org/Portal/Main.aspx?PageID=4001 (retrieved July 6, 2008).

Many professional health and medicine associations now provide measurement tools on their sites. A well-respected site is the Institute of Medicine at www.iom.edu, with lists of reports, projects, and topics. The abstracts of some of the projects describe measurement tools that might be available for use.

The Medical Library Association offers the course, *Measure for Measure: Locating Information on Health Measurement Tools*, developed and taught by Ester Saghafi, MEd, MLS, and Rebecca Abromitis, MLS, from the Health Sciences Library System of the University of Pittsburgh. This course was first taught at the annual meeting in Chicago, Illinois, in May 2008. If you are interested in taking this half-day class, you may email Ester at esaghafi@pitt.edu to find out where and when it will be taught. The syllabus, which includes PowerPoint slides of screen shots of searches, pictures of books described, and lists of Web sites, may be available for purchase as well from the authors or from the Medical Library Association at http://www.MLANET.org.

Corporate Web Sites

■ The Health Measurement Research Group has some standard instruments, some free, others for purchase. The URL for the group is http://www.healthmeasurement.org/Measures.html (retrieved June 15, 2008). For example, a copy of the Minnesota Living with Heart Failure Questionnaire (MLHFQ) is available free, along with scoring information.

- ProQolid: Patient-Reported Outcome and Quality of Life Instruments Database. Go to the URL http://www.qolid.org (retrieved June 19, 2008) to learn about this database. Two access points are available on this Web site. A free access section shows an alphabetical list of instruments available, listed by author's name, by targeted population, and by pathology/disease. There is a member charge to subscribe (priced in Euros because the database originates in Lyon, France) and an online payment option.
- *Survey Monkey* is a site that helps you develop your own survey and lists other programs available to help do your surveys. Go to the URL http://www.surveymonkey.com (retrieved June 19, 2008).

Government Sites

Some government agencies have sections on their sites that contain useful instruments. Instruments developed by government agencies may be found in the Government Documents departments of university and law libraries. Check with the librarians to help find the publications. Please note the following (all retrieved June 18, 2008):

- **AHRQ** (Agency for Healthcare Research and Quality) Tools and Resources for Better Health Care; URL: http://www.ahcpr.gov/QUAL/tools/toolsria.htm
- **HRSA** (Health Resources and Services Administration) U.S. Department of Health and Human Services Measures for Health Center Grantee Performance Review, Calendar Year 2006; URL: http://www.hrsa.gov/performancereview/clinicalmeasures/detailsheet12b.htm
- **National Guideline Clearinghouse** published by the Agency for Healthcare Research and Quality (AHRQ) of the U.S. Department of Health and Human Services; http://www.guideline.gov. This site has a section on measures and tools relevant to specific health problems. This guideline site is free.
- **National Technical Information Service** (NTIS), a U.S. Department of Commerce clearinghouse of scientific and technical information, is located in Springfield, Virginia; URL: http://www.ntis.gov/search/index.aspx. This database is free and contains many reports of government-supported research. Typing in

"health surveys" in the search engine of the database yielded over 200 references. This database is a stretch for finding a copy of an instrument, but may be worthwhile to check.

SUMMARY

In locating instruments, a search on Google occasionally may retrieve a copy of an instrument or scale. Librarians refer to such searches as a "quick and dirty" way of finding what is needed. Searching through the print books suggested is a good starting point for standard instruments. Many of the books cited in the text and in the Suggested Reading lists should be readily available in major university libraries.

The databases suggested (CINAHL, HaPI, PubMed, Cochrane Databases, PsycINFO, and ERIC) may all need to be searched methodically to find articles on validity and reliability. It is to be hoped that with the step-by-step instructions given in this chapter, the APN may practice basic search strategies and use the techniques in other databases to construct meaningful strategies. Luckily, some authors include the instrument within the article. If a dissertation contains an instrument, the document may be ordered online or through library service.

In using the Internet Resources section, take time to look at the university library Web sites to supplement the information in this chapter. It is worthwhile looking at these for more step-by-step approaches that are not covered here. And finally, medical librarians are usually good resources to help find measurement instruments.

SUGGESTED READING—BOOKS

Aday, L. & Cornelius, L. J. (2006). *Designing and conducting health surveys* (3rd ed.). San Francisco, CA: Jossey-Bass.

American Psychiatric Association. (2000). *Handbook of psychiatric measures.* Washington, DC: Author.

Bowling, A. (2001). *Measuring disease: A review of disease-specific quality of life measurement scales.* Philadelphia, PA: Open University Press.

Bowling, A. (2005). *Measuring health: A review of quality of life measurement scales.* New York: Oxford University Press.

Clayton, G. M. (1989). *Instruments for use in nursing education research* [Publ. No. 15-2248]. New York: National League for Nursing.

Dana, R. H. (2005). *Multicultural assessment: Principles, applications, and examples.* Mahwah, NJ: Lawrence Erlbaum.

Directory of unpublished experimental mental measures, published by the American Psychological Association since 1970, is edited by B. A. Goldman and D. F. Mitchell. Washington, DC: American Psychological Association; latest volume published: 2007.

Frank-Stromborg, M. (2004). *Instruments for clinical health-care research*. Boston: Jones and Bartlett.

Kleinpell, R. M. (Ed.) (2001). *Outcome assessment in advanced practice nursing* (1st ed.). New York: Springer Publishing Company. (2nd edition in press, 2009)

Lewis, C. B. (1997). *The Functional tool box: Clinical measures of functional outcomes.* 2 vols. McClean, VA: Learn Publications. [Tools to aid in measuring patient outcomes in rehabilitation interventions. Each tool has simplified instructions with population, descriptions, completion time, interpretation, reliability, validity, and complete references.]

McDowell, I. (2006). *Measuring health: A guide to rating scales and questionnaires* (3rd ed.). New York: Oxford University Press.

Measurement of nursing outcomes (2nd ed.) (3 vols.). [Vol. 1: Waltz, C. F., & Jenkins, L. (Eds.). (2001). *Measuring nursing performance: Practice, education, and research*; Vol. 2: Strickland, O. L., & DiIorio, C. (Eds.). (2003). *Client outcomes and quality of care*; Vol. 3: Strickland, O. L., & DiIorio, C. (Eds.). (2003). *Self-care and coping*]. New York: Springer Publishing Company.

Miller, D. C., & Salkind, N. J. (2002). *Handbook of research design and social measurement* (6th ed.). Newbury Park, CA: Sage Publications.

Murphy, L. L., Spies, R. A., & Plake, B. S. (Eds.). (2007). *Mental measurements yearbook* (17th ed.). Lincoln, NE: Buros Institute of Mental Measurements. (Published every 2 years.)

Peterson, K. W., Travis, J. W., Dewey, J. E., Framer, E. M., Foerster, J. J., & Hyner, G. C. (Eds.). (1999). *SPM handbook of health assessment tools*. Pittsburgh, PA: Society of Prospective Medicine, & Irving, TX: Institute for Health and Productivity Management (published jointly). [This book discusses and lists various types of scales; also has addresses and validity/reliability remarks about them; contains lifestyle tools.]

Redman, B. K. (2003). *Measurement tools in patient education*. New York: Springer Publishing Company.

Schutte, N. S., & Malouff, J. M. (1999). *Sourcebook of adult assessment strategies*. New York: Plenum.

Shelton, P. J. (2000). *Measuring and improving patient satisfaction*. Gaithersburg, VA: Aspen Publishers, Inc. [Appendices include: Appendix A—Focus Group Moderator's Guide; Appendix B—Patient Satisfaction Survey Instrument; Appendix C—Principles of Continuous Quality Improvement: Presentation Slides.]

Test critiques (1984–present; 10 vols.). Kansas City, MO: Test Corporation of America. [This multivolume set is the companion to *Tests* and includes reliability and validity information. For a complete description of *Test Critiques*, see the American Psychological Association's Web site at http://www.apa.org/science/testing.html]

Tests: A comprehensive reference for assessments in psychology, education and business (2002; 5th ed.; edited by T. Maddox). Austin, TX: PRO-ED, Inc. [Includes descriptions of tests, purpose of tests, cost, and availability; does not contain evaluative critiques of data on reliability and validity.]

Tests in print (2006; 7th ed.; published irregularly). Lincoln, NE: Buros Institute of Mental Measurement.

Thompson, C. (1989). *Instruments of psychiatric research.* Somerset, NJ: John Wiley. [Note: This is a $595 book.]

Waltz, C. F., Strickland, O. L., & Lenz, E. R. (2005). *Measurement in nursing and health research* (3rd ed.). New York: Springer Publishing Company.

SUGGESTED READING—INTERNET RESOURCES

The American Psychological Association has an excellent section on their home page titled "Frequently Asked Questions (FAQ) / Finding Information About Psychological Tests" at http://www.apa.org/science/testing.html

Educational Testing Service (ETS) Test Collection Database (corporate Web site URL: http://www.ets.org/testcoll/index.html) contains descriptions of over 10,000 tests and research instruments, with information indicating either a person or institution to contact or a journal citation for an article describing or including the test.

SUGGESTED READING—UNIVERSITY LIBRARY WEB SITES

Consider checking a local university Web site to start your search for instruments. Many librarians have created extensive, detailed guides to finding instruments because this is a common question asked of librarians. Below is a list of some good sites, but by no means is this an exhaustive list. These may be starting points, and a Google search may retrieve many other university sites. These sites were all active when accessed/retrieved June 18, 2008. If Web sites have gone inactive by the time you access them, try to do a Google search of the university library named.

Hough, H. (Ed.). (2002). *Tests and measures in the social sciences: Tests available in compilation volumes.* Arlington, TX: University of Texas at Arlington. URL: http://libraries.uta.edu/Helen/test&meas/testmainframe.htm (updated July 9, 2008; retrieved October 11, 2008).

San Diego State University Library Web site has a section called "SDSU Test Finder." It was developed by librarian M. Stover and may be accessed at http://www-rohan.sdsu.edu/~mstover/tests. On this site, you will find an index of complete tests and instruments found in scholarly journal articles.

Teno, J. M., Okun, S. N., Casey, V., Rochon, T., & Welch, L. C. (2000). *Toolkit of instruments to measure end-of-life care (TIME). Resource guide: Achieving quality of care at life's end.* Providence, RI: Brown University Center for Gerontology and Health Care Research. URLs: http://www.chcr.brown.edu/pcoc/toolkit.htm & http://www.chcr.brown.edu/pcoc/resourceguide.htm (retrieved October 11, 2008).

University of Maryland Libraries. *Tests and measurements guide.* URL: http://www.lib.umd.edu/guides/tests.html. [This guide is designed to serve as a tool to help one get information about published and unpublished educational, psychological, and vocational tests and measurements. It is worth looking at for helpful information. This site has a step-by-step description of the process of finding tests.]

University of Michigan Social Work Library. *Resources for psychological and educational tests and measurements.* URL: http://www.lib.umich.edu/socwork/rescue/testresources. html. [This site has a description of the 5-volume set of *Compendium of Quality of Life Instruments*, among many others.]

University of Michigan Taubman Medical Library. *Tests and measurement instruments.* URL: http://www.lib.umich.edu/hsl/resources/tests. Last updated, August 18, 2008.

University of Pennsylvania. *Tests and measurements—Research guide.* URL: http://get help.library.upenn.edu/guides/educ/tests.html. Last updated, February 15, 2008.

University of Pittsburgh Health Sciences Library System. *Finding information on psychological and psychiatric testing instruments.* URL: http://www.hsls.pitt.edu/guides/tests

University of Washington. *Quick tips for finding measurement tools.* URL: http://health links.washington.edu/howto/measurement/quicktips

6

Measuring Outcomes in Cardiovascular Advanced Practice Nursing

ANNA GAWLINSKI AND KATHY McCLOY

National health care policymakers and professionals have increasingly advocated for the measurement and monitoring of patient safety, quality improvement, and health care outcomes. The development and implementation of national practice guidelines that are based on the best available research have provided clinicians with interventions that can improve patients' outcomes (Dykes, 2003; Titler, 2004). Yet these practice guidelines are not consistently used, and variability in practices varies from clinician to clinician and institution to institution resulting in poor outcomes for patients (Centers for Medicare & Medicaid Services, 2008; Institute of Medicine, 2001; McGlynn et al., 2003; Titler, 2008; Ward et al., 2006).

This emphasis on accountability has resulted in increased focus and incentives for those institutions and providers that perform well on indicators of safety and quality, with measurable outcomes. For example, the Joint Commission on Accreditation of Healthcare Organizations has set standards for performance measurement that include measures of research-based therapies such as aspirin, beta-blockers, and levels of low-density lipoprotein (LDL, with evaluation and treatment until the LDL goal is reached) in patients after hospitalization for myocardial infarction (The Joint Commission, 2008).

Cardiovascular (CV) disease in particular lends itself to measurement of such quality indicators and outcomes. The reasons include:

- High volume and high cost of care
- Chronicity and acuity of CV diseases
- Published practice guidelines (both locally and nationally) outlining "best practices" for treatment of CV disease (Deaton, 2001; Paul, 2000)

Although a great deal of effort has been devoted to the development of CV evidenced-based practice guidelines, more data are needed to demonstrate how these guidelines can be translated into practice and to determine their subsequent effect on outcomes in everyday practice settings. CV advanced practice nurses (APNs) are in a key position to couple their expert knowledge of research-based practices and outcomes measurement to generate data demonstrating successful translation of these guidelines into practice.

This chapter presents an overview of outcomes measurement in advanced practice nursing and describes the role of the CV APN in outcomes measurement. Through two specific case examples, APNs will be exposed to systematic, structured approaches that can be used in the process of making evidence-based practice changes and measuring outcomes. It is the hope of the contributors that the examples and processes shared in this chapter can be replicated in other facilities to reduce variations in practice and improve outcomes in CV patients.

OUTCOME MEASURES USED
IN ADVANCED PRACTICE NURSING

APNs are often faced with the dilemma of what constitutes an outcome and which outcomes should be measured. Outcomes are defined as the "consequences of treatment or interventions"(Oermann & Floyd, 2002; Urden, 1999). They are "the end result of care" (Oermann & Floyd, 2002; Urden, 1999). The outcomes that best reflect clinical practice and the goals of treatment are most meaningful and most amenable to measurement (Gawlinski, 2007; Kleinpell & Gawlinski, 2005). For example, in evaluating the effect of advanced practice nursing in managing heart failure (HF) patients, important outcomes to be measured may include:

- Patients' knowledge of their medications and dietary guidelines, followed by adjustment of diuretics based on daily weight
- Symptom management
- Functional status pre- and posttherapy
- Patients' perceptions of quality of life
- Resource utilization (diagnostic and laboratory tests, procedures, medications)
- Number of inpatient admissions
- Overall length of stay
- Overall cost per case

Historically, the classification of outcomes used medical definitions known as the "five Ds"—death, disease, disability, discomfort, and dissatisfaction (Lohr, 1988; Nolan & Mock, 2000; Urden, 1999). But outcomes have also been categorized in other ways, such as patient- or care-related, system-related, practitioner- or performance-related, and cost/financial-related outcomes (Kleinpell-Nowell & Weiner, 1999). Other categories of outcomes are clinical-, psychological-, functional-, cost/fiscal-, and satisfaction-related (Urden, 1999).

Several publications provide APNs with excellent resources on specific outcome measures and instruments (Kleinpell, 2003, 2007; Kleinpell-Nowell & Weiner, 1999). For example, Fulton and Baldwin (2004) published an annotated bibliography reflecting clinical nurse specialist practice and outcomes. Urden (1999) published a list of a broad spectrum of outcomes using clinical, physiologic, psychological, functional, fiscal, and satisfaction categories. The author also posed a list of *nurse-sensitive* outcomes (defined as sensitive enough to measure the effect of nursing practice) and collaborative outcomes (measuring the effect of an integrated approach of several disciplines to practice). Kleinpell (2003) provided a list of sources for identifying outcome measures and outcome instruments for analyzing the impact of APN care. Table 6.1 provides a listing of outcome measures that can be used by APNs based on these published literature reviews.

Generally, outcome measures in the cardiac population have focused on phenomena such as: (a) the effect of an aggressive cholesterol-

Table 6.1

OUTCOMES FOR ADVANCED PRACTICE NURSING

Clinical (care-related) outcomes

- Mortality
- Morbidity
    - Infection: Nosocomial, urinary tract infection, ventilator or line related
    - Medical conditions (e.g., heart failure)
    - Physiological response
        - Blood pressure, heart rate
        - Temperature
        - Lung sounds
        - Hemodynamic pressures
        - Weight and weight management
        - Serum/urine glucose
        - Wound healing; skin integrity
        - Loss of mobility
- Symptom management
    - Pain
    - Fatigue
    - Nausea, vomiting
    - Constipation
- Nutritional status/management
- Sleep maintenance
- Restraint use
- Smoking cessation
- Low birth weight; preterm infants
- Rates of adherence to best practices
- Hand hygiene compliance rates

Psychosocial outcomes

- Coping; stress management
- Mentation
- Return to work
- Role functioning
- Family functioning/coping
- Anxiety
- Sexual functioning
- Caregiver strain/burden
- Knowledge: medications, diet, treatment regime, motor skills, condition specific
- Staff nurse knowledge

(Table 6.1 continued)

Functional outcomes

- Quality of life
- Self-care: bathing, eating, dressing self, nonparenteral medication administration
- Mobility
- Communication
- Return to:
  - Work
  - School
  - Normal activity/social interaction
- Symptom control

Fiscal outcomes

- Length of stay
- Readmission rates to hospital, home care, other services
- Emergency department visits
- Health care services utilization
- Cost per episode of care
- Resource utilization: ancillary services, community/other services
- Staff nurse retention rates

Satisfaction

- Consumer
  - Care provided
  - Services provided
  - Care provider
- Family
  - Care provided to family member
  - Services provided/available
- Payor
- Provider

Sources: Adapted from Urden (1999) and Kleinpell-Nowell and Weiner (1999).

---

management program implemented by an APN; (b) the effect of applying evidenced-based practices to management of HF; and (c) the effect of APN practice on management of postoperative complications, on interventions to promote quality of life, and on evaluation of a spectrum of physiologic responses to APN interventions (e.g., blood pressure, heart rate, hemodynamics, urine output, daily weight, nutrition, and symptom control) (Meyer & Miers, 2005; Paul, 2000). Outcome measures that are of concern in the CV population are listed in Table 6.2 and will be used in the examples that follow.

There are several approaches that can be used for outcomes measurement in advanced practice nursing. The approach can span the spectrum of scientific rigor, as depicted in Figure 6.1.

For example, various research designs can be used in outcomes measurement, including experimental, quasi-experimental, and comparative designs. These research designs result in a more rigorous scientific process than other methods (e.g., performance-improvement processes) and increase the degree of confidence one can have when drawing conclusions from data. Table 6.3 lists select research designs, the type of questions the design helps to answer, and the degree of control or rigor over factors (or covariates) that can affect the outcome (Clochesy, 2002).

APNs may opt to use existing research to make a practice change and evaluate the effects of implementing a new evidence-based innovation on specific outcomes. This type of project would use a research-utilization or evidence-based practice approach or framework, as described in Table 6.4.

Finally, a performance-improvement process can be chosen. The APN can use any of these approaches to evaluate the impact of a new evidence-based intervention on patient, system, and fiscal outcomes. Each of these approaches has its advantages and disadvantages. The APN must choose among these approaches depending on the variables under study, the outcome measures under study, the instruments used for measurements, and the clinical feasibility (time, resources, and the ultimate goal).

Although the design and method of an outcome project are important with respect to the level of confidence that one can have in the results, the use of valid and reliable measures and instruments is even more important (Clochesy, 2002). There are many valid and reliable instruments to measure common health care outcomes, such as quality of life and functional status (Clochesy, 2002), and there are a growing number of instruments, such as self-report questionnaires, scales, symptom checklists, visual analog scales, and numeric rating scales (Kleinpell, 2003; Nolan & Mock, 2000).

Planning for the implementation of an outcomes project starts with the development of a timeline (Figure 6.2). Components of a timeline

Table 6.2

SELECTED OUTCOMES FOR CARDIOVASCULAR POPULATION

Cardiac risk-factor-reduction outcomes

- Hypertension control (blood pressure)
- Diabetes control (blood glucose, hemoglobin A$_{1c}$)
- Weight loss
- Lipid (cholesterol [LDL, HDL], triglycerides)
- Frequency of aerobic exercise
- Fat intake
- Knowledge: medications, diet, treatment regime, motor skills, condition specific
- Risk control
    - Chest pain/angina
    - Activity level
    - Smoking cessation
    - Alcohol-consumption status

Acute myocardial infarction outcomes

- Cardioprotective medication regimen
    - Frequency prescribed
    - Frequency of reaching target lipid levels
- Chest pain
- Arrhythmias
- Resource utilization
    - Electrocardiograms, blood tests, chest X-ray, etc.
- Length of stay
- Cost per case
- Functional status
- See *Risk-factor-reduction outcomes*

Heart failure outcomes

- Readmission rates
- Symptom management
- Evidenced-based practices and medications
    - Frequency prescribed
    - Compliance with medication regimen
    - Daily weight
    - Fluid limit
- Compliance with low-sodium diet
- Functional status
- See *Risk-factor-reduction outcomes*

(continued)

(Table 6.2 continued)

Post-PTCA/stent outcomes

- Reocclusion rates
- Hematoma rates
- Bleeding requiring transfusion
- Other vascular complications
- Evidenced-based practice meds
  - Antiplatelet and antilipid therapy
- Functional status pre- and post-stent
- Sheath removal techniques and products
- See *Risk-factor-reduction outcomes*

Post-CABG outcomes

- Pain management
- Sedation
- Hemodyanmic management
- Early extubation
- Blood transfusion
- Early extubation
- Early mobility (fast track)
- Infections (sternal, nosocomial pneumonia)
- Wound healing; skin integrity
- Cardioprotective meds
  - Prescribed
  - Compliance
- Functional status
- Quality of life

PTCA = percutaneous transluminal coronary angioplasty; CABG = coronary artery by-pass graft.

include (1) forming the team, (2) identifying the processes or new practices initiated or led by the APN and the outcome measures that are sensitive to them, (3) collecting baseline data, (4) reviewing relevant literature to develop a practice document that reflects the process or new practice change, (5) implementing the APN initiative, and (6) collecting data after implementation of the practice change to evaluate the impact of the change. Although the timeline appears linear, often there is overlap among the various phases of the project. For example, the sample timeline shows that an in-depth review of the literature is done after baseline data is collected; often, however, a review of the

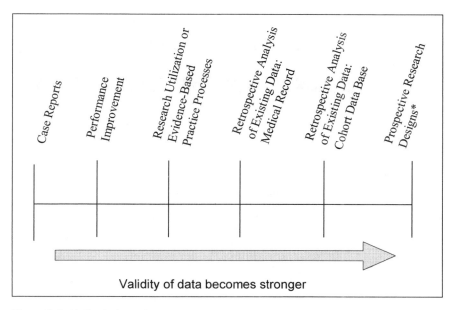

Figure 6.1 Methods for outcomes measurement.

Table 6.3

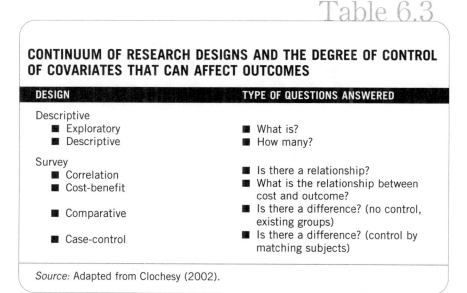

CONTINUUM OF RESEARCH DESIGNS AND THE DEGREE OF CONTROL OF COVARIATES THAT CAN AFFECT OUTCOMES

DESIGN	TYPE OF QUESTIONS ANSWERED
Descriptive	
■ Exploratory	■ What is?
■ Descriptive	■ How many?
Survey	
■ Correlation	■ Is there a relationship?
■ Cost-benefit	■ What is the relationship between cost and outcome?
■ Comparative	■ Is there a difference? (no control, existing groups)
■ Case-control	■ Is there a difference? (control by matching subjects)

Source: Adapted from Clochesy (2002).

Table 6.4

STEPS OF THE RESEARCH UTILIZATION AND EVIDENCE-BASED PRACTICE PROCESS

RESEARCH UTILIZATION	EVIDENCE-BASED PRACTICE
■ Systematically determining patient care problems	■ Identification of a clinical problem or potential problem
■ Finding and assessing research-based knowledge to solve those problems	■ Gathering of best evidence
■ Adopting and designing nursing practice innovations that come from the research-based knowledge	■ Critical appraisal and evaluation of evidence; when appropriate, determination of a potential change in practice
■ Conducting a clinical trial and evaluating the innovation	■ Implementation of the practice change
■ Deciding whether to adopt, alter, or reject the innovation	■ Evaluation of practice change outcomes, both in terms of adherence to processes as well as planned outcomes (e.g., clinical, fiscal, administrative)
■ Developing the means to extend the new practice beyond the trial unit	■ Developing the means to extend the new practice beyond the trial unit
■ Developing mechanisms to maintain the innovation over time	■ Developing mechanisms to maintain the innovation over time

Sources: Adapted from Horsley et al. (1983) and Gawlinski and Rutledge (2008).

literature is also initiated during the early phases of an outcomes project to identify whether the current practice or new process being evaluated affects the selected outcomes or whether a relationship exists between the aspect of APN practice indicators and the identified outcomes.

Following are two examples of outcomes measurement projects. Each aspect of the project is described, such as the cardiac population, the evidence supporting the new innovation, the outcome measure, the methodology used, and the role of the APN. The first case is an illustration of a theoretical example of an outcomes measurement project; the

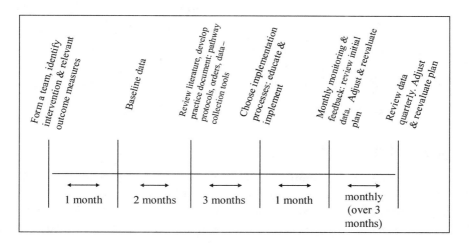

Figure 6.2 Timeline for outcomes measurement.

second case reflects an actual outcomes measurement project. APNs can use these examples as a model to replicate in their own practice.

CASE 1: CARDIAC POPULATION— ADVANCED HEART FAILURE PATIENTS

Outcome Project

Effect of a nurse-implemented diuretic protocol for diuretic management of hospitalized patients with heart failure

Outcome Variables

- Amount of diuresis (liters per day)
- Time to reach hemodynamic goal
- Duration of use of pulmonary artery (PA) catheter
- Hypokalemic and hyperkalemic events
- No. of staffing days with 1:2 nurse:patient ratio staffing days
- Length of stay (LOS) in the hospital, in the cardiac care unit (CCU), and in the advanced cardiac evaluation (ACE) unit

APN

Clinical nurse specialist

Outcomes Measurement Method

Randomized controlled research method

Scope of the Problem

Diuretic therapy is a mainstay of treatment in advanced HF patients. The literature supports the use of intravenous loop diuretics in high doses for patients with severe HF because oral gastrointestinal absorption is impaired by gut edema in patients with decompensated HF (Gawlinski & Stevenson, 2003; Gerlag & van Meijel, 1888; Task Force on Acute Heart Failure of the European Society of Cardiology, 2005; Vasko, Cartwight, Knochel, Nixon, & Brater, 1985). Furosemide is commonly used as the initial loop diuretic. Intravenous diuretics are administered to reduce preload or to reduce right and left ventricular end-diastolic volume and myocardial wall tension.

The reduction in left ventricular end-diastolic volume decreases the stretching of the mitral valve annulus and results in less mitral regurgitation. In general, administration of diuretics should be continued until clinical evidence of congestion is resolved (including jugular venous pressure < 8 mmHg) or the pulmonary capillary wedge pressure (PCWP), if measured, is = 15 mmHg and right atrial pressure (RA) = 7 mmHg (Fonarow et al., 1992; Gawlinski & Stevenson, 2003; Stevenson, 1999).

When the patient approaches the hemodynamic goal and dry weight, the patient may begin treatment with an oral loop diuretic.

Although our institution's advanced HF protocol requires diuretic therapy to be administered to achieve PCWP = 15 mmHg and RA = 7 mmHg, serendipitous observation revealed patients receiving less than ideal doses and frequencies of intravenous furosemide to achieve these hemodynamic goals. Factors contributing to the delays in diuretic orders included: (a) the workload of the house staff, (b) competing clinical needs of other patients, (c) difficulty in decision making, (d) lack of knowledge by house staff regarding importance of diuretic adjustment, and (e) perceived need of house staff to consult with physicians "higher in the chain of command." The result was less diuresis per day, longer times to achieve hemodynamic goals, longer PA catheter days, potentially longer intensive care unit and hospital LOS, and longer times on 1:2 staff ratios.

The clinical nurse specialist of the CCU and ACE unit (used for electively admitted HF patients) collaborated with the HF multidisciplinary team to develop and implement a protocol for diuretic management and an order set for in-hospital HF patients. The clinical nurse specialist was aware of previous research demonstrating positive clinical outcomes when using practice protocols that were integrated into clinical practice and nursing staff routines (Burns & Earven, 2003; Hoffman, Tasota, Zullo, Scharfenberg, & Donahue, 2005; Russell et al., 2002). Although a literature review showed limited research on the effectiveness of diuretic protocols with furosemide in HF patients (Lahav, Regev, Ra'anani, & Theodor, 1992; Schuller, Lynch, & Fine, 1997; van Meyel et al., 1994), the team thought that a protocol would provide a consistent approach to the management of diuretics and could have an effect on clinical outcomes (more diuresis and shorter times to achieve hemodynamic goals, shorter PA catheter days, fewer hypokalemic and hyperkalemic events) as well as on system outcomes (shorter duration on 1:2 staffing ratios, decreased LOS in specialized unit and hospital). The purpose of this outcomes project was to compare the effect of a diuretic management protocol that was based on literature plus the expertise of the multidisciplinary team with non-protocol-directed diuretic therapy for in-hospital advanced HF patients. The hypothesis was that the diuretic protocol would result in more diuresis and shorter times to achieve hemodynamic goals, shorter PA catheter days, shorter duration of 1:2 staffing ratios, fewer hypokalemic and hyperkalemic events, and decreased LOS in specialized unit and hospital.

Methods and Design

Randomized controlled experimental design

Sample and Setting

Heart failure patients between 18 and 80 years of age, admitted to the CCU and ACE unit in a University Medical Center who were instrumented with a PA catheter for medical management.

Data Collection Procedure

Upon patient consent, HF patients who were instrumented with a PA catheter (per our standard of practice) for medical management and hemodynamic guided therapy were randomly assigned to have their diuretic therapy managed by a diuretic protocol (experimental group) or the traditional nonprotocol approach (control group). Randomization was accomplished using sealed envelopes, which were opened at the time each patient was enrolled in the study. The primary clinical outcome measures were the amount of diuresis (liters per day), time to reach hemodynamic goal (days), duration of PA catheter days, and hypokalemic and hyperkalemic events. System outcome measures included length of time on 1:2 staffing and LOS in specialized unit and hospital.

Intervention (Diuretic Protocol and Diuretic Order Set)

A diuretic protocol and diuretic order set were developed by the APN in collaboration with the HF team (physicians, pharmacists, and nurses) for use in advanced HF patients upon instrumentation with a PA catheter. The diuretic orders were initiated by the physicians during morning rounds. The nurse implemented the orders and administered diuretics and potassium replacement according to the guidelines and parameters documented in the orders and protocol. This eliminated the need to obtain an order each time diuretics were necessary or potassium supplementation was needed. Nurses were educated in the protocol and order set and followed parameters for these interventions listed in the protocol and orders (Appendix A).

Data Collection Procedure

Heart failure patients who were instrumented with a PA catheter for medical treatment were randomly assigned to receive either the diuretic protocol ($n = 104$) or non-protocol diuretic therapy ($n = 102$). Upon randomization, if the patient was randomized to the diuretic protocol group, the protocol was initiated by the house staff in conjunction with APN during morning rounds; the staff nurse would implement the protocol based on written protocol parameters as described in Appendix A (such as PCWP, RA and amount of diuresis, potassium, and creati-

Table 6.5

BASELINE PATIENT CHARACTERISTICS STRATIFIED ACCORDING TO DIURETIC PROTOCOL (MEAN ± *SD*)			
VARIABLE	CONTROL GROUP (NONPROTOCOL) (*N* = 102)	EXPERIMENTAL GROUP (PROTOCOL DIRECTED) (*N* = 104)	*p*
Age, yrs	58.1 ± 10.1	57.8 ± 10.2	.895
Gender, No. (%)			
Male	75 (73.53)	83 (79.81)	.466
Female	27 (26.47)	21 (20.19)	
Diagnosis, No. (%)			
Dilated CM	45 (44.12)	44 (42.31)	.55
Ischemic CM	55 (53.92)	57 (54.81)	.81
Restrictive CM	2 (1.96)	3 (2.88)	.86

CM = cardiomyopathy.

nine). If patients were randomized to the nonprotocol-directed HF group (control group), all aspects of diuretics were ordered by the treating house staff physicians. Nurses could not make changes in the diuretic regimen without a physician's written or verbal order each time. Nurses could, however, communicate their opinions and observations about a patient's diuretic need to the house officers. These were the standard methods by which diuretic orders were obtained for HF patients.

Results

Because this theoretical case is used to illustrate an examplar of an outcomes measurement project, the results that follow are not real and are intended as an example for APNs to demonstrate how outcome data can be graphically presented in tables and figures. One hundred and four patients were randomized to receive the diuretic protocol ($n = 104$), and 102 patients received nonprotocol diuretic therapy. There were no differences between the demographic or clinical characteristics of the sample (Table 6.5).

Table 6.6

CLINICAL OUTCOME MEASURES (MEAN ± *SD*)

OUTCOME	CONTROL GROUP (NONPROTOCOL DIRECTED) (*N* = 102)	EXPERIMENTAL GROUP (PROTOCOL DIRECTED) (*N* = 104)	*p*
Urine output (liters/PA-catheter day)	2.2 ± 1.5	3.4 ± 1.4	< .001
Days to hemodynamic goal	4.0 ± 1.9	2.9 ± 1.3	.032
Duration of PA catheter (days)	4.8 ± 3.1	3.5 ± 2.0	.003
Hypo K⁺ events	21 ± 3.1	14 ± 2.0	.043
Hyper K⁺ events	6 ± 3.1	3 ± 2.0	.213
1:2 nurse:patient ratio (days)	6.5 ± 4.5	5.4 ± 3.1	.013
Length of CCU/ACE unit stay (days)	6.5 ± 4.5	5.4 ± 3.1	.013
Length of hospital stay (days)	10 ± 4.2	7.0 ± 3.0	<.001

Hemo = hemodynamic; Hypo K⁺= hypokalemic; HyperK+ = hyperkalemic; PA = pulmonary artery; CCU = cardiac care unit; ACE = advanced cardiac evaluation.

The median duration of time to achieve hemodynamic goals was 2.9 days for the patient managed with the diuretic protocol therapy and 4.0 days for the patients who received nonprotocol diuretic therapy. Kaplan-Meier analyses demonstrated that patients in the diuretic protocol group had statistically shorter times to reach hemodynamic goals than did patients in the nonprotocol diuretic group (Table 6.6). There was a statistically significant increase in the mean amount of diuresis in the nurse-implemented diuretic protocol group (3.4 L/day); in the nonprotocol diuretic group the mean amount of diuresis was 2.2 L/day ($p < .001$). Patients in the diuretic protocol group had statistically shorter PA catheter days (3.5 days in the protocol group, 4.8 days in the nonprotocol group). Patients in the diuretic protocol group had fewer days on 1:2 nurse:patient staffing ratios (mean: 5.4 days in the unit) than the nonprotocol group (mean 6.5 days), and fewer episodes of hypokalemia (14 events in 104 patients in the diuretic protocol group, compared with 21 events in the 102 nonprotocol diuretic group).

LOS in both the specialized unit and hospital were shorter in the diuretic protocol group (5.4 days in the unit and 7.2 days in the hospital, respectively) than in the nonprotocol group (6.5 days in the unit and 10.0 days in the hospital, respectively).

Conclusion

The use of a diuretic protocol can increase diuresis, reduce the time to reach hemodynamic goals and the duration of PA catheter days, decrease the number of hypokalemic and hyperkalemic events, decrease the need for 1:2 staffing ratios, and shorten length of stay in hospitalized patients with HF.

Summary of Case Example

This case example shows the effect of an APN collaborating with a multidisciplinary team to facilitate implementation and evaluation of a new approach in clinical practice (diuretic protocol) and a system change (expanding the staff nurse's role to include protocol-directed administration and titration of diuretics based on the protocol-derived parameters). Improved outcomes occurred in clinical practice (care-related outcomes) and system and fiscal outcomes because cost of care decreased with a decrease in the need for 1:2 nurse:patient staffing ratios and length of stay.

CASE 2: CARDIAC POPULATION— PATIENT ANTICOAGULATED WITH WARFARIN

Outcome Variables

- Therapeutic level of international normalized ratio (INR) level
- Bleeding events
- Clinic processes
- Patient satisfaction

APN

Acute care nurse practitioner (ACNP)

Outcomes Measurement Method

Evidence-based practice process

Background

Warfarin is the mainstay of anticoagulant use for a variety of clinical conditions, including atrial fibrillation, mechanical heart valves, and deep vein thrombosis (Ansell et al., 2004; Bonow et al., 1998). Warfarin can be a difficult medication for health care practitioners to use when treating patients, on account of its narrow therapeutic window and potential complications. With over 2.5 million patients currently taking warfarin in the United States, significant challenges are faced by the prescribing clinician in managing these patients (Singer et al., 2004). Literature supports the benefits of using evidence-based anticoagulation-management protocols, knowledgeable health care practitioners, and specialized clinics to effectively manage patients on oral anticoagulant therapy and prevent adverse events such as emboli or bleeding (Jaffer & Bragg, 2003).

By virtue of the expert knowledge of APNs in clinical care, research, and organizational systems, the APN is ideally suited for identifying and rectifying barriers to delivering quality care while managing these high-risk patients. The following section describes an evidence-based change project that consisted of a structured protocol and monitoring system for anticoagulation management and new processes of care (i.e., an ACNP-managed anticoagulation clinic) that resulted in an increased number of patients having a therapeutic INR level.

Scope of the Problem

Our team of six cardiologists managed a large number of patients taking warfarin. There was variability in practices among the cardiologists. Patients used various clinical laboratories in the community for obtaining their INR levels. A formal tracking system for consistent follow-up on patients' laboratory results was lacking. Thus, patients were often confused regarding their dosage regimens, had delays in waiting for lab results, were lost to follow-up and, in some cases, presented with complications related to overdosing and underdosing of warfarin, such as bleeding and cerebral vascular accidents. The ACNPs were often called upon to troubleshoot clinical problems and subsequently manage patients who telephoned the clinic for INR results or who were confused about their dosing regimens. It became increasingly apparent to the ACNPs that there was a need to optimize the care of patients who were being anticoagulated with warfarin. The ACNPs identified the existing challenges to more effective management of these patients. These challenges included the following:

- Variable management practices among the six physicians
- Inconsistencies in laboratories' reporting practices
- Use of numerous laboratories in the community that were not affiliated with our office
- Variable documentation of INR results and dosing regimens
- Lack of regular follow-up by the patients on their test results
- Lack of written evidence-based guidelines for titrating doses of warfarin based on the basis of INR levels
- Lack of a patient tracking system
- A predominantly elderly population with difficulty following and understanding the dosing regimen

It was essential to address the clinical problem by reviewing the literature for research and other evidence-based information on effective anticoagulation-management protocols and processes. Thus, the ACNPs embarked on an evidence-based change project to determine whether implementing a standardized anticoagulation-management protocol and new processes of care (i.e., an ACNP-managed anticoagulation clinic) that were literature-based (rather than variable practices) could improve the number and percentage of patients with therapeutic INR levels.

Evidence-Based Literature

A primary goal of anticoagulation therapy with warfarin is to maintain a therapeutic INR based on the clinical indications for anticoagulation

(Ansell et al., 2004; Hirsch, Fuster, Ansell, & Halperin, 2003; Salem et al., 2004). Achieving and maintaining a therapeutic INR can prove challenging on account of factors that may alter the patient's ability to comply with a given dosing regimen. A review of selected relevant literature demonstrates consensus among investigators that patients with nonvalvular atrial fibrillation who are anticoagulated with warfarin are, on average, in the INR therapeutic range of 2 to 3 only approximately 60% of the time (Connolly et al., 1991; Gullov et al., 1998; Pengo et al., 1998; Reynolds et al., 2004). Approximately 25% of the time, these patients have a mean INR that is below the minimum target INR of 2 and, therefore, are not adequately protected against stroke (Reynolds et al., 2004); 13% of the time, patients have an INR that exceeds the maximum INR limit of 3 and are at risk for major bleeding events (Reynolds et al., 2004).

Published literature supports the association between the incidence of adverse events and specific nontherapeutic INR ranges. For example, lower ranges (i.e., an INR of 1.1 to 2.1) are associated with higher incidence of stroke, whereas higher values (i.e., up to 4.5) have been associated with bleeds (Reynolds et al., 2004). A few studies have demonstrated that the method by which anticoagulation is managed can affect the level of INR achieved and patient outcomes (Matchar, Samsa, Cohen, Oddone, et al., 2002). For example, when patients were managed via specialized coagulation clinics, the time patients were in a therapeutic INR range were higher than those reported during routine medical management (Chiquette, Amato, & Bussey, 1998; Matchar et al., 2002). Franke and colleagues (2008) demonstrated that a standardized protocol for anticoagulation management plus point of care (POC) testing in a family medicine practice setting improved the frequency of patients with a therapeutic INR range, compared with usual care.

Pharmacists have also been used as frontline clinicians to improve anticoagulation management of patients with positive results. Although differences were modest, an anticoagulation clinic run by clinical pharmacists, compared with usual care provided by family practice physicians, improved anticoagulation control, reduced bleeding events, and improved costs associated with reduced hospitalizations and emergency department visits (Chiquette et al., 1998). Other investigators (Wilson et al., 2003) demonstrated improved outcomes with a pharmacist-run anticoagulation clinic, including a modest improvement in achieving and maintaining therapeutic INR, significantly fewer patients having high-risk INR values (INR less than 1.5 and greater than 5.0) and increased patient satisfaction in the anticoagulation clinic arm of the study, compared with usual care. Additionally, multidisciplinary teams using pharmacists, physicians, and nurses for anticoagulation management have also resulted in improved patient care and outcomes.

However, the role of the ACNP in anticoagulation management is less known. In a descriptive study by Kornblit and associates (1990), a 19-month evaluation demonstrated that anticoagulation managed by a family nurse practitioner–run clinic resulted in safe and effective patient care. Gill and Landis (2002) examined the impact of a registered nurse–managed mobile, multisite, office-based anticoagulation-management program that operated among seven different cardiology offices. Patients made office visits to the nurse and received patient education, POC INR testing, and medication adjustment based on a physician-approved algorithm. The percentage of in-range INRs increased from 40.7% to 58.5%, respectively, after 1 year of implementation of the anticoagulation-management program. Francavilla (2008) describes the development of a multidisciplinary team consisting of a physician, three registered nurses, and a clerical support staff person to comprise a registered-nurse–managed anticoagulation clinic. Three registered nurses managed the anticoagulation clinic using evidence-based consensus guidelines and demonstrated improved compliance with INR target in a subset of 20 patients from 59% (preclinic) to 73% (postclinic) after 1 year.

Thus, these descriptive comparative studies provide some support from the literature for anticoagulation clinics and their role in providing a more coordinated and efficacious approach to anticoagulation monitoring. These anticoagulation clinics may have standardized processes that reduce the variability among health care providers. However, additional large-scale, long-term randomized controlled clinical trials are needed to strengthen the evidence for anticoagulation clinics and to assess the impact of ACNP management.

Interventions

The first intervention was to develop and standardize a protocol for the management of patients' anticoagulation. Originally, warfarin was managed on an individual basis by each patient's cardiologist. Variations in practice occurred and were not consistently based on the latest research and evidence-based guidelines. In an effort to facilitate and standardize anticoagulation management among the team of ACNPs and cardiologists, an anticoagulation management protocol that was literature-based was developed and approved.

The anticoagulation management protocol was written according to the format of a standardized procedure, which is a document that guides ACNP practice. This format was chosen because the change process included managing the transition of care of patients who were taking warfarin from the individual cardiology practice to an ACNP-managed anticoagulation "clinic." With the anticoagulation management protocol written as a standardized procedure, the ACNPs had a document that was required legally and broadened their scope of practice to include the evaluation and management of patients on warfarin (California Board of Registered Nursing, 2004) (Appendix B). The content of evidence-based anticoagulation management protocol and standardized procedure provided the ACNPs with specific guidelines regarding (1) adjustment of warfarin dosage, (2) management of warfarin based on the INR (in or out of therapeutic range), (3) management of bleeding, and (4) criteria for physician consultation and referral (Appendix C). The anticoagulation management protocol was created based on evidence-based recommendations from the Seventh American College of Chest Physicians Conference on Antithrombotic and Thrombolytic Therapy: Evidence Based Guidelines (Ansell et al., 2004). Published reports support the use of these guidelines as a standard for anticoagulation management with warfarin (Franke et al., 2008; Hirsh et al., 2003; Jaffer & Bragg, 2003).

The second intervention was to implement a process whereby cardiologists could refer their patients to the clinic for anticoagulation management by the ACNP. Physicians started this process by completing the Anticoagulation Clinic Enrollment Form for their patients. This form specified the patient's demographic information, diagnosis, rationale for anticoagulation therapy, warfarin dose at the time of enrollment, and the therapeutic INR target range (Appendix D). The form provided an important mechanism for communication between the physician and the ACNP regarding the clinical management of patients.

To reduce delays in laboratory reporting times, the third intervention was to implement POC testing for INR and prothrombin time (PT) levels. POC testing consisted of obtaining a blood sample by a finger stick rather than a venipuncture so that immediate INR results and warfarin dose could be determined during the patient's clinic visit. The literature supports the accuracy and reliability of POC testing for INR and PT results (Kaatz et al., 1995; Lizotte et al., 2002; Rochon, 2006). Measuring INR on site eliminated many telephone calls to outside laboratories to obtain INR results, and then to patients to communicate changes in medication dosing regimen. On-site POC testing also allowed the ACNP to assess the patient at the time of the clinic visit for (1) risk factors that could lead to complications, such as bleeding, and (2) clinical indications that required special instructions, such as preparation for surgical procedures requiring cessation of warfarin.

The fourth intervention was to identify the unique roles and responsibilities of each team member involved in the new anticoagulation clinic. The roles and responsibilities were delineated in a document that described the administrative duties by clinic staff, such as the frequency of scheduling patients, and clinical duties by the clinic staff nurses, such as performing finger sticks. Clinical therapeutic anticoagulation targets and subsequent actions of each team member were also addressed in the document, as well as interventions for the presence or absence of bleeding.

The ACNP's roles and responsibilities included supervision of the anticoagulation clinic staff so that clinic efficiency was maximized and so that patients received their INR results and instructions for warfarin dosing adjustments at the same visit. To achieve this goal, the ACNPs implemented a process for assessment of a patient's current anticoagulation regimen at each visit and for an expanded role of the clinic staff nurses. This process consisted of patients completing a 3-item questionnaire when they arrived at the clinic. The questionnaire asked about the patient's current anticoagulation regimen and included questions regarding tablet strength of warfarin, weekly dose schedule, and the presence or absence of bleeding since the last visit. After the patient completed the questionnaire, the patient's INR was measured. The clinic staff nurse then reviewed the patient's completed questionnaire for any high-risk or abnormal occurrences and reported these to the ACNP with the INR value.

Initially, all patients were seen by the ACNP. However, as clinic staff nurses became more knowledgeable and skillful, the role of the clinic staff nurse was expanded. Patients with a therapeutic INR requiring no medication adjustment and who were without complications were given protocol-derived written instructions for dosing and follow-up appointment by the clinic staff nurse. To assure safe practice for these patients, a second page, outlining the patient's recommended medication dosing schedule, was added to the patient questionnaire, but was completed by the clinic staff nurse. One copy was given to the patient and the original was placed in the medical record. Complex cases were automatically referred to the ACNP. Criteria for complex patient referrals to the ACNP included:

- An INR value that was out of range
- Complications (such as bleeding) from anticoagulation
- New clinical issues, such as future surgical or dental procedures
- Need for more in-depth education
- Noncompliance with dosing regimen for one or more clinic visits
- Patient request to see the ACNP, regardless of INR level

The fifth intervention was to begin to implement the new change. This process required education of all team members, as well as one-to-one coaching, mentoring, and feedback. Staff training occurred on a variety of levels, both formally and informally. Our clinic's staff nurses were trained to use the CoaguChek S (Roche Diagnostics, Inc., 2001). POC monitoring by the company representative and subsequent skill laboratories were run by the ACNP on a quarterly basis. Monthly meetings were scheduled to review processes within the clinic, troubleshoot problems, and obtain feedback for recommended changes. In addition, cases were reviewed to enhance the clinic staff nurse's knowledge and skill in using data from the patient questionnaire and in selecting an appropriate action.

Factors that increased clinic efficiency were also discussed. Feedback regarding timing of appointments led to scheduling patients at shorter intervals so that more patients could be accommodated. Clinic nurses also were given access to the appointment system to schedule the next follow-up appointments, which eliminated the wait time at the front desk for scheduling subsequent INR visits.

As practice changes were made, it was clear that many patients were uncertain about why they were prescribed or were taking warfarin and why frequent INR tests were needed. Patient education materials were revised to reflect this information and a formalized process for educating patients was implemented. Revised education materials outlined the indications for, risks of, and benefits of warfarin; INR testing; and dietary and medication interactions. A patient education visit was required for all patients when warfarin was started or when the patient enrolled in the anticoagulation clinic. Subsequent patient education sessions were scheduled as needed, depending on the patient's adherence to the prescribed regimen.

A Patient Agreement Form was also developed and given to each patient at the time of his/her clinic visit. The Patient Agreement Form outlines the benefits and risks of warfarin and the importance of adhering to clinic visits (Appendix D). A copy of the Patient Agreement Form was given to the patient and the original was filed in the patient's medical record.

The final intervention was to set up a database so that outcomes could be tracked over time. The ACNPs began collecting data that included patients' demographics, weekly warfarin dosage(s), INR results, and visit notes. The ACNPs entered all pertinent information from the patient questionnaire into the database. They used the information in the database to inform their clinic practice during patient visits and to check on the progress of their clinic staff nurses in providing protocol-derived counseling to the stable patients. For example, for patients who were seen by the clinic staff nurse, the ACNP periodically reviewed the patients' INR results and their responses to the questionnaire. Data on important variables and indicators of the clinic's success, such as the number of missed appointments and the percentage of patients with INR levels in and out of range, were shared with all team members. Each cardiologist was able to access reports of these outcomes for his or her respective patients.

Results Postproject Implementation

After implementing the new structure and process for patient anticoagulation management, the ACNP evaluated the effects of the change on areas that had been identified as problematic or outcomes identified in

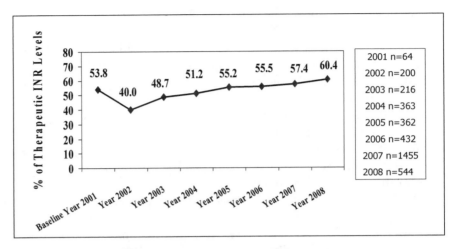

Figure 6.3 Results: Percentage of patients with therapeutic INR levels.

the literature. Outcomes included (1) the percentage of patients with INR levels within therapeutic range, (2) streamlining processes of care, and (3) patient satisfaction. During the first 6 months of the change process, the clinic was in a transition period and processes were being "fine tuned." Initially, outcome data were reviewed quarterly to evaluate the number and percentage of patients with INR results that were in and out of range. After several years of operating the clinic, annual outcome data has shown a steady increase in the percentage of patient visits with therapeutic INR levels from a baseline of 53.8% to 60.4% (Figure 6.3). These results exceed data reported in selected published studies that ranged from 34% to 60% (Samsa et al., 2000; van Walraven, Jennings, Oake, Fergusson, & Forster, 2006). Published clinical trials have reported even higher numbers of patients with therapeutic INR ranges (CARS Inverstigators, 1997; Stroke Prevention in Atrial Fibrillation Investigators, 1991).

Bleeding is a major risk factor associated with use of warfarin (Cortelezzo, 1993; Jacobs, 2005; Levine, Raskob, Beyth, Kearon, & Schulman, 2004). The role of the ACNP in the management of complications related to warfarin is comprehensive because the ACNP is often the first health care provider to detect that patients have complications such as bleeding. The type and severity of all bleeding events are assessed by the ACNP at each clinic visit. High-risk patient characteristics are evaluated, including prior history of bleeding, hypertension, recent surgery, recent cerebrovascular accident or myocardial infarction, renal insufficiency (serum level of creatinine < 1.5), and concomitant medications that potentiate bleeding (Jaffer, 2005; Jaffer & Bragg, 2003; Levine et al., 2004). The ACNP often initiates treatment plans and referrals are often initiated by the ACNP for further evaluation and treatment, including diagnostic tests (e.g., prothrombin time, INR, complete blood count), evaluation in the emergency department for unstable bleeding, and evaluation by a primary care physician or specialized health care provider for less significant bleeding. Physician consultation is required for all bleeding events and all INR values of 5.0 or greater, regardless of the presence or absence of bleeding. Specific guidelines for the management of supratherapeutic INRs and bleeding are outlined in the anticoagulation management protocol (Appendix C).

Satisfaction of patients was informally monitored on the basis of feedback patients gave the office manager, clinic staff nurses, ACNPs, and physicians. Patients reported preferences for blood testing via finger stick as opposed to venipuncture. Patients expressed increased satisfaction with receiving results of laboratory tests and instructions for dosing immediately rather than waiting for phone calls.

Additional benefits of the anticoagulation management clinic are numerous for the patient and the provider. These benefits include seamless POC testing for patients taking warfarin, early communication and intervention for complications associated with the use of warfarin, and increasing the number of patients seen while enhancing patient satisfaction. Follow-up of patients has improved dramatically with the use of the clinical database and the streamlined appointment system. The number of patients seen at the clinic has increased from approximately 50 patients to 300 active patients over time. This change represents a fivefold or 500% increase in number of patients seen compared with when the clinic started, with the clinic now having approximately 350 to 400 patient visits per month and approximately 4,500 visits annually. Complication rates of significant bleeding are rare and are less than the 1% to 3% rates reported in clinical trials with similar patient populations (Reynolds et al., 2004). Communication with the attending cardiologist has improved as a result of quarterly and event reporting. Thus, the ACNP-managed anticoagulation clinic has delivered safe and effective care to patients taking warfarin.

Limitations

Our new structure and process for anticoagulation patient management were designed on the basis of the current best available evidence and the needs of our patients. Consequently, this evidence-based practice project may be applicable only to similar anticoagulation clinics and office-type clinical settings. Despite this limitation, the results of this practice change indicated that our newly developed standardized anticoagulation management protocol and processes have been effective in achieving our goals. We increased the percentage of patients with therapeutic INR levels and improved patient satisfaction with new structures and processes for care delivered by an ACNP-managed anticoagulation clinic.

Our standardized anticoagulation management protocol was timely and enhanced communication between our physician and ACNP and improved quality of patient care. Furthermore, team members have stated that this evidence-based practice project has resulted in greater cohesiveness among the team members, expansion of their roles, and an increase in their job satisfaction.

Discussion

This evidence-based practice change project involved the development and implementation of an anticoagulation management protocol and new processes that were based on published reports. The percentage of patients with theraupeutic INR values increased after the intervention.

These findings build on the evidence-based literature on anticoagulation management and effectiveness of ACNP care because (1) a template of a standardized anticoagulation management protocol was developed from recommendations in the literature, (2) a new structure and processes for care delivered by an ACNP-managed anticoagulation clinic were implemented and, (3) these interventions were tested on important patient outcomes related to the number and percentage of patients who achieved therapeutic INR levels.

This project provided an opportunity for ACNPs to influence care for large numbers of patients in their clinic as well as throughout their office and hospital practice. As physician colleagues noted the improved anticoagulation management of their patients, the standardized protocol was gradually adopted throughout the office practice and system-wide to ensure continuity of care and safety of patients. Acute care nurse practitioners who are at the point of the delivery of care were able to identify a clinical practice issue that required an evidence-based practice solution. This evidence-based practice project provides support for the ACNPs to lead multidisciplinary teams that involve physician colleagues and staff nurses in the process of using research and other levels of evidence to develop, implement, and test new innovations in the clinical setting. The use of the standardized anticoagulation management protocol has been expanded first beyond the clinic to the entire office practice, and has led to more uniform anticoagulation of patients who are hospitalized from our practice as well as system-wide. Our health care system has adopted this new protocol and these new practices for implementation of an anticoagulation clinic on a system-wide basis.

Strategies were implemented to ensure that the practice change would be sustained. These strategies include incorporating the standardized anticoagulation management protocol in the orientation of new medical, nursing, and office staff and incorporation of key elements of the new processes, such as the POC testing, into annual assessments of skills competencies and dissemination of the results internally.

Summary of Case Example

Structures and processes for anticoagulation management can be improved by assessing current management practices, developing an evidence-based intervention to improve structures and practices related to anticoagulation management, and evaluating the effects on outcomes. Creation of a specialized ACNP-led anticoagulation clinic practice allowed ACNPs at the point of delivery of care to implement a standardized protocol and processes for anticoagulation management that increased the number and percentage of patients who achieved therapeutic INR levels and the number of patients seen.

REFERENCES

Ansell, J., Hirsh, J., Poller, L., Bussey, H., Jacobson, A., & Hylek, E. (2004). The pharmacology and management of the vitamin K antagonists: The Seventh ACCP Conference on Antithrombotic Therapy and Thrombolytic Therapy. *Chest, 126*(3 Suppl.), 204S–233S.

Bonow, R. O., Carabello, B., de Leon, A. C., Jr., Edmunds, L. H., Jr., Fedderly, B. J., Freed, M. D., et al. (1998). ACC/AHA guidelines for the management of patients with valvular heart disease: A report of the American College of Cardiology/American Heart Association Task Force on Practice Guidelines (Committee on Management of Patients With Valvular Heart Disease). *Journal of the American College of Cardiology, 32*, 1486–1588.

Burns, S. M., & Earven, S. (2003). Improving outcomes for mechanically ventilated medical intensive care unit patients using advanced practice nurses: A 6-year experience. *Nursing Clinics of North America, 14*(3), 231–243.

California Board of Registered Nursing. (2004). *Nursing Practice Act: Rules and Regulations.* Publication No. 23550. Sacramento, CA: Department of Consumer Affairs.

CARS Investigators. (1997). Randomised double-blind trial of fixed low-dose warfarin with aspirin after myocardial infarction. Coumadin Aspirin Reinfarction Study (CARS) investigators. *Lancet, 350*(9075), 389–396.

Centers for Medicare and Medicaid Services. (2008). Retrieved June 2008 from http://www.cms.hhs.gov/

Chiquette, E., Amato, M. G., & Bussey, H. I. (1998). Comparison of an anticoagulation clinic with usual medical care: Anticoagulation control, patient outcomes, and health care costs. *Archives of Internal Medicine, 158*, 1641–1647.

Clochesy, J. M. (2002). Research designs for advanced practice nursing outcomes research. *Critical Care Nursing Clinics of North America, 14*, 293–298.

Cortelazzo, S., Finzaai, G., Viero, P., et al. (1993). Thrombotic and hemorrhagic complication in patients with mechanical heart valves attending an anticoagulation clinic. *Thrombosis and Hemostasis, 69*, 316–320.

Deaton, C. (2001). Outcomes measurement and evidence-based nursing practice. *Journal of Cardiovascular Nursing, 15*, 83–86.

Dormans, T. P., van Meyel, J. J., Gerlag, P. C., et al. (1996). Diuretic efficacy of high dose furosemide in severe heart failure: Bolus injection versus continuous infusion. *Journal of the American College of Cardiology, 28*, 376–382.

Dykes, P. C. (2003). Practice guidelines and measurement: State-of-the-science. *Nursing Outlook, 51*, 65–69.

Fonarow, G. C., Chelimsky-Fallick, C., Stevensen, L. W., et al. (1992) Effect of direct vasodilation with hydralazine versus angiotensin-converting enzyme inhibition with captopril on mortality in advanced heart failure: The Hy-C Trial. *Journal of the American College of Cardiology, 19*, 842–850.

Francavilla, C. (2008). Registered nurse-managed anticoagulation clinic: Improving patient outcomes. *Nursing Economic$, 26*, 130–132.

Franke, C., Dickerson, L., & Carek, P. (2008). Improving anticoagulation therapy using point of care testing and standardized protocol. *Annals of Family Medicine, 6*(Suppl. 1), S28–S32.

Fulton, J., & Baldwin, K. (2004). An annotated bibliography reflecting CNS practice and outcomes. *Clinical Nurse Specialist, 18*, 21–39.

Gawlinski, A. (2007). Evidence-based practice changes: Measuring the outcome. *AACN Advanced Critical Care, 18*, 320–322.

Gawlinski, A., & Rutledge, D. (2008). Selecting a model for evidence-based practice changes: A practical approach. *AACN Advanced Critical Care, 19*, 1–10.

Gawlinski, A., & Stevenson, L. (2003). Treatment goals for heart failure in critical care. In M. Jessup & K. McCauley (Eds.), *How to provide the best care to heart failure patients* (pp. 81–95). New York: Future Media Services, Inc.

Gerlag, P. G., & van Meijel, J. J. (1988). High-dose furosemide in the treatment of refractory congestive heart failure. *Archives of Internal Medicine, 148,* 286–289.

Gill, J., & Landis, M. (2002). Benefits of a mobile, point of care anticoagulation therapy management program. *The Joint Commission Journal on Quality Improvement, 28,* 625–630.

Hirsch, J., Fuster, V., Ansell, J., & Halperin, J. (2003). American Heart Association/American College of Cardiology Foundation guide to warfarin therapy. *Circulation, 107,* 1692–1711.

Hoffman, L. A., Tasota, F. J., Zullo, T. G., Scharfenberg, C., & Donahue, M. P. (2005). Outcomes of care managed by an acute care nurse practitioner/attending physician team in a subacute medical intensive care unit. *American Journal of Critical Care, 14,* 121–130.

Horsley, J. A., Crane, J., Crabtree, M., & Wood, D. (1983). *Using research to improve practice: A guide.* New York: Grune and Stratton.

Institute of Medicine. (2001). *Crossing the quality chasm: A new health system for the 21st century. Report from the Committee on Quality of Health Care in America.* Washington, DC: National Academy Press.

Jacobs, L. (2005). Warfarin pharmacology, clinical management, and evaluation of hemorrhagic risk for the elderly. *Clinics in Geriatric Medicine, 22,* 17–32.

Jaffer, A. (2005). Issues in anticoagulant therapy: Recent trials start to answer the tough questions. *Cleveland Clinic Journal of Medicine, 72,* 157–163.

Jaffer, A. K., Brotman, D. J., & Chukwumerije, N. (2003). When patients on warfarin need surgery. *Cleveland Clinic Journal of Medicine, 70,* 973–984.

Jaffer, M., & Bragg, L. (2003). Practical tips for warfarin dosing and monitoring. *Cleveland Clinic Journal of Medicine, 70,* 361–371.

The Joint Commission. (2008). *Facts about the 2008 National Patient Safety Goals.* Retrieved June 6, 2008, from http://www.jointcommission.org/PatientSafety/NationalPatientSafetyGoals/08_npsg_facts.htm.

Kaatz, A., White, R., Hill, J., Mascha, E., Humphries, J. E., & Becker, D. M. (1995). Accuracy of laboratory and portable monitor internationalized ratio determinations. Comparisons with a criterion standard. *Archives of Internal Medicine, 155,* 1861–1867.

Kleinpell, R. M. (2003, February). Measuring advanced practice nursing outcomes: Strategies and resources. *Critical Care Nurse,* Suppl., 6–10.

Kleinpell, R. M. (2007). APNs: Invisible champions? *Nursing Management, 38*(5), 18–22.

Kleinpell, R. M., & Gawlinski, A. (2005). Assessing outcomes in advanced practice nursing practice: The use of quality indicators and evidence-based practice. *AACN Clinical Issues, 16,* 43–57.

Kleinpell-Nowell, R., & Weiner, T. (1999). Measuring advanced practice nursing outcomes. *AACN Clinical Issues, 10,* 356–368.

Lahav, M., Regev, A., Ra'anani, P., & Theodor, E. (1992). Intermittent administration of furosemide vs continuous infusion preceded by a loading dose for congestive heart failure. *Chest, 102,* 725–731.

Levine, M., Raskob, G., Beyth, R., Kearon, C., & Schulman, S. (2004). Hemorrhagic complications of anticoagulant treatment: The seventh ACCP conference on antithrombotic and thrombolytic therapy. *Chest, 126*(3 Suppl.), 287S–310S.

Lizotte, A., Quessy, I., Vanier, M.-C., Martineau, J., Caron, S., Daraveau, M., et al. (2002). Reliability, validity and ease of use of a portable point of care coagulation device in a pharmacist managed anticoagulation clinic. *Journal of Thrombosis and Thrombolysis, 14,* 247–254.

Lohr, K. N. (1988). Outcome measurement: Concepts and questions. *Inquiry, 25,* 37–50.

Matchar, D. B., Samsa, G. P., Cohen, S. J., et al. (2002). Improving the quality of anticoagulation of patients with atrial fibrillation in managed care organizations: Results of the managing anticoagulation services trial. *American Journal of Medicine, 113:* 42–51.

McGlynn, E. A., Asch, S. M., Adams, J., et al. (2003). The quality of health care delivered to adults in the United States. *New England Journal of Medicine, 348,* 2635–2645.

Meyer, S. C., & Miers, L. J. (2005). Cardiovascular surgeon and acute care nurse practitioner collaboration on post-operative outcomes. *AACN Clinical Issues, 16,* 149–158.

Nolan, M. T., & Mock, V. (2000). *Measuring patient outcomes.* Thousand Oaks, CA: Sage.

Oermann, M. H., & Floyd, J. A. (2002). Outcomes research: An essential component of the advanced practice nurse role. *Clinical Nurse Specialist, 16,* 140–146.

Paul, S. (2000). Impact of a nurse-managed heart failure clinic: A pilot study. *American Journal of Critical Care, 9,* 140–146.

Reynolds, M., Fahrbach, K., Hauch, O., Wygant, G., Estok, R., Cella, C., et al. (2004). Warfarin anticoagulation and outcomes in patients with atrial fibrillation: A systematic review and metaanalysis. *Chest, 126,* 1938–1945.

Roche Diagnostics. (2001). *CoaguChek™ S System Policies and Procedures Manual* (pp. 1–73). Author.

Rochon, A., & Shore-Lesserson, L. (2006). Coagulation monitoring. *Anesthesiology Clinics, 24,* 839–856.

Russell, D., VorderBruegge, M., Burns, S., et al. (2002). Effect of an outcomes-managed approach to care of neuroscience patients by acute care nursing practitioners. *American Journal of Critical Care, 11,* 353–362.

Salem, D. N., Stein, P. D., Al-Ahmad, A., Bussey, H. I., Horstkotte, D., Miller, N., et al. (2004). Antithrombotic therapy in valvular heart disease—native and prosthetic: The Seventh ACCP Conference on Antithrombotic and Thrombolytic Therapy. *Chest, 126*(3 Suppl.), 457S–482S.

Samsa, G. P., Marchar, D., Goldstein, L., et al. (2000). Quality of anticoagulation management among patients with atrial fibrillation: Results of a review of medical records from 2 communities. *Archives of Internal Medicine, 160,* 967–973.

Schuller, D., Lynch, J. P., & Fine, D. (1997). Protocol-guided diuretic management: Comparison of furosemide by continuous infusion and intermittent bolus. *Critical Care Medicine, 25,* 1969–1975.

Singer, D. E., Albers, G. W., Dalen, J. E., Go, A. S., Halperin, J. L., & Manning W. J. (2004). Antithrombotic therapy in atrial fibrillation: The seventh ACCP conference on antithrombotic and thrombolytic therapy. *Chest, 126*(3 Suppl.), 429S–456S.

Stevenson, L.W. (1999). Tailored therapy to hemodynamic goals for advanced heart failure. *European Journal of Heart Failure, 1,* 251–257.

Stoke Prevention in Atrial Fibrillation Investigators. (1991). Stroke Prevention in Atrial Fibrillation study: Final results. *Lancet, 84,* 527–539.

Task Force on Acute Heart Failure of the European Society of Cardiology. (2005). Executive summary of the Guidelines on the Diagnosis and Treatment of Acute Heart Failure. *European Heart Journal, 26,* 384–416.

Titler, M. G. (2004). Methods in translation science. *Worldviews on Evidence-Based Nursing, 1,* 38–48.

Titler, M. G. (2008). The evidence for evidence-based practice implementation. In R. G. Hughes (Ed.), *Patient safety and quality: An evidence-based handbook for nurses* (chap. 7). Retrieved April 7, 2008, from http://www.ahrq.gov/qual/nurseshdbk/

Urden, L. D. (1999). Outcome evaluation: An essential component for CNS practice. *Clinical Nurse Specialist, 13,* 39–46.

van Meyel, J. J., Smits, P., Dormans, T., et al. (1994). Continuous infusion of furosemide in the treatment of patients with congestive heart failure and diuretic resistance. *Journal of Internal Medicine, 235,* 329–334.

van Walraven, C., Jennings, A., Oake, N., Fergusson, D., & Forster, A. J. (2006). Effect of study setting on anticoagulation control: A systemic review and metaregression. *Chest, 129,* 1155–1166.

Vasko, M. R., Cartwright, D. B., Knochel, J. P., Nixon, J. V., & Brater, D. C. (1985). Furosemide absorption altered in decompensated congestive heart failure. *Annals of Internal Medicine, 102,* 314–318.

Ward, M. M., Evans, T. C., Spies, A. J., et al. (2006). National Quality Forum 30 safe practices: Priority and progress in Iowa hospitals. *American Journal of Medical Quality, 21,* 101–108.

Wilson, A., Wells, P., Kovacs, M., Lewis, G., Martin, J., Burton, E., et al. (2003). Comparing the quality of oral anticoagulant management by anticoagulation clinics and by family physicians: A randomized controlled trial. *Canadian Medical Association Journal, 169,* 293–298.

Appendix A. Diuretic Protocol and Order Set

Cardiac Care Unit and ACE Unit
Advanced Heart Failure
Diuretic Orders

<u>Furosemide* KCL and Urine Output Orders:</u>

❏ Administer furosemide ____ mg IVP q ____ hrs until PCW pressure < ____ or RA < ____ (usual goal PCW ≤ 15, RA ≤ 7, with SBP > 80 mmHG) or _____ liters net negative/day.

❏ Increase dose of furosemide by ____ mg each dosing interval (to maximum 200 mg per dose) if **urine output < _____ ml/hr after prior dose.**

❏ Continuous IV furosemide drip, start at _____ mg/hr (straight drug in buretrol)

❏ KCL with each furosemide dose (consider current K level, serum creatinine, and UO)

❏   KCL 20 meq (extended-release tab) po with each furosemide dose
(hold for K > 4.5, UO < 50 ml/hr)

OR

❏ KCL 40 meq (extended-release tab) po with each furosemide dose
(hold for K > 4.5, UO < 50 ml/hr)

<u>Metolazone Orders:</u>
Consider adding metolazone if UO < 500 cc negative 4 hrs after furosemide dose of ≥ 160 mg IVP:
❏ Add metolazone 5 mg po ❏ qd or ❏ bid (maximum dose 20 mg/ day); give 30 minutes prior to furosemide dose.
If patient is started on metolazone for diuresis, serum K must be checked within 4 hrs of PO administration

For prepulmonary artery catheter diuresis:

❏ Administer furosemide _____ mg IVP q __ hrs until __ liters negative over 24 hrs, with SBP > 85 mmHG

Electrolyte Replacement Orders:

❐ Check serum K (❐ q 6, ❐ q 12 hrs) @ (times) _____ and if UO > _____.

❐ Check serum Mg q 24 hrs @ times _____

❐ KCL Replacement: Based on serum K level, please replace K as indicated below. (Indicate route of administration.)

RANGE SERUM K LEVEL	KCL REPLACEMENT
>5.0 mmol/L	Call HO
4.0–4.5 mmol/L	None
3.5–4.0 mmol/L	❐ KCL 20 meq (extended-release tab) po x 1 OR ❐ KCL 20 meq IVPB over 2 hrs (via central line)
3.0–3.4 mmol/L	❐ KCL 40 meq (extended-release tabs) po x 1 OR ❐ KCL 40 meq IVPB over 4 hrs (via central line)
<3.0 mmol/L	call HO

❐ $MgSO_4$ Replacement: Based on serum $MgSO_4$ level, please replace $MgSO_4$ as indicated below.

❐ If $MgSO_4$ 1.6–1.8 meq/L, replace Magnesium sulfate 1 Gram/50cc D5W IVPB over 1 hour.

❐ If $MgSO_4$ ≤ 1.5 meq/L, replace Magnesium sulfate 2 Grams/50cc D5W IVPB over 2 hours.

❐ **If $MgSO_4$ < 1.5 or > 2.5 meq/L notify HO.**

❐ Prior to administration of the a.m. furosemide and KCL dose, check a.m. serum creatinine.

   Baseline/current serum creatinine level is _____.

   If serum creatinine level > __ hold next furosemide and KCL dose and call HO.

❐ Call HO @ 2000 to review protocol plans for diuresis and K replacement during night shift.
   *These furosemide orders replace previous furosemide orders.
   *Subsequent furosemide orders will cause cancellation of this protocol.

_____   _____   _____
Physician's   Beeper   Date and Time
Signature

_____   _____
RN Signature   Date and Time

Appendix B.   Standardized Procedure for Anticoagulation Management

Management of Oral Anticoagulation Therapy

I. Policy
    A. As described in the General Policy Component.
    B. Covers only those nurse practitioners identified in the General Policy Component.

II. Purpose
    A. This Standardized Procedure serves as a supplement to the General Policy Component. It establishes the guidelines for the participation of the Cardiology Nurse Practitioner (NP) in the evaluation and management of patients in the UCLA-Santa Monica Cardiology practice requiring anticoagulation therapy.

III. Protocol
    A. Definition: This protocol covers the management of oral anticoagulation therapy in the outpatient setting at UCLA-Santa Monica Cardiology for cardiac-related diagnoses that include, but are not limited to, atrial fibrillation, atrial flutter, prosthetic (mechanical) valves, and left ventricular thrombus.

    B. Setting: This protocol covers the Cardiology NP in the care of patients requiring anticoagulation management who have a leading cardiology diagnosis and a cardiologist at UCLA-Santa Monica Cardiology.

    C. Database
    Subjective: May include but is not limited to:
    1. Relevant history of present illness and past medical history
    2. Medication history
    3. Social history
    4. Family history
    5. Review of systems

    Objective Data: May include but is not limited to:
    1. Physical examination appropriate to the subjective findings and past medical history
    2. Laboratory tests or procedures to assist in monitoring of oral anticoagulation including but are not limited to pro-

thrombin time, international normalized ratio (INR), complete blood count, and electrocardiogram

Assessment: May include:

1. Diagnosis or diagnoses most consistent with subjective and objective findings; if diagnosis is not clear, assessment to level of surety plus differential diagnosis
2. Status of existing condition(s)

D. Plan
   1. Treatment
      a. Goals of therapy include:
         i. Attaining and maintaining a therapeutic INR
         ii. Maintaining a steady state INR with monthly surveillance
         iii. Prevent complications related to Coumadin
         iv. Educate the patient and family through collaboration and empowerment
      b. Warfarin dosing (see Addendum I)
      c. Treatment of supratherapeutic INR and use of vitamin K (see Addendum II)
      d. Use of Lovenox in patients requiring invasive procedures (see Addendum III)
      e. Assessment of high-risk patients including:
         i. Age >75
         ii. History of falls
         iii. Gait instability
         iv. History of bleeding
         v. Cognitive impairment
      f. Further lab or other studies as appropriate
      g. Diet and exercise prescription as indicated by disease process and patient condition
      h. Patient education and counseling appropriate to the disease process and patient condition (see Addendum IV: Coumadin and diet information handout)
      i. Follow-up appointments for further evaluation and treatment if indicated
      j. Consultation and referral as appropriate
      k. Furnish medications following the Drugs and Devices protocol

2. Documentation
   a. Specific patient records will include diagnosis, initial Coumadin dosing, and goal range for INR (see Addendum V: Coumadin Enrollment Sheet)
   b. Records include the Coumadin flowsheet and Coumadin database
   c. Nonlicensed staff will be supervised per protocol

3. Physician Consultation: As described in the General Policy Component
   a. INR not reaching goal
   b. INR >5.0
   c. Patient noncompliance
   d. Active bleeding
   e. Patients status post valve replacement with INR >5.0

4. Referral to physician or specialized clinic
   a. Conditions for which the diagnosis and/or treatment are beyond the scope of the nurse's knowledge and/or skills
   b. For those conditions that require consultation
   c. Inability to attain goal INR

5. Evaluation will be done through quarterly review of:
   a. Subtherapeutic and supratherapeutic INR
   b. Hospital admissions related to Coumadin
   c. Adverse reactions secondary to Coumadin

Note: Used with permission from the University of California Los Angeles-Santa Monica Cardiology, Division of Cardiology, Los Angeles, California.

Appendix C. Anticoagulation-Management Protocol

Warfarin Dosing Protocol: This protocol is to be used only as a guideline in the dosing of warfarin as the individual patient and clinical situation should be taken into account.

International normalized ratio (INR) below therapeutic range:	Increase total weekly warfarin intake by 10% to 20% and monitor more frequently; or a one-time larger dose can be given followed by frequent monitoring, without change in the total weekly intake.
INR therapeutic:	No change in dosing.
INR above therapeutic range but < 5.0; no significant bleeding:	Hold warfarin for zero or one dose, monitor more frequently, and decrease total weekly warfarin intake by 10% to 15%. If only minimally above therapeutic range, no dose reduction may be required.
INR > 5.0 but < 9.0; no significant bleeding:	Hold warfarin for one or two doses, monitor more frequently, and decrease total weekly intake by 10% to 15%. Vitamin K can be given if at an increased risk of bleeding.*
INR > 9.0; no significant bleeding:	Hold warfarin and give vitamin K, monitor more frequently and resume therapy at a lower dose when INR therapeutic.*
Serious bleeding at any elevation of INR:	Hold warfarin and give vitamin K, supplemented with fresh frozen plasma. Vitamin K can be repeated every 12 hours.*
Life-threatening bleeding:	Hold warfarin and give prothrombin complex concentrate supplemented with vitamin K; repeat if necessary depending on INR.*

*See *Treatment of Supratherapeutic INR and Use of Vitamin K.*

Note: Used with permission from University of California Los Angeles-Santa Monica Cardiology, Division of Cardiology, Los Angeles, California.

■ For dose adjustments within the 10% change limit, the INR will be rechecked in 1 to 14 days.

- Once the INR is within the target range on two consecutive laboratory tests, a monthly surveillance schedule can be started.
- The decision to recheck an INR prior to dosage adjustments can be made on an individual basis.

Source: Adapted from Ansell et al. (2004).

Treatment of Supratherapeutic INR and Use of Vitamin K Protocol: This protocol is to be used only as a guideline for the treatment of INRs above the therapeutic range, as the individual patient and clinical situation should be taken into account. The physician will be notified of all supratherapeutic INRs above 6.0.

Recommendation for Management of Excessive Prolongation of the INR in the Outpatient Setting:

INR >5.0 but <9.0; no significant bleeding:	Vitamin K (1 to 2.5 mg) can be given orally if the patient is at an increased risk of bleeding. Monitor levels frequently. If the INR is still high, additional oral vitamin K (1 to 2 mg) can be given.
INR >9.0; no significant bleeding:	Administer vitamin K (5 to 10 mg) orally with the expectation that the INR will be reduced substantially in 24 to 48 hours. Monitor levels frequently and use additional vitamin K if necessary.
Serious bleeding at any elevation of INR:	Administer vitamin K (10 mg) by slow IV infusion supplemented with fresh frozen plasma or prothrombin complex concentrate, depending on the urgency of the situation. Vitamin K can be repeated every 12 hours.
Life-threatening bleeding:	Administer prothrombin complex concentrate or recombinant factor VIIa supplemented with vitamin K 10 mg by slow IV infusion. Repeat if necessary, depending on the INR.

In the clinic:

- The patient's physician will be immediately notified if the INR is > 6.0.

- The single dose of vitamin K orally will be administered to the patient while in the clinic.
- The patient will return to the clinic the following business day for a recheck of the INR, and more frequent monitoring of the INR will be established.
- Patients with signs/symptoms of active bleeding are not candidates for oral vitamin K and should be seen in the emergency department.

Use of vitamin K:
- By administering oral vitamin K and withholding warfarin, the INR will fall into a safe range in approximately 24 to 48 hours.
- High doses of vitamin K, though effective, may lower the INR more than necessary and may lead to warfarin resistance for a week or more.
- The response to vitamin K administered subcutaneously (SC) is less predictable compared to oral vitamin K and is sometimes delayed. Thus oral vitamin K will be given when possible.

Source: Adapted from Ansell et al. (2004).

Lovenox Protocol: Patients on long-term anticoagulation who are undergoing invasive procedures may require the use of Lovenox to bridge the gap in protection against thromboembolism when warfarin is stopped. This protocol is to be used only as a guideline as the individual patient and clinical situation should be taken into account.

Before the procedure/surgery:
1. Stop warfarin 4 to 5 days prior to the procedure/surgery.
2. Start Lovenox 36 hours after last warfarin dose (approximately 2 days prior to the procedure) at 1 mg/kg subcutaneously every 12 hours.
3. Give the last dose of Lovenox 24 hours prior to the procedure/surgery.
4. Check INR the morning of the procedure. Surgery is considered safe when the INR <1.5.

After the procedure/surgery:
1. Restart Lovenox 24 hours after the procedure at 1 mg/kg subcutaneously every 12 hours.

2. Start warfarin at the patient's preoperative dose on postoperative day 1.
3. Monitor the PT/INR daily until the INR is in the therapeutic range.
4. Discontinue the Lovenox when the INR is 2 to 3 for 2 consecutive days.
5. Monitor CBC including platelets on days 3 and 7.

The strategy for managing perioperative anticoagulation is dependent upon the risk for thromboembolism. Patients at risk may require heparin or Lovenox as a bridge while off warfarin.

A. Patients at high risk for thromboembolism, bridging advised:
- Venous or arterial thromboembolism within the preceding 1–3 months
- Atrial fibrillation plus mechanical heart valve in any position
- Atrial fibrillation with history of cardioembolism
- Acute intracardiac thrombus visualized by echocardiogram
- Older mechanical valve (single-disk or ball-in-cage) in mitral position
- Recently placed mechanical valve (< 3 months)

B. Patients at intermediate risk for thromboembolism, bridging individualized:
- Cerebrovascular disease with multiple (2 or more) strokes or TIAs without risk factors for cardiac embolism
- Newer mechanical valve model in mitral position
- Older mechanical valve in aortic position
- Atrial fibrillation without a history of cardiac embolism but with multiple risk factors for cardiac embolism (i.e., ejection fraction < 40%, diabetes, hypertension, nonrheumatic valvular disease, transmural myocardial infarction within preceding month)
- Venous thromboembolism > 3 to 6 months ago

C. Patients at low risk for thromboembolism, bridging not advised:
- Atrial fibrillation without multiple risks for cardiac embolism
- Newer model prosthetic valve in aortic position
- Intrinsic cerebrovascular disease without recurrent strokes or TIAs
- One remote venous thromboembolism (> 6 months ago)

D. Procedures in which warfarin can be continued:
- Ophthalmic procedures: cataract extraction
- Gastrointestinal endoscopy: upper endoscopy with or without biopsy, flexible sigmoidoscopy with or without biopsy, colonoscopy with or without biopsy, endoscopic retrograde cannulation of the pancreatic duct without sphincterotomy
- Dental procedures: restorations, prosthetics, uncomplicated extractions, dental hygiene treatment, periodontal therapy
- Other procedures: joint and soft-tissue aspirations and injections, minor podiatric procedures

Lovenox Dosing:
1. Lovenox dosing is based on weight and creatinine, usually 1 mg/kg twice daily for normal kidney function.
2. For renal insufficiency, defined as creatinine clearance < 30 mL/min, reduced dosing is required. A dose of 40 mg daily is preferable to the 30-mg twice-daily dose.

A Lovenox patient assistance program is available.

Sources: Adapted from Ansell et al. (2004) and Jaffer, Brotman, & Chukwumerije (2003).

Appendix D. Physician Referral Form ACNP-Managed Anticoagulation Clinic

(PATIENT LABEL)

UCLA—Santa Monica Cardiology
PHYSICIAN REFERRAL FORM ACNP-MANAGED ANTICOAGULATION CLINIC

Alternate Contacts:

Name: _____

Phone: _____

Phone: _____

MD Contacts:

Name: _____

Phone: _____

Phone: _____

Indication for Anticoagulation (circle one):

		High-Risk Patient (Circle One):
Atrial fibrillation	INR 2.0 – 3.0	I. Age > 75
Aortic Valve Replacement	INR 2.0 – 3.0	II. H/O falls
Mitral Valve Replacement	INR 2.5 – 3.5	III. Gait instability
DVT	INR 2.0 – 3.0	IV. H/O bleeding
PE	INR 2.0 – 3.0	V. Cognitive Impairment
OTHER: _____	INR _____	VI. Other: _____

Will need enoxaparin bridge if stops coumadin?
❑ Yes   ❑ No

Coumadin Start Date: _____

Coumadin Start Dose: _____

Additional medications (circle one):

Amiodarone
_____

Digoxin

Complications:

Date: _____

Complication: _____

ASA 325 mg po daily until therapeutic INR
   Date: _____
ASA 325 mg _____ 81 mg _____
   Complication: _____
Plavix
Other: _____

Cardioversion instructions:

   ❏ Weekly INR 2.0–3.0 x one month pre-Cardioversion
   ❏ Weekly INR 2.0–3.0 x one month post-Cardioversion

Physician's
   Signature: _____   Date: _____

Note: Used with permission from University of California Los Angeles-Santa Monica Cardiology, Division of Cardiology, Los Angeles, California.

Appendix E. Patient Responsibility Agreement Form

UCLA Santa Monica Cardiology
Warfarin (Coumadin) Patient Responsibility Agreement Form

I, (patient's name): _____, have been counseled on
the use of warfarin (Coumadin), including the following:

- I understand the risk and benefits of taking and not taking warfarin (Coumadin).
- I agree to take warfarin (Coumadin) per the dosing schedule provided by my healthcare provider.
- I understand the importance of:
  - Noting and reporting to my healthcare provider any signs and symptoms of bleeding or bruising.
  - Reporting to my healthcare provider any changes in medications, both over-the-counter and prescription medications, as well as any herbal remedies.
  - Maintaining a consistent diet and reporting any changes in diet, including changes relating to vitamin K-containing foods.
  - Reporting to my healthcare provider how I actually have taken warfarin (Coumadin), especially reporting changes from the recommended dosing schedule.
- Regular PT/INR lab tests to properly monitor warfarin (Coumadin) therapy.
- Going to the clinic/lab on time and on the appropriate day for PT/INR blood tests as instructed by my healthcare provider.
- I agree to notify my healthcare provider promptly of any changes in address or telephone number.
- I understand that if I am unable to keep my appointment for PT/INR testing it is my responsibility to call and reschedule another appointment within the appropriate time frame.

■ I understand that warfarin (Coumadin) causes birth defects when taken during pregnancy. For female patients of childbearing age: I agree to contact my healthcare provider immediately when I become pregnant.

■ I understand the contents of this form and have received a copy.

PATIENT _____ DATE _____
                    (Signature)

NURSE PRACTITIONER _____ DATE _____

Note: Used with permission from the University of California Los Angeles-Santa Monica Cardiology, Division of Cardiology, Los Angeles, California.

7

Ambulatory NP Outcomes

MARY JO GOOLSBY

The potential outcomes of ambulatory care match the broad range of conditions and patients encountered in these settings, whether primary or specialty care. Nurse practitioners (NPs) in primary care settings manage patients with both chronic and acute conditions, while also addressing health promotion and disease prevention for their patients. The incidence of many chronic conditions, such as hypertension, chronic obstructive pulmonary disease (COPD), and diabetes, is increasing and many of these patients routinely seek care in primary care settings, where patients with acute conditions, such as pneumonia, urinary tract infections, and upper respiratory infections, are also likely to receive care. The clinical specialty specifies which NPs are more likely to encounter women, men, children, or older adults in their primary care settings. In subspecialty practices, the clinical focus sets the expectations on types of patients seen, yet NPs will want to measure outcomes of routine management as well as exacerbations.

In the early 1980s, a newly prepared NP assigned to a military internal medicine clinic maintained an index-card box that held a one-page form on each patient she saw. Patients usually were referred for management of a chronic condition such as hypertension or diabetes. The forms allowed quick access to specific clinical information, such as blood pressure, lipids, blood glucose, and/or weight, recorded immediately following each encounter, since the patients' health records were not maintained in the clinic. It was not long before curiosity promoted comparisons of the data over time. Because the NP was, in effect, the primary care provider for adult patients with chronic health conditions such as hypertension, diabetes, COPD, and heart failure, these forms allowed for extraction of clinical comparison information over time— and the NPs' outcome measurement practice was born. The data collected soon found their way into administrative reports describing the practice and benefits associated with referrals to the NP. Over the years, the NP's sophistication in measuring and analyzing outcomes of practice improved; however, these early activities in her initial NP position were as satisfying and rewarding as subsequent, more detailed efforts. This tale describes how this author's interest in outcome measurement developed.

While some, like the author, fall into outcome measurement in a gradual way, it can be intimidating for others who contemplate the need to establish a formal process for measuring outcomes. This chapter builds on the early chapters of this textbook by providing a practical framework that ambulatory care NPs can use in implementing outcome measurement in their practices. A practical way for NPs to develop the skills necessary to move on to a formal outcome research practice is to start by participating in performance improvement (PI) or program-evaluation activities.

This chapter will (a) review the purpose and importance of measuring and documenting outcomes of individual NP practices, (b) briefly summarize some of the literature on NP outcomes, (c) describe the categories and examples of outcome measures relevant to ambulatory NPs, (d) discuss practical considerations for selecting outcomes and a measurement approach, (e) provide examples of how to approach outcome measurement in practice, and (f) discuss available resources relevant to primary care outcome measurement (see Table 7.1).

IMPORTANCE/PURPOSE OF PRIMARY CARE OUTCOME MEASUREMENT

As noted in earlier chapters, there are many reasons for conducting outcome measurement in practice. Outcomes research should ultimately improve the health of our patients. Further, there are many stakeholders interested in how and to what degree we improve the health of those

Table 7.1

AMBULATORY OUTCOME MEASURES

OUTCOME CATEGORY	OUTCOME EXAMPLES
Physiological status	Vital signs Physical examination findings Laboratory studies
Psychosocial status	Mentation Mood and affect Coping status Social function
Functional status	ADL function IADL function
Behavioral activities and knowledge	Performance of therapeutics Problem-solving ability Knowledge test scores
Symptom control	Pain Fatigue Dyspnea Nausea Incontinence
Patient perception	Quality of life Satisfaction with care
Resource utilization	Hospital readmission rates Emergency visits Unplanned office visits Health care costs
Performance measures	Availability of recommended resources Implementation of recommended practices

ADL = (routine) activities of daily living; IADL = instrumental activities of daily living.

we serve, including our patients, employers, colleagues, payors, policy-makers, and others. In addition to knowing how much NP care costs and saves, they are interested in knowing what precisely NPs do in their patient encounters and the objective patient-centered benefits of that care. As practitioners of a relatively new role created in the mid-1960s, NPs must continue to document the outcomes of their care.

Moreover, evaluation of clinical outcomes is an expectation of the NP role. The National Organization of Nurse Practitioner Faculties lists a number of competencies relative to outcome measurement in *Domains and Core Competencies of Nurse Practitioner Practice* (National Organization of Nurse Practitioner Faculties, 2006). Examples of outcome-related competencies are evident throughout the domains, including (a) "evaluates outcomes of care," (b) "incorporates access, cost effectiveness, and quality when making care decisions," and (c) "evaluates the impact of the health care delivery system on care." Domain 6 (of 7) is specific to monitoring and ensuring the quality of health care practice and lists three related competencies: (a) "monitors quality of care," (b) "assures accountability for practice," and (c) "engages in continuous quality improvement (CQI)." Clearly, at least the CQI outcome measurement is an expected competency for all NPs.

SUMMARY OF EXISTING PRIMARY CARE NP OUTCOME LITERATURE

The published research on NP outcomes has consistently supported the quality and cost-effectiveness of NP practice. In 1974, a classic report of the Burlington Trial documented outcomes in mortality, as well as physical, emotional, and social function, concluding that NP and physician outcomes were comparable (Spitzer et al., 1974). The Congressional Budget Office reviewed studies on NP practice and outcomes in 1979, with the conclusion that the NPs' outcomes, diagnoses, and management were at least as good as those of physicians. In 1986, the Office of Technology Assessment came to the same conclusions. Later meta-analyses of NP care had similar findings (Brown & Grimes, 1995; Horrocks, Anderson, & Salisbury, 2002; Laurant et al., 2006), as have additional review articles (Cunningham, 2004). Mundinger et al. (2000) and Lenz et al. (2004) described primary care outcomes of patients assigned to either physician or NP, finding equivalent outcomes for both sets of patients. Regarding cost-effectiveness of NP care, studies have also consistently demonstrated that NPs provide quality care efficiently with reduced cost, compared with physicians (Burl, Bonner, & Rao, 1994; Chenowith et al., 2005; Office of Technology Assessment, 1981; Paez & Allen, 2006; Roblin et al., 2004).

MEASURES RELEVANT TO AMBULATORY CARE PRACTICE

The outcomes selected by a given NP will depend on the type of practice, areas of interest, and available resources. Even in a focused subspecialty-type practice, there are several options to measure. Outcomes can be categorized in many ways. One categorization would classify outcomes as best demonstrating one of the following: physiological status, psychosocial status, functional status, behavioral activities, and knowledge, symptom control, patient perception, or resource utilization. Within each category, there are likely measures relevant to any area of practice. Another common area of measurement that does not fit the definition of outcome, but which must be considered relevant to contemporary ambulatory care, involves performance measures.

Physiological status involves those biomarkers that are usually readily available in the course of routine patient care. They include routinely collected vital signs such as blood pressure, pulse, and temperature; physical exam findings such as lung sounds and weight; and laboratory values such as glucose and lipid levels. Abnormal findings in these physiologic markers are often the defining characteristics of health problems and the targets of care; thus, they provide a means of later following response to and outcomes of treatment. For instance, the outcomes of diabetes, hypertension, or hyperlipidemia management should include measurement of blood glucose/glycosylated hemoglobin, blood pressure, or lipids, respectively. A feature of physiologic measures such as vital signs and laboratory findings is that they are objective and quantified. Laboratory studies, in particular, are usually validated against some control procedure. The quality of vital signs and physical examination findings is dependent on the quality of the equipment and technique used in obtaining the measures.

Psychosocial status includes measures that are often identified during the history of the patient and which are qualitative in nature. Even psychosocial measures can be quantified and this process involves some added effort beyond what the routine history may reveal. Examples of psychosocial outcomes include mentation, mood and affect, attitude, coping status, and general social functioning. While psychosocial status outcomes often involve some degree of subjectivity, there are a number of validated and quantitative scales available, depending on the focus of concern. For instance, there are validated scales to measure depression and anxiety, confusion, and dementia. The Mini-Mental State Examination (MMSE) is well published and validated.

Specific functional status involves ability to achieve routine activities of daily living (ADL) and instrumental activities of daily living (IADL) and can be measured with global functional scales or measures more specific to select abilities such as mobility and communication. A number of measures of functionality exist, including the Physical Activities of Daily Living and Instrumental Activities of Daily Living scales, as well as the 10-minute Screener for Geriatric Conditions. Others include the Functional Independence Measure Scale (FIMS) and the Barthel Scale.

Behavioral activities and knowledge include areas of both therapeutic competence and understanding of treatments. Therapeutic competence involves the ability to perform the skills necessary to carry out prescribed or recommended treatments as well as the ability to problem solve related to therapeutic guidance. Understanding is related to basic knowledge regarding recommended diet, medications, and treatments without a behavioral component. Knowledge tests have been developed and described in the literature for select conditions. Measurement of behavioral activity competence is more complex to assess than knowledge, by comparison.

Symptom control is another area of outcomes where the history often includes the basic related details, but requires further quantification to serve as an outcome measurement. Examples of the symptoms that could be quantified as outcome measures include level of pain, fatigue, dyspnea, nausea, constipation, diarrhea, and incontinence. There are a number of validated scales to measure many symptoms, and pain scales are perhaps among the better known. One means of assessing specific symptoms would be to use a 10-centimeter visual analog scale (VAS), where the poles of the scale represent symptom extreme (complete absence of the symptom versus worst possible degree of the symptom), or having the symptom similarly rated using a numerical scale.

Patient perceptual category includes areas such as a patient's perceived quality of life (QOL) and expressed satisfaction with care. QOL refers to patients' satisfaction with their life circumstances and sense of well-being. It can further relate to a more narrowed focus of satisfaction with specific components of the patient's life, for instance, with how a specific symptom affects life quality. There are general and condition-specific QOL scales, and a VAS can also be used to measure perceived QOL. In contrast, satisfaction refers to satisfaction with the patient experience and care received. Patient perceptions also include a patient's determination of progress toward meeting goals. For instance, patients can identify their personal goals for treatment, then subsequently rate the degree to which they are able to accomplish the goal over time.

Resource utilization involves a range of outcomes, such as numbers of hospitalizations, length of stay for any admission, the cost of care, and any unplanned office or emergency visits. In many cases, it is difficult to accurately identify all hospitalizations or emergency visits, along with the cost for each, as the patient's history must often be relied upon. However, within a well-defined system such as a managed care organization or hospital-anchored system, and so on, pulling records of other visits, admissions, and associated costs is more easily accomplished. In addition to identifying any change in resource utilization associated with care, cost analysis of the actual care provides another outcome indicator. (An earlier chapter described approaches to conducting economic analysis of practice.) Vincent (2002) describes the application of cost analysis involving staff compensation, overhead, and supplies involved in managing specific patient populations, compared with the revenue associated with the same group of patients.

Performance measures are receiving increased interest, primarily with respect to their role in a number of quality initiatives and the growing "pay for performance" (P4P) role, although they do not necessarily measure outcomes of care. Performance measure may be seen as a surrogate for actual outcomes, with the increasing availability of electronic health records, which provide queries of coded procedures, to readily identify the performance of certain activities. Certainly, current P4P mandates are based primarily on documenting the resources available and the processes implemented, as opposed to actual improved outcomes, so that incentives are based on providers documenting activities such as making appropriate referrals, monitoring of suggested laboratory studies, and administration or ordering of recommended treatments (e.g., pneumonia vaccines for persons over 65 years of age or beta blockers for patients experiencing a myocardial infarct). Although recommendations often imply that if specific activities are carried out as recommended, then improved outcomes would result, it would be ideal to document the results of the performance measures, as well as the performance itself.

There are currently many resources available to provide guidance on performance measurement. Sources include the National Quality Measures Clearinghouse (NQMC), the Agency for Healthcare Research and Quality (AHRQ), the National Committee for Quality Assurance (NCQA), the National Quality Forum (NQF), the Centers for Medicare and Medicaid Services (CMS), and the Ambulatory Care Quality Alliance (AQA).

SELECTING PRACTICAL OUTCOMES OF INTEREST

With the broad range of potential outcomes of primary care NP practice, the dilemma becomes determining what should and can be measured. It is advisable to start with an answerable question and then proceed to select the available measures and/or type of data that will contribute to the answer. Certainly, one deciding factor should be the provider's own areas of interest and questions. Other considerations will include the context in which the care is delivered, the resources available to support outcome measurement, and anticipated patient variables.

The decision to measure outcomes of practice may be based on questions the NP has regarding how his or her practice outcomes compare to some benchmark or published report. In practices with an established PI process, there may be baseline data that support the need for improvements and that trigger outcome measures. Just as PI activities typically focus on conditions of large volume, high cost, and high risk, these same three criteria are helpful in guiding decisions on where to expend energy in outcome measures.

The practice context is important. The practice may have limited resources helpful to outcome measures or a wealth of resources. Practices with electronic health records may enhance ability to automate queries to pull data specific to identified outcomes or activities. Breslin, Burns, and Moores (2002) describe issues related to extracting data from existing records, particularly related to the need for specific and accurate coding. If an electronic health record system either does not capture data on the unique outcome variables of interest or is coded in such a way as to not serve as an outcome measure, the NP will have to implement added manual recording of outcomes or consider alternative measures.

Another type of resource specific to practices is the type of economic resources available for patient care. If a practice has a largely indigent population, the type of measures readily available may differ from one with a more affluent patient population, unless the practice has additional sources of funding to support patient care needs. Another organizational consideration involves any philosophical expectation or mission that could mandate select measures used for outcomes. Since it is rare for a health care provider to be the sole provider in an ambulatory clinic, it is often helpful for the team of providers to collaborate and select clinical topics and outcomes of interest. Moores, Breslin, and Burns (2002) describe the process of talking through problems with peers as a means of bringing the issue into focus as an answerable question.

Patient-specific variables must be considered. If an NP has patients who tend to seek episodic care and are not easily followed over time, shorter term outcomes will be important. Of course, efforts to enhance continuity could be implemented and then long-term follow-up included as a measure itself. Similarly, NPs who primarily treat acute and episodic conditions will select different outcomes of care than those who treat more chronic ones, which can be measured over time. Finally, the outcome measures should be culturally sensitive to the patient population served (Breslin et al., 2002).

Published clinical recommendations or guidelines provide an excellent source for outcome selection. These often identify a number of outcomes that could be used to track response to treatment, including recommended tools. For example, when focusing on a specific condition, it is often favorable to use condition-specific measures that will be more sensitive to change with treatment of that select condition, whenever possible. For instance, while asthma affects psychosocial and functional outcomes, these may also be affected by a number of other comorbid conditions, so that these other conditions confound the response to care. By measuring specific asthma variables, outcomes are more easily attributed to treatment of that specific condition. In considering relevant outcome measures, the NP must also consider what is recommended for the condition of interest. For varied conditions, generic outcomes could be used. For instance, generic functionality measures, or SF-36, are broadly used. Scales of quality of life could be responsive to a number of health changes, as would pain scales. However, there are a number of condition-specific measures, many of which are described in clinical recommendations. There are scales to assess outcomes of treatment of conditions such as arthritis, asthma, fibromyalgia, and benign prostatic hyperplasia, in addition to the relevant physiologic markers such as pulmonary functions, blood glucose, hypertension, etc.

⟩ When the topic of interest has been identified, feasible outcome measures based on the characteristics of the practice, patient population, and providers should be identified and a plan should be written to guide the continuing effort. While most NPs may be more comfortable with associating the outcome measurement process with CQI or PI than with more formal "research," outcome measurement is a form of exploratory research (Breslin et al., 2002) and the methodological issues are important considerations. An important benefit of establishing a written plan early in the planning process is that the plan will help to identify any related costs as well as added resources needed. Additionally, even with CQI/PI projects, it is advisable to discuss the plans with a representative from the affiliated institutional review board or research board, to determine whether a formal application and approval are expected.

CASE EXAMPLES

The Shotgun Approach

The first case is an example of how using a "shotgun" approach to outcome measurement can "backfire." An NP inherited a position involving oversight of a clinic created to provide disease management for patients with asthma and/or COPD. Her predecessor had created the clinic and had developed a very detailed plan for measuring the outcomes of the practice. At the baseline initial visit and again at 3, 6, 12, and 18 months, patients would be assessed with a focused history and physical, as well as by completing the following measures: the Center for Epidemiology Depression Scale, the State-Trait Depression and Anxiety Scale, the SF-36 Medical Outcomes Scale, the Modified Dyspnea Index, a record of peak flow usage, history of tobacco usage, medication list, a number of VASs (quality of life, dyspnea), and a 6-minute walk with pulse oximetry, breath sounds, peak flow, and pulmonary functions before and after. Additionally, the system's records were queried at these intervals for any emergency room visits and hospitalizations, as well as the costs and charges for each. Needless to say, even in a 1-hour visit, it was hard to conceive how anyone would accomplish all of the necessary outcome measures, if time were to be spent on patient problem solving, support, and education. The clinic NP provider had recently resigned and a temporary part-time NP was filling in. Further, it was noted that patients rarely returned after the second visit.

Very quickly, the NP manager and interim NP provider reviewed the process, what outcomes were feasible given the available system, and comments from patients. The outcome measures had become the focus of the clinic, not the delivery of care that would have achieved the outcomes. The process was changed so that necessary outcomes would be embedded in the encounter record, and the number of outcomes was definitely abbreviated. Patient interviews ascertained that patients saw little benefit in participating in all of the multi-item scales and that they also found the numerous depression, anxiety, medical outcomes, and dyspnea scales difficult to understand. What did seem feasible was to record responses of the dyspnea VAS, develop a rating scheme for anticipated symptoms (shortness of breath, cough, interrupted sleep, etc.), peak flow averages, tobacco use, and some other select outcomes, as well as to quarterly pull records to support a cost analysis of resources used. When changes were implemented, the continuity of care immediately improved: patients remained in the clinic, and the outcomes improved as patients were being educated on their conditions.

The physiologic measures showed improvement. The population's emergency room visits were cut in half and the number of hospitalizations was decreased to approximately 15% of the historical data following enrollment to the clinic. On an ongoing basis, the clinic has been able to demonstrate positive outcomes and to serve as a model for other disease-managed clinics.

Triangulation

A chapter in the first edition of this book (Kleinpell, 2001) describes combining quantitative and qualitative efforts in outcome measurements to provide for triangulation. An NP involved in pulmonary management monitored tobacco use in her patients. Instituting the "5A" approach (ask about patient's habits, advise of consequence of smoking, assess willingness to quit, assist with cessation plan development, arrange for follow-up) and providing support based on her patient's level of readiness, she wanted to measure the outcomes of the process.

As part of the plan, she determined that she would ask all newly referred patients whether or not they smoked and, for those who did smoke, the number of cigarettes used per day. The measure would be tobacco use "Yes/No" and number of cigarettes. The measure would be collected from each patient on his/her first visit and again at 3, 6, and 12 months. At baseline and at 3 and 6 months, the percentage who smoked was 45%, 43%, and 49%, respectively, and the number of packs per day for patients who smoked was .91, .65, and .60, respectively. Certainly, the decrease in amount of tobacco used per smoker was positive, but the anticipated outcome had included a decreasing percentage of smokers, not an increase.

The NP instituted a series of interviews with the patients to explore the tobacco use. For instance, she realized that, prior to the first appointment, a number of patients might have "quit" smoking, but have been unable to maintain abstinence. Instead, she found that the percentage of her patients who smoked was actually stable over time; some patients indicated that they had not been forthright in identifying whether or not they smoked, concerned that their care might be affected or that they would be lectured for the practice. Only after they developed a comfort with the new provider were they more likely to be open about their tobacco use. The series of interviews also identified a number of other issues related to tobacco use for her patients and the NP was able to use the findings to obtain funding for an individualized tobacco-cessation program, based on the fact that while the amount smoked decreased, the number who smoked did not. The funded program, which provided a range of resources for patients during the process, did result in a decreased percentage of smokers. However, without the qualitative interviews, the quantitative data would not have provided the necessary information to further improve practice and later outcomes.

APPROACHES TO OVERCOMING POTENTIAL BARRIERS TO OUTCOME MEASUREMENT

There are many barriers to beginning the process of outcome measurement. These include lack of confidence, time, and support, as well as limited data analysis resources. Primary care NPs are likely to have confusion over where to start with outcome measures and to be intimidated by the concept. Primary care is fraught with many competing demands and the need to remain current on the recommended approach to many conditions. This may leave little time for the individual NP to prepare himself or herself for practice in outcome measures. Depending on the practice setting, there may not be a significant level of support for outcome measures or the emphasis may be on the basic performance measures rather than actual outcomes. Finally, given availability of outcome measures, many NPs will lack the initial knowledge of how to analyze the data.

Luckily, there are several resources that will facilitate the outcome measurement process. Resnick (2006) provides a four-step process to implementing outcomes research. While her discussion is directed toward implementation of projects that will develop new and generalizable knowledge rather than limited findings to one practice setting, the steps provide examples of how to go about the process as well as encouragement for NPs contemplating the process. The other resources cited earlier also provide guidance.

Key facilitators include the NP's desire to improve practice and to optimize the outcomes of care. Another strength is the clinical expertise of NPs; a sound knowledge of a clinical area supports understanding of expected outcomes of care, which should provide direction on how to proceed in measurement activities.

Finally, it can be very helpful for NPs to establish a collaborative process either with the other providers within the same practice or with providers in other settings who have similar needs. Through collaboration, the providers are able to work together to establish outcome processes. If there are no other colleagues in the practice setting with whom to collaborate, an external mentor can be sought to coach through the process. Alternatively, there are networks for practice-based research in which providers can participate to become involved in the research process.

REFERENCES

Breslin, E., Burns, M., & Moores, P. (2002). Challenges of outcomes research for nurse practitioners. *Journal of the American Academy of Nurse Practitioners, 14*, 138–143.

Brown, S., & Grimes, D. (1995). A meta-analysis of nurse practitioners and nurse midwives in primary care. *Nursing Research, 44*, 332–339.

Burl, J., Bonner, A., & Rao, M. (1994). Demonstration of the cost-effectiveness of a nurse practitioner/physician team in primary care teams. *HMO Practice, 8,* 156–157.

Chenowith, D., Martin, N., Penkowski, J., & Raymond, I. (2005). A benefit-cost analysis of a worksite nurse practitioner program. First impressions. *Journal of Occupational and Environmental Medicine, 47,* 1110–1116.

Congressional Budget Office. (1979). *Physician extenders: Their current and future role in medical care delivery.* Washington, DC: U.S. Government Printing Office.

Cunningham, R. (2004). Advanced practice nursing outcomes: A review of selected empirical literature. *Oncology Nursing Forum, 31,* 219–232.

Horrocks, S., Anderson, E., & Salisbury, C. (2002). Systematic review of whether nurse practitioners working in primary care can provide equivalent care to doctors. *British Medical Journal, 324,* 819–823.

Kleinpell, R. (Ed.). (2001). *Outcome assessment in advanced practice nursing.* New York: Springer Publishing Company.

Laurant, M., Reeves, D., Hermens, R., et al. (2006). Substitution of doctors by nurses in primary care. *Cochrane Database of Systematic Reviews,* Issue 1.

Lenz, E. R., Mundinger, M. O., Kane, R. L., Hopkins, S. C., & Lin, S. X. (2004). Primary care outcomes in patients treated by nurse practitioners or physicians: Two-year follow-up. *Medical Care Research and Review, 61,* 332–351.

Moores, P., Breslin, E., & Burns, M. (2002). Structure and process of outcomes research for nurse practitioners. *Journal of the American Academy of Nurse Practitioners, 14,* 471–474.

Mundinger, M., Kane, R., Lenz, E., Totten, A., Tsai, W., Cleary, P., Friedewald, W., Sui, A., & Shelanski, M. (2000). Primary care outcomes in patients treated by nurse practitioners or physicians: A randomized trial. *Journal of the American Medical Association, 283,* 59–68.

National Organization of Nurse Practitioner Faculties. (2006). *Domains and core competencies of nurse practitioner practice.* Retrieved June 23, 2008, from http://www.nonpf.org/NONPF2005/CoreCompsFINAL06.pdf

Office of Technology Assessment. (1981). *The cost and effectiveness of nurse practitioners.* Washington, DC: U.S. Government Printing Office.

Office of Technology Assessment. (1986). *Nurse practitioners, physician assistants, and certified nurse midwives: A policy analysis.* Washington, DC: U.S. Government Printing Office.

Paez, K., & Allen, J. (2006). Cost-effectiveness of nurse practitioner management of hypercholesterolemia following coronary revascularization. *Journal of the American Academy of Nurse Practitioners, 18,* 436–444.

Resnick, B. (2006). Outcomes research: You do have the time! *Journal of the American Academy of Nurse Practitioners, 18,* 505–509.

Roblin, D., Howard, D., Becker, E., et al. (2004). Use of midlevel practitioners to achieve labor cost savings in the primary care practice of an MCO. *Health Services Research, 39,* 607–626.

Spitzer, W., Sackett, D., Sibley, J., Roberts, R., Gent, M., Kergin, D., Hacket, B., & Olynich, A. (1974). The Burlington randomized trial of the nurse practitioner. *New England Journal of Medicine, 290,* 252–256.

Vincent, D. (2002). Using cost-analysis techniques to measure the value of nurse practitioner care. *International Nursing Review, 49,* 243–249.

8

Assessing Outcomes in Clinical Nurse Specialist Practice

NANCY DAYHOFF AND BRENDA LYON

Clinical nurse specialists (CNSs) work on an advanced level of practice in three spheres of influence: (a) patient/clients, (b) nurses and nursing practice, and (c) systems/organizations (NACNS, 2004). As a result, CNSs contribute to promoting positive outcomes in a number of ways. Understanding the effect of CNS care on outcomes is important in today's health care system. Furthermore, the shift in the health care delivery system over the past several years to focus on outcomes management requires that CNSs be able to articulate and demonstrate their contributions to outcomes both clinical and economic. Achieving quality outcomes while balancing cost-containment issues is central to the work of CNSs. In a cost-containment environment, communicating information about outcomes of CNS practice is paramount to the survival of the CNS as an advanced practice nurse (Papenhausen & Beecroft, 1990; Scott, 1999). The purposes of this chapter are to: (1)

Throughout this chapter, the term *patient* will be used to refer to either patients or clients. According to *Webster's Dictionary* (1983), the term *patient* means someone under the care of a physician, whereas *client* means someone or group who engages another to act on its behalf. CNSs may provide services to individuals or groups who are not also receiving services from a physician. Therefore, the term *client* is more generic to individuals receiving the services of CNSs. However, the term *patient* is more commonly used and this convention will be followed.

describe important historical barriers to identifying and measuring CNS-related outcomes; (2) describe the core components of CNS practice, regardless of specialty and setting; (3) discuss the findings of selected outcome studies related to CNS practice; and (4) recommend outcomes that could be assessed, with suggested documentation strategies. The chapter is not meant to describe specific tools that CNSs could use to assess outcomes for specific client-care problems. The chapter will provide CNSs with a framework to identify potential outcomes for their specialty area as well as to provide examples of the current state of assessments.

CNS ROLE AND OUTCOME ASSESSMENTS

While CNSs have a long history as health care providers, a number of factors have contributed to professional stakeholders and patients/clients not understanding the unique contributions CNSs bring to the health care delivery system (Cannon & Beare, 1999; Wilson-Barnett & Beech, 1994; Wong, 1998). Two of the major contributing factors are: (a) CNSs describing the practice as occurring in various subroles; and (b) CNSs not clearly articulating their unique contributions to the cost-effective care of patients and the resultant nurse-sensitive outcome(s).

As early as the 1970s, CNSs were defined by multiple subroles: practitioner, educator, consultant, researcher, and administrator (Hamric, Spross, & Hanson, 2008; Menard & Wabschall, 1987). This subrole orientation contributed to CNSs defining their advanced practice by processes inherent in each of the subroles rather than by their contributions to client outcomes. Consequently, evaluations of outcomes of the work of CNSs focused on how well the CNSs performed subrole processes rather than on what effect their practice had on clinical and fiscal outcomes. For example, when the Oncology Nursing Society undertook development of an advanced practice certification examination, they reported that the first step in the process was the conduct of a role-delineation study based on subroles in order to define advanced clinical practice (McMillan, Heusinkveld, & Spray, 1995).

Three articles demonstrate the tendency to measure role activities rather than outcomes. Scott (1999) identified 42 advanced practice psychomotor and psychosocial nursing activities and then described the relative amount of time 724 CNSs spent in the subroles, but data were not reported about outcomes. CNSs have used subrole descriptions (standards) as the basis of developing an evaluation tool, such as the one described by Hill, Ellsworth-Wolk, and DeBlase (1993) that was used as the basis of performance appraisals. Performance-level definitions for each standard were developed that enhanced the use of the tool, not only for evaluations, but to guide goal setting for improvement. Houston and Luquire (1991) also described the development of a performance-appraisal tool using the four traditional subroles and adding seven additional performance criteria. Each criterion was then scaled, from 0 to 20, with 0 meaning "not met" and 20 meaning "ideal performance." However, neither of these two tools included data about influence on either clinical or economic outcomes. When subroles are used to define practice, outcome measures tend to describe how well the CNS performs the subroles rather than or in addition to what effect the performance had on clinical and economic outcomes. For example, what are the clinical outcomes of a CNS participating in interdisciplinary care conferences as a provider of care, or the CNS consulting as a change agent, or the CNS conducting staff education, or the CNS disseminating research findings to staff nurses? As long ago as 1975, Bloch pointed out that measuring *only* role activities is insufficient; clinical outcomes must also be measured. Assuming that the results of participation in these subroles are improved clinical and fiscal outcomes, it is incumbent upon CNSs to document the influence the activities have had on outcomes. Not to do so may lead to devaluing the contributions of CNS in this health care environment.

Another factor that contributed to difficulty in identifying the unique contributions of CNSs to outcomes was the fact that prior to 1998 the nature of CNS practice was not clearly articulated. While other advanced practice nurses may define their advanced practice as expansion into another discipline, CNSs are experts in the discipline of nursing. Their practice expertise is the differential diagnosis of non-disease-based etiologies of symptoms and functional problems, in the presence or absence of disease—disease that nursing has the primary responsibility to treat while expertly assisting with medical diagnosis and treatment, as appropriate (NACNS, 1998, 2004). The unique contribution of nursing, as a discipline, was first described by Florence Nightingale (1859/1992), when she proposed that disease and illness/suffering were two distinctly different phenomena. Illness is the experience of somatic discomfort in conjunction with a functional ability below the individual's perceived capability (Lyon, 1990, 1996; NACNS, 2004). Somatic discomfort may be physical or emotional. Illness may be disease-based, and thus the target of the medical discipline, or non-disease-based, the target of the nursing discipline. Examples of categories of non-disease-based etiologies include disturbances in physiological, psychological, or emotional processes as well as environmental factors. Wellness is the experience of somatic comfort and a functional ability at or near perceived capability level. The goals of nursing are to assist clients in preventing and resolving illness experiences and promoting wellness, in the presence or absence of disease (Lyon, 1990). While there may be a number of staff nurses, in addition to CNSs, who expertly assist with medical diagnosis and treatment, the differential diagnosis of and treatment for client problems with non-disease-based etiologies are the functions that set CNSs apart from other advanced practice nurses. Describing the unique contributions of practice activities clearly differentiating the practice of CNSs, as compared with those of other advanced practice nurses and other providers, is requisite to assessing outcomes of CNS practice and documenting the unique clinical and fiscal outcomes of that practice. In summary, the distinguishing characteristics of the clinical practice of CNSs is that they are experts in the diagnosis and treatment of illness and promotion of wellness with non-disease-based etiologies and, in certain specialties, are experts in assisting with the medical diagnosis and treatment of disease.

Because there are few research studies describing outcomes within and across CNS specialties and few measures developed for use of the practicing CNS to document outcomes of practice, CNSs have not systematically incorporated outcome measures in their activities to demonstrate what they offer to clients and delivery systems. However, assessment and documentation of how the multidimensionality of CNS practice contributes to quality clinical outcomes, advancement of nursing practice, and systems issues, including cost-effectiveness, is an important and crucial measure of practice and not just extraneous work (Boyle, 1995). Recent research, however, has focused on the effect of CNS practice on specific outcomes, including the impact of structured interventions on clinical pain management (Barnason, Merboth, Pozehl, & Tietjen, 1998; White, 1999); delirium recognition (Lacko et al., 2000); length of stay and complications for orthopedic patients (Wheeler, 1999); foot care practices for diabetic patients (Willoughby & Burroughs, 2001); reduced complications for patients with atrial fibrillation (McCabe, 2005); improved patient satisfaction for hospitalized medical patients (Forster et al., 2005); attendance rates at support groups for patients with implantable cardioverter defibrillators (Dickerson, Wu, & Kennedy, 2006); quality-of-life outcomes for patients in an outpatient anemia-management program (Hamilton & Hawley, 2006); bleeding complications after cardiac surgery (Ley, 2001); falls, activity levels, and pressure ulcers for nursing home patients (Rantz et al., 2001); early extubation for cardiac surgery patients (Jacavone, Rick, & Tyner, 1999); and clinical pathways for patients with sickle cell pain (Larsen, Neverett, & Larsen, 2001). Fulton and Baldwin (2004), in a review of the literature on outcomes of CNS practice, emphasize that a wide number of outcome measures have been used to evaluate CNS outcomes. While recent publications have served to showcase additional areas of influence for CNS practice, continued research on CNS outcomes is needed to further demonstrate the impact of CNS practice on the spheres of influence of the role.

FRAMEWORK FOR MEASURING CNS OUTCOMES

Historically, there has been no one model developed to articulate the outcomes of CNSs practice across populations and settings to guide assessment of outcomes. In 1998, however, after 3 years of reviewing literature, surveying CNSs across geographic regions and practice areas, reviewing numerous job descriptions, and receiving feedback from its own members as well as numerous external reviewers, the National Association of Clinical Nurse Specialists (NACNS) published the *Statement on Clinical Nurse Specialist Practice and Education* (Lyon, 1998; NACNS, 2004). Within this statement are descriptions of core CNS competencies and outcomes of practice. The competencies and outcomes are articulated, not in terms of the typical subroles used to describe CNS practice (Hamric & Spross, 1983; Hamric, Spross, & Hanson, 1996), but in terms of spheres of influence that clearly differentiate the practice and outcomes of CNSs from other advanced practice nurses. This conceptualization will be used as the framework to describe the assessment and documentation of CNS clinical outcomes. Lastly, the economic impact of CNS practice will be discussed as it applies across the three CNSs practice domains.

The term *outcomes* typically means the consequences or results of care, especially when it applies to clinical and fiscal outcomes. According to Nies et al. (1999), the defining attributes of *outcomes* are the end results; some action is required to produce the results, and that action precedes the results. Consistent with these attributes, the definition of outcomes used to describe outcomes of CNS practice is focused on the influence or consequences of purposeful CNS activities, including initiating and facilitating change or transformation actions as well as the effect of CNS care on direct patient outcomes, patient and family education, and nursing care practices and education (NACNS, 2004).

CONCEPTUALIZATION OF CNS CORE PRACTICES AND OUTCOMES

CNS practice spans three spheres of influence—patient/client, nursing personnel, and health care organization/network. It is through these three spheres that CNS practice influences outcomes. While the balance of CNS practice across the three spheres may vary by speciality, job description, and setting, the CNS's work is always purposed toward the cost-effective improvement of client outcomes. Improvements in cost-effective clinical outcomes are the raison d'etre for CNSs to advance the practice of other nursing personnel and contribute to policy and programmatic changes for the system. (Table 8.1 lists examples of outcomes across the three spheres of influence.) It is for these reasons that CNSs' work needs to focus on activities that influence outcomes and not on work-related process activities such as orientation of new nursing personnel.

When considering assessment and documentation issues, it is incumbent upon the CNS and the employing system to clearly negotiate and understand the expected balance between the CNS's practice activities within each sphere of influence. For example, within one system it may be expected that the CNS's major emphasis would be in the patient sphere of influence, with less time devoted to nursing personnel and system issues (Wells, Erickson, & Spinella, 1996). Another system may need the CNS's practice activities to be primarily targeted on advancing the practice of nursing personnel or on influencing client outcomes through systems-related activities. From a survey of 742

Table 8.1

CATEGORIES OF OUTCOMES OF CNS PRACTICE AND ROLES ACROSS THREE SPHERES OF INFLUENCE*

CATEGORIES OF OUT-COMES IN PATIENT/ CLIENT SPHERE	CATEGORIES OF OUT-COMES IN NURSING PER-SONNEL SPHERE	CATEGORIES OF OUT-COMES IN ORGANIZATION/ NETWORK SPHERE
1. Programs of care are designed for specific populations (e.g., oncology, specific ethnic groups).	1. Knowledge and skill development needs of nursing personnel are profiled.	1. Clinical problems are articulated within the context of the particular organization or network.
2. Phenomena of concern with etiologies requiring nursing interventions are identified.	2. **State-of-the-art knowledge and skills are reflected in registered nurse practice.**	2. Patient care processes reflect continuous improvements that benefit the system.
3. **Nursing therapeutics target specific etiologies.**	3. The research base for innovations is articulated, understandable, and accessible.	3. Policies are evidence-based and enhance the practice of nurse providers and multidisciplinary teams.
4. **Nursing therapeutics, in combination with medical therapeutics, where appropriate, result in achievement of goals for prevention, alleviations, or reduction of symptoms, functional problems, or risk behaviors.**	4. **Nurses articulate nursing's unique contributions to patient care and expected nurse-sensitive outcomes.**	4. **Innovative models of practice are developed, piloted, evaluated, and incorporated as appropriate across the continuum of care.**
5. Health care plans are appropriate for meeting client needs within available resources.	5. **Nurses solve patient care problems at the care-delivery level.**	5. Innovations in practice contribute to the achievement of quality, cost-effective outcomes for populations of patients.
6. **Real and potential unintended consequences and errors are prevented.**	6. **Desired patient outcomes are achieved through the synergistic effect of collaborative practice between nursing and other providers.**	6. Stakeholders (nurses, other health care professionals, and management) share a common vision of practice outcomes.

(continued)

(Table 8.1 continued)

CATEGORIES OF OUT-COMES IN PATIENT/CLIENT SPHERE	CATEGORIES OF OUT-COMES IN NURSING PER-SONNEL SPHERE	CATEGORIES OF OUT-COMES IN ORGANIZATION/NETWORK SPHERE
7. Nurse-sensitive outcomes are explicated.	7. Nursing career enhancement programs are ongoing, accessible, innovative, and effective.	7. Decision makers within the institution are informed regarding practice problems, factors contributing to the problems, and the significance of those problems with respect to outcomes and costs.
8. Effective interventions are incorporated into guidelines for practice.	8. Nursing personnel experience enhanced self-efficacy in patient care.	8. Nursing care initiatives and programs are aligned with the organization's strategic imperatives, mission, and vision.
9. Interventions that do not meet evaluation standards are discontinued.	9. Nursing personnel experience job satisfaction.	
10. Collaboration with patient/client as well as physicians and other health care professionals occurs as appropriate.	10. Competent nursing personnel are retained.	
11. Innovative educational programs for patients, families, and groups are developed, implemented, and evaluated.	11. Nursing personnel are engaged in learning.	
12. Transitions across the continuum of care are smooth.	12. Educational programs for nursing personnel focused on advancing the practice of nursing are developed, implemented, and evaluated.	

(Table 8.1 continued)

CATEGORIES OF OUT-COMES IN PATIENT/ CLIENT SPHERE	CATEGORIES OF OUT-COMES IN NURSING PER-SONNEL SPHERE	CATEGORIES OF OUT-COMES IN ORGANIZATION/ NETWORK SPHERE
13. Reports of new clinical phenomena and/ or interventions are published.	13. **The overall cost of care is reduced through judicious purchase and use of resources that enhance quality of patient care outcomes.**	

*Outcomes directly associated with CNS practice are in boldface; other outcomes are reflective of subroles CNSs may use to indirectly influence practice outcomes.
Source: Adapted from NACNS (2004).

CNSs, Scott (1999) found that the primary targets of their practice were patients (29% to 91% of their time) and the nursing personnel/system (18% to 96% of their time).

GENERAL ASSESSMENT STRATEGIES

A variety of measures may be used to provide general indices of the work of CNSs. These general indices include time and activities documentation and process evaluations. These general indices are measures of what the CNS does, not of what outcomes result from the deliberative work of the CNS.

Time on Activities

Several authors propose using "time on activities" documentation to assess CNS practice. Data from daily records are aggregated to profile time on categories of activities for weeks or months. CNSs may use a combination of appointment books/journals and/or completion-of-activity summary documentation to assess and document activities on a daily basis. For example, Aikin, Taggart, and Tripoli (1993); Buchanan

(1992); Hill, Ellsworth-Wolk, and DeBlase (1993); and Robichaud and Hamric (1986) used "time on activity summaries" to document CNS job performance. These authors devised tools for CNSs to hand-record amounts of time spent on a variety of activities each day as well as places to record qualitative documentation to describe activities more fully. The basis for the tools were position descriptions of the health care facility, typically described in generalities using a subrole framework, and the activity or process components associated with the description.

Picella (1996) describes the use of a computerized database of CNS activities that could run on either a personal computer or a laptop. This system provides periodic evaluations of the amount of time a CNS spent in each of the five major CNS subroles. Additionally, relational databases are configured so that CNS activities can be linked to client information. While the database included practice activities within the patient sphere, there was not a link with patient outcomes. However, as the author reported, "It is, however, a critical first step toward demonstrating whether or not the CNS is performing appropriate functions and establishing a foundation of critical information for future process and outcome evaluations" (p. 306). CNS productivity logs and database programs such as Microsoft Access can, however, be used to capture standardized sets of CNS activities and interventions, such as clinical interventions, educational offerings, consultations, research projects, advanced procedures, and specific cost-saving interventions (Prevost, 2001).

Regardless of whether a CNS hand-records or uses a computerized system, weekly and monthly summaries can then be used to provide one source of evidence documenting the breadth of CNS activities during a given time frame. These evaluations may be useful in helping employers and others understand the diversity of CNS work; however, they fall short in guiding the assessment and documentation of the CNS's contributions to clinical and fiscal outcomes.

Process Measures

Process measures, unlike "time on activities" documentation measures, typically use external sources to evaluate the competencies of CNS activities in the various subroles. Evaluations frequently assess how well others perceive that the CNS performs components of the subroles that are reflective of the job description. Such measures may include peer reviews, evaluations by staff nurses and other health care professionals, as well as clients' perceptions of care and the fulfillment of an internal contract between a CNS and an administrator (Malone, 1986; Nuccio et al., 1993; Peglow et al., 1992; Wilson-Barnett & Beech, 1994). Buchanan (1994) attempted to extend the process measurement by developing a tool for measuring outcome abilities of CNSs, using the nursing process as a framework. However, again, the abilities assessed through this tool do not link with client outcomes; it is important for CNSs to clearly differentiate measuring their own competencies and processes from measuring the client's clinical outcomes. Clinical outcomes are the end products of what happens to the client as the result of the purposeful CNS activities and not as a result of how well the CNS performs competencies. However, CNSs could assemble a portfolio of products developed during practice activities that may be used during self-evaluations and evaluations with administrators to articulate the outcomes. Contents of the portfolio could include examples of outcomes within each sphere influenced by the CNS, such as (a) discharge destination to appropriate sites as a result of discharge plans for a client or groups of clients, (b) decrease in falls or infection rates linked to staff education offerings, or (c) cost reductions with equal or better clinical outcomes associated with a product evaluation initiative.

ASSESSMENT OF OUTCOMES IN THE PATIENT/CLIENT SPHERE

General Outcomes: Changes in Disease State

The hallmark of CNS practice is the diagnosis and treatment of illness/wellness experiences with etiologies that are treatable through nursing therapeutics (Lyon, 1990, 1996). However, depending on the specialty, the CNS may also be an expert in assisting with medical diagnosis and treatment, and in these situations outcomes within the medical domain may serve as surrogate indicators of the CNSs' practice. Such indicators include physiologic changes in a client's disease status (including laboratory results), anatomic changes (such as changes in X-rays), and aggregate health care data (such as morbidity and mortality data). However, as Deyo (1998) points out, these outcome measures are considered "surrogate outcomes." Surrogate measures are typically influenced by medical practice patterns and therefore may mask the contributions of the CNS. While they are assumed to be linked with outcomes of interest to clients, such as symptom relief and improved functional abilities—both outcomes associated with CNS practice—they may be poor markers for these outcomes. It is important that outcome measures be selected that are reflective of the "deliberative activity" of the CNS, whenever possible, rather than using surrogate measures.

Hospital Aggregate Data

Morbidity, mortality, and length of hospital stay have historically been used as indicators of clinical outcomes. These measures may be useful in comparing outcomes of health care across systems, but have limitations as indicators of the advanced practice of a CNS. For example, morbidity indices, such as infection rates, reflect the practices of all health care workers involved in patient care as well as the general condition of the clients, such as nutritional status. It is difficult to explicate the specific contributions of CNS practice to morbidity indices without accounting for the multiplicity of factors that contribute to morbidity. However, if a decrease in complications such as infection rates can be linked to deliberate CNS activities, assessing changes in infection rates is appropriate. Naylor, Munro, and Brooten (1991) argue that in many cases mortality is not an appropriate measure of quality of nursing care; that mortality is more of a gross indicator of medical care and communication between nurses and physicians. Lastly, length of stay may be an indicator of nursing care if data on rehospitalizations, postdischarge acute care visits, and caregiving burden are factored into the data.

Nurse-Sensitive Outcomes

Outcomes that are clearly influenced by nursing care should be targeted for assessment of CNS practice. Such outcomes include clients' perceptions of symptom relief, improved physical and cognitive functioning, effective coping with situational stress contributing to illness, minimizing the burden of care by family members and other lay caregivers, ability to perform self-care, and avoidance of risk behaviors (Lyon, 2000; Naylor, Munro, & Brooten, 1991; Peglow et al., 1992). Outcomes also include nurse-sensitive indicators of pain control and prevention of complications such as skin breakdown, falls, and infection (Duffy, 2002; Johnson, Maas, & Moorhead, 2000).

Within the patient/client sphere, described in the NACNS Statement, there are at least 16 core outcomes that CNSs may use to measure products of practice. The practices within this sphere that are unique to CNSs as advanced practice nurses include expertise in integrating knowledge of disease and medical treatment in a holistic assessment of persons while focusing on the differential diagnosis of illness experiences (such as symptoms or functional status) as well as implementing population-based programs of care by integrating nursing interventions and treatments to enhance patient outcomes (NACNS, 2004).

Outcomes of CNS practice within this sphere may include: (1) programs of care designed for specific populations that either replace existing programs found not to yield effective clinical outcomes in a cost-effective manner or initiating programs new to the cohort of clients in need of services; (2) development of care plans, care maps, or pathways that are evidence-based and improve clinical fiscal outcomes; (3) client reports of improvement in symptoms, functional problems, or decreased performance of risk behaviors and improved self-care behaviors, as compared to data obtained prior to CNS interventions; (4) nursing therapeutics, in combination with medical therapeutics where appropriate, that result in better client outcomes than occurred prior to CNS interventions; (5) development of innovative educational programs for clients, families, and groups that are implemented and evaluated; (6) desired outcomes are achieved without increasing the demand on health care services; (7) prevention of complications, unintended adverse outcomes, and errors as clients transition across the continuum of care; and (8) barriers to clinical practice are identified and appropriate resolutions are implemented to improve clinical and fiscal outcomes (Fleschler & Luquire, 1998; NACNS, 2004).

Strategies that may be used to assess the above outcomes include:

- Use of an effectiveness worksheet, describing outcomes associated with direct client care (Bakker & Vincensi, 1995).
- Surveys or interviews (verbal assessments with documentation) to assess the client's perception of symptom relief or improved

functioning. Two questions could be used to focus on assessing how a client is feeling and doing (functioning) as compared to before he or she was hospitalized or received a specific nursing therapeutic modality. Some health care providers use the SF-36 to examine outcomes of care; however, the tool is limited in the range of discomforts and functional problems measured (Hayes, Sherbourne, & Mazel, 1993).

- Chart reviews to document the incidence of complications such as pressure ulcers, hospital-acquired pneumonia, falls, and infection
- Documentation of the number of referrals of complex clients received by the CNS from other providers as well as the number and type of clients cared for as the primary provider. An example of caseload outcomes is discussed by Brieger, Smith, and Muenchau (1989) in which they recommend tracking referrals to the CNS by staff and determining whether the referrals were consistent with preestablished criteria (e.g., clients with anticipated extended length of stays or outliers from clinical paths that might require the competencies of a CNS). These authors recommend a monthly report be used by the CNS to document all aspects of their practice and roles.
- Review of risk-management data and tracking of sentinel events (JCAHO, 1996) as well as the typical data tracked by systems, such as rehospitalizations, recidivism, repeat visits to emergency rooms, length of stay, postdischarge morbidity, discharge destinations, and functional assessments at the time of discharge. Benchmarking using internal criteria as well as external standards for a specific population could also provide evidence of the effects of CNS practice within the client sphere.

Sources to help CNSs identify nurse-sensitive outcomes include reference books compiling potential outcome measures for the above phenomenon. For example, *Measures for Clinical Practice* (Corcoran & Fisher, 1987), *Measurement Tools in Patient Education* (Redman, 1998), *Instruments for Clinical Health-Care Research* (Frank-Stromborg & Olsen, 2004), and *Nursing Outcomes Classification (NOC)* (Johnson, Maas, & Moorhead, 2000) are references from which CNSs may either select or design outcome measures at the client level. A review of research literature associated with a specific phenomenon could yield clinically useful outcome measures. During the writing of the NACNS

Statement, 47 research reports documenting CNS outcomes on various client populations were reviewed and summarized; the summary is included in the Appendix. The tools used to assess outcomes in these reports may be useful for CNSs in the service arena.

Designing, implementing, and evaluating innovative psychoeducational interventions are important components of most CNSs' practice, regardless of specialty. Outcome measures of psychoeducational interventions could include changes in clients' knowledge about their self-care regimen, attitudes toward performing behaviors, improvements in self-efficacy for performing health-related behaviors or changes in perceived threat, and improvements in emotions or coping effectiveness (Bennett, Puntenney, Walker, & Ashley, 1996; Redman, 1998). Examples of assessments used to document changes in symptom experiences include: perceived health, symptom distress, pain measures, and measures specific to the symptom being treated. Examples of assessments used to document functional outcomes include: activities of daily living (ADL) scales appropriate to the population, functional measures, that capture how clients perceive they are functioning with respect to their desired functional level discharge destination—to home or to a facility because of needing assistance with ADLs.

Web sites are excellent sources for helping to identify outcomes and assessments. Examples include outcomes from the client and family perspective (e.g., Picker.org), outcome information across the continuum of care (e.g., caredata.com), the National Guideline Clearinghouse (guideline.gov), and the NACNS organization (NACNS.org). The site for the "best practice" network that provides information on benchmarking as well as practical and practice issues is best4health.org. Measures of outcomes of CNS practice in the patient/client sphere must be specific to the problems of the population of patients that receive the services of the CNS. The more specific the measure to the patient problem being treated, the more sensitive the outcome measurement to the deliberative CNS services. The chapter by Schwartz et al. in this book outlines additional Web-based resources for identifying outcomes as well as tools for assessing outcomes of APN practice.

Assessing Outcomes in the Nursing Personnel Sphere

One of the defining characteristics of CNS practice is providing leadership to advance the practice of nursing personnel to achieve quality, cost-effective outcomes within a specialty population and as appropriate across populations (NACNS, 2004). Assessing and documenting client outcomes sensitive to total nursing care is important. Through role modeling of practice, consultation with nursing personnel, research utilization, and formal educational programs, CNSs change the practice of nurses and other personnel (Brieger, Smith, & Muenchau, 1989; Heinemann et al., 1996; McCaffrey, 1990; Vollman & Stewart, 1996). Clinical outcomes of such strategies should be reflected in the nursing personnel's practice and indirect measures should be reflected in the climate among the nurses.

Examples of outcomes of the CNS practice through nursing personnel include: (a) nurses solving client care problems at the care-delivery level, (b) nursing personnel experiencing improved job satisfaction with improved job retention, and (c) overall cost of care being reduced through judicious use of resources and selection of products that enhance quality patient care outcomes.

Because nurses' notes in patient charts may be used to assess outcomes of care, it is important that the notes contain important data and consistently reflect clients' responses to interventions. One kind of evidence that may be used to assess the influence of CNS practice in advancing nursing care is that the nursing documentation system contains relevant and reliable information (Wilson-Barnett & Beech, 1994). Examples of the influence of CNSs in advancing nursing practice are reported by Gryfinski and Lampe (1990). A CNS chaired a task force to implement focus charting. Evaluation data confirmed that through the changes: (a) the implemented program met standard charting criteria at higher rates than before implementation; (b) nurses spent less time charting, thereby increasing nursing productivity and reduced overtime; and (c) data retrieval was enhanced, thereby increasing productivity in other settings.

A number of delivery systems are implementing electronic records that include nursing documentation. CNSs can make important contributions to the development of the nursing documentation systems because of the competencies they bring to the table. For example, as change agents targeting quality, cost-effective outcomes, they would be able to synthesize relationships between documentation of critical information and information needed to track clinical and fiscal outcomes.

Patient outcomes discussed in the client/patient sphere of influence could also be used to track the outcomes of groups of patients. For example, if a CNS designed a patient education program to be delivered by staff nurses, outcomes such as return visits to clinics or emergency rooms or decreased lack of compliance to preoperative instructions at the time of admission for surgery could be assessed. Improved immunization rates among school-age children, decreased risk behaviors, and increased participation in health programs are additional examples of outcomes of programs designed by CNSs for implementation by nurses and other providers.

Assessing Outcomes in the Organization/Network Sphere

Through institutional responsibilities, CNSs may also affect clinical and fiscal outcomes. While it may be important to document the numbers of nursing, multidisciplinary, and administrative committees of which the CNS is a member, CNSs need to assess and document outcomes associated with participation on those committees. Examples of such outcomes include: (a) contributions to establishing benchmarks for care of aggregates of patients that occur because of multidisciplinary care, (b) changes in policies and procedures that are evidence-based, (c) development of critical paths with improved clinical and fiscal outcomes, (d) decrease in complications and adverse events, and (e) product evaluations and purchases with improved clinical outcomes and associated cost-avoidance or cost-reduction.

Fleschler and Luquire (1998) suggest (a) documenting instances of sharing critical reviews of research and expert opinion literature with multidisciplinary teams to guide the development of team plans of care and (b) raising questions concerning predictors of care and risk stratification. A recurring theme of outcomes of CNS practice at all levels of influence is providing leadership in the development of innovative solutions to problems or gaps in clinical and fiscal outcomes. Innovations might include a solution that is totally novel; but innovations may also be adapting a solution currently used with one group of patients to the situation of another group not currently receiving the interventions, or using and adopting interventions across providers when the intervention is only used by one provider on a multidisciplinary team. Because some practices vary by geography, innovation may also include the testing of a solution used by one system for adoption, with or without modifications, to the CNSs' employing system. One of the outcomes of any change project in which a CNS is involved is that the change process and outcome are evidence-based. Examples of assessments and outcomes of evidence-based practice could include bibliographic references with appropriate research literature cited, attached to policies and procedures and care maps.

Another example is that new products and evaluation of current products for use with client care are systematically evaluated for clinical efficacy and usability by staff before decisions are made to purchase new products. There are few strategies described in the literature to guide CNS conduct of product evaluation, especially since most products involve a multidisciplinary team and are frequently the purview of a purchasing department. One strategy is described by Oates (1997). A pediatric CNS led a multidisciplinary team to compare the clinical effects of two different devices. The team was guided in the product evaluation by the Iowa Model for Research-Based Practice to Promote Quality Care and the algorithm is presented within the article. While the strengths of this model are that it clearly links research literature review to guiding the process, it does not specifically direct steps to follow that are unique to product evaluation.

One model, *Product Evaluation and Selection: A Nursing Model for Product Review*, was developed by M. A. Underhill (1993) and incorporated into the product evaluation process of a large midwestern hospital. Included in the 10 steps of product evaluation, in addition to a review of the literature, are questions specific to products, such as Step 1 (identifying a need to change or buy a new product vs. a "want" on the part of a provider to purchase a product) or Step 2 (determining specifications of the needed product using structure, process, and outcome criteria). Additional steps include: designing methodology to evaluate products, selecting a product that meets specifications, developing an implementation plan, and periodic monitoring of the use and outcomes once the product is implemented. Because of the clinical expertise of the CNS, the CNS is an appropriate leader of product evaluation committees to assure that quality outcomes are achieved with purchases while being mindful of fiscal considerations as well as the usability by nursing personnel and other providers. Health care systems have found that the least expensive product is not necessarily the cheapest if desired clinical outcomes are not achieved, if nursing personnel have difficulty providing care using the product, and if adverse clinical outcomes are not avoided.

Data from patient satisfaction surveys may be especially informative if the data are available both before and after a CNS is involved in the care of a population of patients. Patients' descriptions of quality care are important as hospitals compete for consumers (Heinemann et al., 1996; Oermann, 1999). Patients' perceptions of whether nurses were competent and skilled, talked effectively with them, and educated them about the care are factors related to their satisfaction. While most health care systems do not track clinical data concerning symptoms and functioning, they do track patient satisfaction data, which serves as a proxy for factors important to the patients and clients. Additionally, data concerning readmissions, repeat visits to emergency rooms, and other surrogate indicators may suggest that clinical outcomes were affected by inserting a CNS into the organizational system (Deyo, 1998; Forster et al., 2005; McCabe, 2005; Naylor, Munro, & Brooten, 1991; Rantz et al., 2001; Wong, 1998).

"Nursing report cards" are being developed to provide data-based evidence of nursing's contributions to patient outcomes. Report cards serve to aggregate data about patient outcomes as well as about staffing statistics and quality indicators of care (Lowe & Baker, 1997; Sheehy et al., 2000). The reports were initially designed to examine the impact of workforce restructuring and redesign on outcomes of patient care. Ten core indicators comprised the initial report cards; the indicators include patient, nursing personnel, and organizational measures. Report cards could be used to examine the influence of CNS practice in all three spheres of influence, especially if the report card data are collected before and after a CNS is involved in solving problems of a population of patients, if CNSs deliberately influence the care of nursing personnel, or if deliberative actions are taken at the organizational level. While report cards are in the developmental stages, they may provide data supporting the work of CNSs.

In summary, when a CNS is integrated into an organizational system, unit, or problem-solving situation, changes in patient outcomes are indicative of the impact of the CNS practice through influencing nursing personnel. Measures may be direct assessments of changes in patients' symptom experiences, functioning, and avoidance of complications, or they may be indirect, such as with patient satisfaction indicators.

Economic Outcomes

As Edmunds (1992) and Edwardson (1992) point out, the economic impact of services of nurse anesthetists, midwives, and, more recently, nurse practitioners is relatively easy to measure. CNS services, however, may be more difficult to measure. While CNSs are typically not responsible for fiscal management of client care, they do need to have a working knowledge of such management. This knowledge enables them to communicate with financial staff and others to assure that the fiscal analysis of clinical outcomes is relevant to the nursing diagnoses and treatments, changes in care by nursing personnel, and changes at the systems level.

Most CNS activities are not billable to third-party payors, so they can be tracked through a financial system. However, things such as a CNS clinic for older adults, a foot clinic, or care for patients with diabetes mellitus may be billable. Although CNS activities at the nursing personnel and system levels in particular may be difficult to track, doing so may enable systems to understand the economic contributions of CNS practice. There are three ways to demonstrate cost-effectiveness: (1) cost savings, (2) cost avoidance, and (3) revenue generation:

- Cost savings occur when a less expensive product or process can accomplish the same or better clinical outcomes. An example of cost savings is the selection of a product for nursing care that is less expensive, but accomplishes desired outcomes.
- Cost avoidance occurs when a new or modified action or process prevents costs. A common example of cost avoidance is teaching clients who are covered by a managed care system to improve self-care behaviors so as to prevent emergency room visits.
- Revenue generation occurs when CNS activities, such as teaching and consulting, produce revenue for the institution. Revenue generation also occurs when CNSs conduct and oversee nursing centers and clinics.

Other examples of cost-saving activities include savings through recruitment and retention of nursing personnel, product evaluation, decreased length of stay, and developing new clinics.

From her survey of 724 nurses, Scott (1999) found that few CNSs were able to identify the influence of their practice on revenue generation or cost reduction through savings and avoidance. Of those CNSs who did specify revenue-generating activities, most attributed them to charges for services, for case management, for providing continuing education, and for legal and clinical consultation.

There are a variety of ways to evaluate economic impact of care that incorporate revenue generation and analysis of cost-benefit and cost-effectiveness. Bakker and Vincensi (1995) proposed a revenue analysis. They proposed using three sources of revenue as outcome measures: (a) gross revenue generated from length of stay; (b) cost savings from decreasing expenses in the delivery of care and the savings in unreimbursable expenses; and (c) other indirect revenue factors, such as the marketing value of patient satisfaction. This model uses indicators from all three spheres, but principally indicators at the systems level, such as acuity level of care, recidivism, and prevention of complications to infer cost savings of care were significant. One of the cautions in using systems indicators such as length of stay is that a shortened stay may not result in cost savings. If a shorter stay contributes to increased demands on lay caregivers, physicians' offices, or other posthospital services within the system, there may simply be a cost shifting rather than a cost savings. Another sensitive issue pertinent to system-level indicators is that such factors as decreased length of stay or decreased hospital or emergency room visits may also decrease revenue. It is particularly important for CNSs to factor into system-level outcomes non-CNS-related influences on outcomes, such as variability in physician practice patterns and cultural differences among units within the same system (Gift, 1992a, 1992b).

Edwardson (1992) describes a cost-benefit analysis and cost-effectiveness analysis. The article describes the formulas for conducting a cost-benefit analysis using all costs and benefits that are usually measured on a monetary scale. Cost-effectiveness analysis is added to the equation when not all costs and benefits can be measured using the same scale or when assigning a dollar value to benefits is not applicable, such as quality of life or patient satisfaction as outcomes.

Gardner, Allhusen, Kamm, and Tobin (1997) compared two methods of analysis, one with evidence of validity and one with an innovative model being tested at the time of the report. Assumptions underlying a cost-effectiveness strategy at this level include: (a) the hospital has accurate variable and fixed costs for each chargeable service; (b) the financial system can capture charges and costs per patient day;

(c) nursing service uses reliable indicators of nursing activities or work-load; and (d) the pathways have been in place long enough to establish consistent outcomes, such as for 6 months. Such an analysis requires the combined efforts of nursing and financial personnel. Gardner et al. (1997) provide examples—of a standardized cost report for one clinical pathway and of a method to determine cost of the nursing component of pathways—that may be useful as guidelines for other CNSs. The value of the second method is to increase the cost sensitivity by using nursing hours per day as an indicator.

The study by Brooten et al. (1988) was one of the first major studies to document the economic outcomes of home care after hospitalization by CNSs. The goal of the randomized clinical trial was to evaluate the cost-effectiveness of an experimental group of low-birth-weight infants whose families received care from a CNS and who were discharged 11 days earlier than a control group. The authors documented an $18,560 mean savings for the early discharge of low-birth-weight infants without compromising quality of care. Neidlinger, Scroggins, and Kennedy (1987) examined the cost-effectiveness of discharge planning by geron-tological CNSs for hospitalized older adults. On average, the hospital costs for the CNS-patient group were $3,069 and the average cost for the 41 in the control group $4,380. Ferraro-McDuffie, Chan, and Jerome (1993) examined the financial benefits of CNSs at a children's hospital. They analyzed the cost-savings and revenue-generating activities of 15 unit-based and specialty-based CNSs. Their analysis demonstrated a financial impact of $1.6 million in 1 year and more than $800,000 a subsequent year.

The ability to link clinical and fiscal outcomes will be enhanced through the use of relational information and data-based systems. Bozzo, Carlson, and Diers (1998) described such a system, by which a CNS tracked clinical outcomes of care for complex clients across the system (such as achieving desired laboratory values and other standards of care) together with length of stay, readmissions, and use of emergency department services. While these indicators reflect the care of a multidis-ciplinary system, this system provides opportunities to track changes in fiscal as well as traditional clinical outcomes on the basis of changes in practices initiated or led by the CNS. What this system does not track is the effects on the clients in terms of improvements in symptoms, functioning, decreased performance of risk behaviors, and avoidance of complications. Prevost (2002) gives examples of capturing CNS impact on cost savings by such measures as tracking the cost of complications that can be averted with CNS care, including aggressive education and research utilization to prevent nosocomial pressure ulcers, as well as cost savings associated with peripheral intravenous central catheter (PICC) line insertions as compared to surgical insertion costs. Demonstrating the cost-effectiveness of CNS care becomes a powerful strategy for documenting the influence of the CNS role.

SUMMARY AND CONCLUSIONS

Although CNSs have a long history of caring for patients and improving outcomes through nursing personnel and multidisciplinary teams, the competencies needed by today's CNSs are greatly expanded from those needed in the 1960s, '70s, '80s, and '90s. During the last decade, changes in the delivery and payment structure for health care were particularly salient for CNSs. Health care delivery systems need CNSs who are focused on both (a) the advancement of nursing practice to maintain and improve clinical outcomes of care important to the patient and (b) cost-effectiveness and revenue generation. Therefore, to be effective, CNSs must be able to identify, evaluate, and document targeted patient-care-related outcomes and to track revenue generation, cost avoidance, cost savings, and/or cost-effectiveness. (See Table 8.2 for summary of examples of outcome assessments.) While CNS practice is complex because the outcomes of practice at the patient, nursing-personnel, and systems levels are so interrelated, it is incumbent on CNSs to specify the outcomes that are sensitive to the deliberative services of the CNS's practice. These are the outcomes that are unlikely to occur if CNSs were not practicing. Additionally, selection of specific clinical outcomes appropriate to the CNS's practice will be determined by the job description, population, and setting. Focusing on the specific outcomes that result from CNS care, including cost savings; the cost benefit of avoiding complications that can be averted; and the consequences of implementing new roles, interventions, or programs, can help to showcase the power of CNS influence (Prevost, 2002). CNSs are masters in nursing care, well positioned to make continued substantial and verifiable contributions to cost-effective achievement of quality outcomes.

Table 8.2

SUMMARY OF ASSESSMENTS OF CLINICAL NURSE SPECIALISTS PRACTICE

FOCUS OF PRACTICE	EXAMPLES OF TYPES OF ASSESSMENTS/DATA	EXAMPLES OF SOURCES OF EVIDENCE
Performance of subroles	Implementation of job expectation as advanced practice clinician, educator, consultant, and utilizer of research	Time on activities logs/journals and summaries Peer review and evaluations of staff nurses and other health care professionals Portfolio of products of practice

Client sphere	Morbidity, mortality data
	    Symptom experience
	    Functional status
	    Mental status
	    Stress level
	    Client satisfaction with care
	    Burden of care
	    Effective self-care behaviors/
	        reduced risk behaviors
	    Avoidance of complications
	Quality of life
		Hospital databases
		Instruments that specifically measure changes in patient problems and achievement of goals/outcomes of care from both nurse and client perspectives
		
		Surrogate indices: Morbidity, mortality, rehospitalization, discharge destination
		Clinical data such as laboratory and X-ray reports
		Chart audits, risk management information

Nursing personnel sphere	Recruitment and retention
	    successes
	Improved job satisfaction
	Improvements in nursing
	    personnel competency
	Decreased cost of products
	    and other resources used in
	    patient care
		Information from human resource department
		Attendance at staff development meetings; chart audit
		Financial data

Systems sphere	Length of stay, recidivism, use
	    of postdischarge health
	    services
	Achievement of benchmarks
	Patient satisfaction
	Workforce redesign/patient care
		Systems databases including data from hospital, post-discharge services, physician offices
		Benchmark data from internal data and comparison data provided by state and national sources
		Satisfaction surveys
		Nursing report cards

REFERENCES

Aikin, J. L., Taggart, J. R., & Tripoli, C. A. (1993). Evaluation and time documentation for the clinical nurse specialist. *Clinical Nurse Specialist, 7*, 33–38.

Bakker, D. J., & Vincensi, B. B. (1995). Economic impact of the CNS: Practitioner role. *Clinical Nurse Specialist, 9*, 50–53.

Barnason, S., Merboth, M., Pozehl, B., & Tietjen, M. J. (1998). Utilizing an outcomes approach to improve pain management by nurses: A pilot study. *Nursing Clinics of North America, 12*, 28–36.

Bennett, S., Puntenney, P. J., Walker, N. L., & Ashley, N. D. (1996). Development of an instrument to measure threat related to cardiac events. *Nursing Research, 45*, 266–270.

Bloch, D. (1975). Evaluation of nursing care in terms of process and outcomes. *Nursing Research, 24*, 256–263.

Boyle, D. M. (1995). Documentation and outcomes of advanced nursing practice. *Oncology Nursing Forum, 22*(8 Suppl.), 11–17.

Bozzo, J., Carlson, B., & Diers, D. (1998). Using hospital data systems to find target populations: New tools for clinical nurse specialists. *Clinical Nurse Specialist, 12*, 86–91.

Brieger, G., Smith, D. F., & Muenchau, T. (1989). One approach to quantifying the CNS role. *Nursing Management, 20*, 80i–80s.

Brooten, D., Brown, L. P., Munro, B. H., York, R., Cohen, S. M., Roncoli, M., & Hollingsworkth, A. (1988). Early discharge and specialist transitional care. *Image— The Journal of Nursing Scholarship, 20*, 64–68.

Buchanan, L. C. (1992). A rehabilitation clinical nurse specialist: Evaluation of the role in a home health care setting. *Holistic Nursing Practice, 6*, 42–50.

Buchanan, L. M. (1994). Therapeutic nursing intervention knowledge and outcome development and outcome measures for advanced practice. *Nursing & Health Care, 15*, 190–195.

Cannon, J., & Beare, P. G. (1999). Hospital and parish (county) utilization of master's-prepared nurses in Louisiana. *Clinical Nurse Specialist, 13*, 199–207.

Corcoran, K., & Fisher, J. (1987). *Measures for clinical practice.* New York: The Free Press.

Cunningham, R. S. (2004). Advanced practice nursing outcomes: A review of selected empirical literature. *Oncology Nursing Forum, 31*, 219–230.

Deyo, R. (1998). Using outcomes to improve quality of research and quality of care. *Journal of the American Board of Family Practice, 11*, 465–473.

Dickerson, S. S., Wu, Y. B., & Kennedy, M. C. (2006). A CNS-facilitated ICD support group: A clinical project evaluation. *Clinical Nurse Specialist, 20*, 146–153.

Duffy, J. R. (2002). The clinical leadership role of the CNS in the identification of nursing-sensitive and multidisciplinary quality indicator sets. *Clinical Nurse Specialist, 16*, 70–76.

Edmunds, M. W. (1992). Should CNSs look at the economic value of their services? *Clinical Nurse Specialist, 6*, 162.

Edwardson, S. R. (1992). Costs and benefits of clinical nurse specialists. *Clinical Nurse Specialist, 6*, 163–167.

Ferraro-McDuffie, A., Chan, J. S. L., & Jerome, A. M. (1993). Communicating the financial worth of the CNS through the use of fiscal reports. *Clinical Nurse Specialist, 7*, 91–97.

Fleschler, R., & Luquire, R. (1998). Linking outcomes management and practice improvement. *Outcomes Management for Nursing Practice, 2*, 54–56.

Forster, A. J., Clark, H. D., Menard A., et al. (2005). Effect of a nurse team coordinator on outcomes for hospitalized medical patients. *American Journal of Medicine, 118*, 1148–1153.

Frank-Stromborg, M., & Olsen, S. J. (2004). *Instruments for clinical health-care research* (3rd ed.). Boston: Jones and Bartlett.

Fulton, J. S., & Baldwin, K. (2004). An annotated bibliography reflecting CNS practice and outcomes. *Clinical Nurse Specialist, 18*, 21–39.

Gardner, K., Allhusen, J., Kamm, J., & Tobin, J. (1997). Determining the cost of care through clinical pathways. *Nursing Economic$, 15*, 213–217.

Gift, A. G. (1992a). Determining CNS cost effectiveness. *Clinical Nurse Specialist, 6*, 89.

Gift, A. G. (1992b). Effectiveness of the CNS as educator and discharge planner. *Clinical Nurse Specialist, 6*, 201.

Gryfinski, J. J., & Lampe, S. S. (1990). Implementing Focus Charting®: Process and critique. *Clinical Nurse Specialist, 4*, 201–205.

Hamilton, R., & Hawley, W. (2006). Quality of life outcomes related to anemia management of patients with chronic renal failure. *Clinical Nurse Specialist, 20*, 139–143.

Hamric, A. B., & Spross, J. A. (1983). *The clinical nurse specialist in theory and practice.* Philadelphia: W. B. Saunders.

Hamric, A. B., Spross, J. A., & Hanson, C. M. (2008). *Advanced nursing practice: An integrative approach.* Philadelphia: Saunders Elsevier.

Hayes, R. D., Sherbourne, C. D., & Mazel, R. M. (1993). The Rand 36-item health survey. *Health Economics, 2*, 217–227.

Heinemann, D., Lengacher, C. A., VanCott, M. L., Mabe, P., & Swymer, S. (1996). Partners in patient care: Measuring the effects on patient satisfaction and other quality indicators. *Nursing Economic$, 14*, 276–285.

Hill, K. M., Ellsworth-Wolk, J., & DeBlase, R. (1993). Capturing the multiple contributions of the CNS role: A criterion-based evaluation tool. *Clinical Nurse Specialist, 7*, 267–273.

Houston, S., & Luquire, R. (1991). Measuring success: CNS performance appraisals. *Clinical Nurse Specialist, 5*, 204–209.

Jacavone, J., Rick, D., & Tyner, I. (1999). CNS facilitation of a cardiac surgery clinical pathway program. *Clinical Nurse Specialist, 13*, 126–132.

Johnson, M., Maas, M., & Moorhead, S. (Eds.). (2000). *Nursing outcomes classification (NOC)* (2nd ed.). St. Louis, MO: Mosby-Year Book.

Joint Commission on Accreditation of Healthcare Organizations [JCAHO]. (1996). *Hospital accreditation standards.* Oakbrook Terrace, IL: Author.

Lacko, L. A., Dellasega, C., Salerno, F. A., et al. (2000). The role of the advanced practice nurse in facilitating a clinical research study. *Clinical Nurse Specialist, 14*, 110–115.

Larson, L. S., Neverett, S. G., & Larsen, R. F. (2001). Clinical nurse specialist as facilitator of interdisciplinary collaborative program for adult sickle cell population. *Clinical Nurse Specialist, 15*, 15–22.

Ley, S. J. (2001). Quality care outcomes in cardiac surgery: The role of evidence based practice. *AACN Clinical Issues, 12,* 606–617.

Lowe, A., & Baker, J. K. (1997). Measure outcomes: A nursing report card. *Nursing Management, 28,* 40–41.

Lyon, B. (2000). Stress, coping & health: An overview. In V. Rice (Ed.), *Handbook of stress, coping, and health: Implications for nursing theory, practice, and interventions* (p. 42). Thousand Oaks, CA: Sage.

Lyon, B. L. (1990). Getting back on track: Nursing's autonomous scope of practice. In N. L. Chaska (Ed.), *The nursing profession: Turning points* (pp. 267–274). St. Louis: C. V. Mosby.

Lyon, B. L. (1996). Meeting societal needs for clinical nurse specialist competencies: Why the clinical nurse specialist and NP roles should not be blended in master's degree program. *Online Journal of Issues in Nursing,* June 15, www.nursingworld.org

Lyon, B. L. (1998). NACNS statement on clinical nurse specialist competencies and education is approved. *Clinical Nurse Specialist, 12,* 3–5.

Malone, B. L. (1986). Evaluation of the clinical nurse specialist. *American Journal of Nursing, 86,* 1375–1377.

McCabe, P. J. (2005). Spheres of clinical nurse specialist practice influence evidence-based care for patients with atrial fibrillation. *Clinical Nurse Specialist, 19,* 308–317.

McCaffrey, D. (1990). Indices of success. *Clinical Nurse Specialist, 4,* 156–157.

McMillan, S. C., Heusinkveld, K. B., & Spray, J. (1995). Advanced practice in oncology nursing: A role delineation study. *Oncology Nursing Forum, 22,* 41–50.

Menard, S. W., & Wabschall, J. M. (1987). *The clinical nurse specialist: Perspectives in practice.* New York: John Wiley & Sons.

National Association of Clinical Nurse Specialists [NACNS]. (2004). *Statement on clinical nurse specialist practice and education.* Glenview, IL: National Association of Clinical Nurse Specialists.

Naylor, M. D., Munro, B. H., & Brooten, D. A. (1991). Measuring the effectiveness of nursing practice. *Clinical Nurse Specialist, 5,* 210–215.

Neidlinger, S. H., Scroggins, K., & Kennedy, L. M. (1987). Cost evaluation of discharge planning for hospitalized elderly: The efficacy of clinical nurse specialist. *Nursing Economics, 5,* 225–230.

Nies, M. A., Cook, T., Bach, C. A., Bushnell, K., Salisbury, M., Sinclair, V., & Ingersoll, G. L. (1999). Concept analysis of outcomes for advanced practice nursing. *Outcomes Management for Nursing Practice. 3,* 83–86.

Nightingale, F. (1859/1992). *Notes on nursing: What it is and what it is not.* Philadelphia: J. B. Lippincott.

Nuccio, S. A., Costa-Lieberthal, K. M., Gunta, K. E., Mackus, M. L., Riesch, S. K., Schmanski, K. M., & Westen, B. A. (1993). A survey of 636 staff nurses: Perceptions and factors influencing the CNS role. *Clinical Nurse Specialist, 11,* 270–273.

Oates, K. (1997). Models of planned change and research utilization applied to product evaluation. *Clinical Nurse Specialist, 11,* 270–273.

Oermann, M. H. (1999). Consumers' descriptions of quality health care. *Journal of Nursing Care Quality, 14,* 47–55.

Papenhausen, J. L., & Beecroft, P. C. (1990). Communicating clinical nurse specialist effectiveness. *Clinical Nurse Specialist, 4,* 1–2.

Peglow, D. J., Klatt-Ellis, T., Stelton, S., Cutillo-Schmitter, T., Howard, J., & Wolff, P. (1992). Evaluation of clinical nurse specialist practice. *Clinical Nurse Specialist, 6,* 28–35.

Picella, D. V. (1996). Use of a relational database program for quantification of the CNS role. *Clinical Nurse Specialist, 10,* 301–308.

Prevost, S. S. (2002). Clinical nurse specialist outcomes: Vision, voice and value. *Clinical Nurse Specialist, 16,* 119–124.

Rantz, M. J., Popejoy, L., Petroski, G. F., et al. (2001). Randomized clinical trial of a quality improvement intervention in nursing homes. *Gerontologist, 41,* 525–538.

Redman, B. K. (1998). *Measurement tools in patient education.* New York: Springer Publishing Company.

Robichaud, A., & Hamric, A. B. (1986). Time documentation of clinical nurse specialist activities. *Journal of Nursing Administration, 16,* 31–36.

Scott, R. A. (1999). A description of the roles, activities, and skills of clinical nurse specialists in the United States. *Clinical Nurse Specialist, 13,* 183–190.

Sheehy, C. M., Saewert, K. J., Bell, S. K., Steinbinder, A., Cromwell, S. L., & McNamara, A. M. (2000). Using clinical models to frame outcomes evaluation: The Arizona Nurses' Association nursing report card project. *Outcomes Management for Nursing Practice, 4,* 13–18.

Tijhuis, G. J., Zwinderman, A. H., Hazes, J. W., et al. (2002). A randomized comparison of care provided by a clinical nurse specialist, an inpatient team, and a day patient team in rheumatoid arthritis. *Arthritis and Rheumatism, 47,* 525–531.

Tsay, S. L., Lee, U. C., & Lee, Y. C. (2005). Effects of an adaptation training programme for patients with end-stage renal disease. *Journal of Advanced Nursing, 50,* 39–46.

Underhill, M. A. (1993). *Product evaluation and selection: A nursing model for product review.* Unpublished manuscript, Community Hospitals of Indianapolis.

Vollman, K. M., & Stewart, K. H. (1996). Can we afford not to have clinical nurse specialists? *AACN Clinical Issues, 7*(2), 315–323.

Webster's new universal unabridged dictionary (deluxe 2nd ed.). (1983). New York: Simon and Schuster.

Wells, N., Erickson, S., & Spinella, J. (1996). Role transition: From clinical nurse specialist to clinical nurse specialist/case manager. *Journal of Nursing Administration, 26,* 23–28.

Wheeler, E. C. (1999). The effect of the clinical nurse specialist on patient outcomes. *Critical Care Nursing Clinics of North America, 11,* 269–275.

White, C. L. (1999). Changing pain management practice and impact on patient outcomes. *Clinical Nurse Specialist, 13,* 166–172.

Willoughby, D., & Burroughs, D. A. (2001). CNS-managed diabetes foot-care clinic: A descriptive survey of characteristics and foot-care behaviors of the patient population. *Clinical Nurse Specialist, 15,* 52–57.

Wilson-Barnett, J., & Beech, S. (1994). Evaluating the clinical nurse specialist. A review. *International Journal of Nursing Studies, 31,* 561–571.

Wong, S. T. (1998). Outcomes of nursing care: How do we know? *Clinical Nurse Specialist, 12,* 147–151.

9

Outcomes Measurement in Nurse-Midwifery Practice

RHONDA ARTHUR, JULIE MARFELL, AND SUZAN ULRICH

In a 2001 report, the Institute of Medicine (IOM) stated that health care today frequently causes harm to patients and routinely fails to deliver its potential benefits. The IOM report asserts that fundamental, sweeping redesign of the entire health care system is needed. In today's culture of limited health care resources and dramatic need for change in health care policy, nurse-midwives are in a unique expert position to write, lobby, and support beneficial health care policies in the arena of women's and infants' health (IOM, 2001).

In order to delineate areas of maternal–child health care that are favorable or need improvement, identification of desired outcomes and effective methods of outcome measurement are essential. Data from clinical outcomes studies in midwifery help to improve the quality of clinical care for patients, enhance cost-effectiveness, define practice guidelines or protocols, manage resources, and establish the basis for contracting with third-party payors. Clinical outcomes data also provide support for health policy changes that will permit nurse-midwives to provide much-needed quality care.

Acknowledgment: The authors would like to acknowledge the authors of the nurse-midwifery chapter in the first edition of this book: Mary Ellen Murray and Kelly Lindgren.

This chapter will discuss outcomes for nurse-midwifery practice. Suggested outcome classifications in midwifery practice that include examples of specific client and aggregate data and outcomes studies regarding nurse-midwifery practice are considered. The definition of health care outcomes and the process of evaluating these in relation to nurse-midwifery practice are also explored.

HISTORICAL PERSPECTIVE

Outcome evaluation of nurse-midwifery practice in the United States is as old as the profession. Mary Breckenridge brought nurse-midwifery to America in 1925 and created the Frontier Nursing Service (FNS). FNS was a demonstration project that provided health care to the rural poor in southeastern Kentucky. Mrs. Breckenridge took the advice of one of her consultants, Dr. McCormack, who said she would be unable to determine the scope of the FNS without a complete assessment of the health status of the community. Her first step in establishing the FNS was to ride over 700 square miles on horseback to obtain health histories of all the area families so that the impact of the nurse-midwives could be measured (Breckinridge, 1981).

Meticulous records were kept at the FNS. The Metropolitan Life Insurance Corporation was asked to analyze the data of the first 1,000 births attended by the nurse-midwives at FNS. The results were incredible. Dr. Louis Dublin reported, "The study shows conclusively that the type of service rendered by the Frontier nurses safeguards the life of mother and Babe. If such service were available to the women of the country generally, there would be a saving of 10,000 mothers' lives a year in the United States. There would be 30,000 less stillbirths and 30,000 more children alive at the end of the first month of life" (Tom, 1982, p. 8). One sees that measuring nurse-midwifery outcomes started with the first nurse-midwifery service in the United States and has been an integral component of establishing nurse-midwifery as a profession in the United States.

The American College of Nurse-Midwives (ACNM) was established in 1929. ACNM is a professional organization for nurse-midwives with the mission of promoting the health and well-being of women and infants. The ACNM defines eight standards for the practice of midwifery. It is no surprise that each of these standards is related to quality and safety outcomes. The ACNM encourages data collection related to these standards for benchmarking. Benchmarking is the process of comparing one's individual practice to the practice of others in the same field. This comparison is useful in the identification of both clinical and operational practices that are the most beneficial so that best practices can be identified and implemented (ACNM, 2005).

In 1998, the University of California at San Francisco Center for the Health Professions convened a task force on midwifery in order to examine the effects of health care market changes on the practice of the profession. The work of the task force resulted in 14 recommendations related to midwifery practice. In discussing research, the task force recommended that research should be strengthened and funded in the following areas that relate to outcome measurement:

- Descriptions and outcome analyses of midwifery methods and processes
- Analyses of midwifery practice outcomes
- Cost-benefit, cost-effectiveness, and cost-utility analyses
- Satisfaction with maternity and midwifery care
- Midwifery practice and benchmarking data (among midwives)

Certified nurse-midwives (CNMs) are driven by a passion for caring for women and babies. Intimate interpersonal relationships and family-centered care characterize their clinical practice. Because nurse-midwives are concerned with quality improvement and want to be included in much-needed health policy reform, nurse-midwives must become even more active in outcome measurement and data collection. Since the time of the UCSF task force, many of these outcomes have been measured. A review of that literature is included in this chapter.

DEFINITIONS OF OUTCOMES

The emphases on outcomes in health care in general are not new. The contemporary process began with Florence Nightingale, who first studied mortality and morbidity statistics in the Crimean War. Since then, multiple definitions of health care outcomes have been put forth in the literature, but all include some common elements. Outcomes on health care have been defined as:

- The end result of a process of care
- A measurable change in the health status or behavior of clients
- The desired and realistic condition of clients recorded at intervals during the care process
- A measurable, expected, client-focused goal

PURPOSE OF OUTCOMES MEASUREMENT IN NURSE-MIDWIFERY PRACTICE

The most compelling rationale for outcome measurement is that it assists in efforts to improve the quality of clinical care for patients. A recent report by the American College of Nurse-Midwives (2008) highlights that high-quality care, which includes high levels of client satisfaction and lower cost, is provided by CNMs with outcomes equal to or better than those of obstetricians or gynecologists.

One approach to initiating an outcome study is to define a care process that leads to identified outcomes at predictable times. This is exemplified in the design of protocols or practice guidelines and/or critical pathways (alternatively called care maps, clinical pathways, or multidisciplinary care plans). In this approach, the plan of care for a certain period of time, usually 24 hours, is carefully laid out by expert clinicians using evidence gathered from the literature. The assessments, medications, interventions, client teaching, and expected clinical outcomes are all listed. While these guidelines still require individualization to meet the needs of unique patients, the wisdom of such a tool is that a link is created between process and outcome. A defined practice process leads to predictable and measurable clinical outcomes. This assures that the care process can be replicated, evaluated, and taught to novices in the profession.

A second reason for outcome measurement is to enhance cost-effectiveness. In cost-effectiveness studies, alternative methods of obtaining the same goal are compared. Clients with similar conditions may be treated with alternative approaches, often with significantly different costs but with very similar outcomes. Studies that document the cost-effectiveness of nurse-midwifery practice while maintaining clinical outcomes have long been documented (Cherry & Foster, 1982; Lubic, 1981; Oakley et al., 1996; Reid & Morris, 1979; Stewart & Clark, 1982). Jackson et al. (2003) discuss collaborative care with CNM versus traditional physician-based care and the decrease in length of stay and in number of emergency room visits documented in women in collaborative care. The safety outcomes in the neonates in this study were similar across both groups.

Alternatively, clients of CNMs and physicians with similar conditions may be treated with different approaches, and one group may experience superior outcomes. An example of this is that physicians more often complete episiotomies, while the CNM might try different approaches such as perineal massage, warm packs, or positioning to reduce the need for episiotomy as well as overall perineal trauma during childbirth (Hastings-Tolsma, Vincent, Emeis, & Francisco, 2007; Robinson, Norwitz, Cohen, & Lieberman, 2000).

A third reason for outcome measurement is that, as independent practitioners, the measurement of clinical and fiscal outcomes aids nurse-midwives in the management of their group or solo practice. Data from clinical outcomes will help to define practice guidelines or protocols. If, for example, one wishes to establish guidelines for hydration during labor, it is necessary to understand what outcomes are associated with alternative means of hydration (intravenous solutions or oral fluids). Is one method more effective in meeting tissue needs? Is one method more satisfactory to clients? These are measurements of clinical outcomes. At another level, the CNM considers the costs associated with each alternative intervention and outcome. Data from fiscal outcome measurement will help to determine charges, manage resources, and establish the basis for contracting with third-party payors.

Finally outcome measurement gives evidence and support to the practice of midwifery. Examples of how quality outcomes can influence and increase appreciation and accessibility of nurse-midwifery practice in the United States include the 2004 Virginia Governor's Task Force on Health Care Reform recommendations for the development and funding of pilot birth centers in rural areas. The purpose of these sites is to demonstrate the effectiveness of midwifery care and increase access to high-quality pregnancy-related care. The recommendations call for collection and annual reporting of data by the pilot sites, using the American Association of Birth Centers Uniform Data Set (Governor's Health Reform Commission, 2007).

Research is the basis of all clinical practice, a guiding principle shared by all disciplines. It is this requirement for evidence-based practice that is another rationale for outcome measurement in nurse-midwifery practice. While outcome measurement is not synonymous with research, the two methodologies both provide empirical support for evidence-based changes in clinical practice.

CLASSIFICATION OF OUTCOMES MEASUREMENT FOR NURSE-MIDWIFERY PRACTICE

There are several approaches to the classification of outcomes within nurse-midwifery practice. Each method provides data for evidence-based clinical practice. The following outcome classification will be discussed: physiological, perceptual, psychosocial, cognitive, functional, and fiscal.

Physiological outcomes are those that have to do with the impact of CNM interventions on the process of birth. The division of physiological outcomes is somewhat arbitrary, since all nurses employ a holistic approach to health care, recognizing the interrelatedness of perceptual and psychosocial outcomes. Physiological outcomes can be further divided into groups of expected birth outcomes as well as adverse outcomes. It may be more helpful in outcome studies to focus on expected birth outcomes and to designate adverse events as variances from the usual and expected outcomes. Both classifications are of interest to CNMs, since this information provides direction for clinical care improvement. Examples of physiological outcomes in midwifery practice include blood glucose levels, iron deficiency anemia, fetal heart rate, maternal breathing patterns, and use of relaxation techniques in labor.

Perceptual outcomes are defined in terms of patient satisfaction. This may include satisfaction with CNMs as providers, with the facilities, with the care received, or with the clinical outcomes. It is important to understand that perception refers to the situation as the client views it or understands it. Whether this is or is not entirely congruent with the provider's reality does not matter. What does matter is that this is the client's perception of reality. Perceptual outcomes are crucial to the marketing and public acceptance of nurse-midwifery service.

Psychosocial outcomes are those that have to do with such things as the client's affective state, self-image, self-esteem, and interpersonal relationships. Examples of psychosocial outcomes that would be of clinical interest to nurse-midwives include: maternal–infant bonding, presence of social support, confidence in ability to care for infant, comfort with pregnant body image, and sense of self-actualization associated with childbirth.

Cognitive outcomes include the knowledge and skills that the client will need to safely and effectively care for herself and/or an infant. These would include the knowledge of prenatal nutrition, breastfeeding skills, and the signs and symptoms of postpartum infection.

Functional outcomes have to do with the maintenance or improvement of physical functioning. While there are standardized measures of functional outcomes, such as various Activities of Daily Living (ADL) or Independent Activities of Daily Living (IADL) scores, most CNM clients are women involved in a healthy childbearing process. There are standardized tools that measure functional outcomes in the postpartum woman; for example, the Childbirth Impact Profile (Tulman, Fawcett, Groblewski, & Silverman, 1990) and the Inventory of Functional Status after (Tulman & Fawcett, 1988). Examples of functional outcomes include the ability to care for the infant and readiness to return to a job outside the home.

Fiscal outcomes involve those having to do with the cost of care. Because many CNMs are in independent or group practice, understanding these outcomes is crucial to the survival of their clinical practice. Fiscal measures include such things as cost per case, hospitalization costs, length of stay, incremental costs of specialized nursing care during labor, reimbursement by payor, and laboratory costs. There are two approaches to the measurement of fiscal outcomes: cost data and charge data.

Charge Data Analysis

Some institutions use charges as a proxy measurement for costs. Charges are defined as the charges appearing on the client's bill. Charges are somewhat arbitrary and do include some profit or mark-up amount added to the cost of producing a service or product. Just as a department store adds a mark-up to the charge for clothing or appliances, so does a health care system add a profit amount to the cost of producing a service. Charges are the same for each client for each procedure and do not reflect policy or group discounts. Because contractual payors often receive a provider discount, it is important that charges be studied before the discounts are applied for the purpose of outcomes measurement. Charges can be collected from both the client billing records and from the provider's professional service records.

Cost Analysis

Other institutions have a cost-accounting system that will permit the measurement of actual costs of client care, that is, the cost of the service being produced. Cost is a complex concept and can be further reduced to a consideration of direct costs (supplies, salaries, rent) and indirect costs (employee benefits, costs allocated by other departments, such as a portion of the building maintenance). Some costs are defined as fixed, that is, they do not change with an increase in client volume. An example of a fixed cost would be heat and light costs. Other costs are variable, meaning that they change with client volume. Laundry and housekeeping costs are examples of variable costs.

What is important in fiscal outcome measurement is that CNMs understand what is included in the costs or charges in order to make appropriate comparisons. Another consideration is that charges in a clinical practice may be "bundled." This means that there is a prospective fee determined by an organization for a particular set of services. For example, hospital charges associated with a normal vaginal delivery may be set at $4,000. This is one all-inclusive fee and there will not be additional charges reflected on the client billing record. This approach does make it difficult to determine variation in fiscal outcomes. If there are no other cost data available when charges are bundled, it is difficult to assess the effect of practice changes on costs.

A decision must be made as to the appropriate interval or timing of charge or cost outcome data collection for nurse-midwifery clients. The purpose of the study will determine the period of measurement. If charges are to represent the entire period of pregnancy, one method to consider is to define the period from the date of determination of pregnancy until 2 months after birth in order to capture the full scope of the charges for the mother. When collecting fiscal data related to infant outcomes, similar decisions regarding the appropriate measurement interval must be made. Because many infants do not remain within the CNM system, but move to pediatric care, this is an important decision.

WRITING CLIENT OUTCOMES

Writing client outcomes is not difficult. It is something that was a part of undergraduate nursing education and included as a step in the nursing process: assessment, analysis, outcome identification, planning, implementation, and outcome evaluation. Now the CNM builds on that foundation and uses the knowledge and skill base of nurse-midwifery practice to identify and write outcomes for clients during the perinatal period. Start by asking two basic questions:

1. What results would you (the CNM) like to see as a result of the care process?
2. When will the results likely be achieved by the client and/or family?

When initiating outcome studies, it is essential to be cognizant of some fundamental principles in outcome analysis. These principles are:

1. *Outcomes must be measurable.* A CNM outcome that states that "client satisfaction will improve" is not measurable. It is necessary to be explicit about the indicators that will be used to measure satisfaction. The CNM in this case must specify the tool to be used to measure client satisfaction. For example, "Scores on the Picker patient satisfaction tool will increase after CNM care" is a specific measurable outcome.
2. *The outcome must relate to the care process or intervention.* Spontaneous pushing during labor can reasonably be expected to relate to the postpartum perineal condition.
3. *The outcome should be realistic for both the client and the CNM.* While improving client nutrition is a desirable outcome, there will be some clients who have no interest in the outcome and no amount of education and teaching material will improve their knowledge of nutrition or alter intake. It is important, however, to study negative outcomes as well as positive ones. There is much to be learned from both.
4. *Outcomes are measured within an accessible time span.* If a CNM wishes to study maternal–infant bonding, comparing attachment indications at 1 week of age to those of 1 year of age for the

same subjects, there will be major difficulties in maintaining the subjects in the study. This is not to negate the value of the study, but to help the CNM anticipate the inherent challenges in such a design.

5. *The risk status of the subject population is described.* Risk is defined as "the presence or absence of selected factors associated with non-optimal outcomes" (Selwyn, 1990). While the typical population of clients of CNMs is described as low to moderate risk, there are clinical differences among midwifery practices as to what constitutes low risk. Many studies use the risk factors that would preclude admission to the midwifery service as descriptors of the status of the population. This might include such things as hypertension requiring medication during pregnancy, serious cardiac disease, chronic renal or lung disease, known multiple gestation, or planned cesarean delivery. While there is debate in the literature regarding the accuracy of obstetric risk-assessment instruments, it is necessary that the risk profile be described so that appropriate comparisons can be made.

6. *All data collection has a cost.* Often novices at outcomes studies ask, "How many subjects are needed?" The only answer is, "It depends." It depends on the size of the population available, the sensitivity of the instrument used to measure outcomes, and the resources available to commit to data collection. More is usually better, but it is necessary to be realistic about the cost of data collection. Some outcomes may be collected for all clients within the midwifery service. At other times, sampling techniques may be used after preliminary analysis of a pilot that would yield sufficient data to conduct a power analysis. Such an analysis is a means of establishing that the study was conducted on a large enough sample to find an effect or relationship among variables, if indeed it does exist.

Here are some examples of individual client outcomes written for a nurse-midwifery practice:

1. *For a client at the first prenatal visit:* Client will verbalize an understanding of 2,200-calorie diet, the food pyramid, and dietary needs in pregnancy such as iron and calcium, and complete a 3-day intake diary by her next visit.

2. *For a client at the 8-month visit:* Client will demonstrate knowledge of signs and symptoms of onset of labor and verbalize when to call CNM.
3. *For a client at her first postpartum visit:* Breastfeeding at least 8 to 12 times per day, starting 1 week after delivery.

Note that all of these outcomes are written for an individual client. It is also important to recognize the importance of individual outcomes as well as the aggregate outcomes. Certified nurse-midwives are concerned with outcome evaluation both on an individual client basis and in aggregate groups. This process helps the CNM to rapidly identify deviations from expected outcomes and to adjust individual client care appropriately.

Outcome measurements on aggregate groups are defined as issues related to a specific, identified population. Outcomes for the aggregate group would be those that are appropriate for all clients within the nurse-midwifery service. These outcomes might include the following:

1. Verbalize signs and symptoms of postpartum endometritis before discharge from birthing center
2. Demonstrate safety in taking infant temperature, bathing infant, and positioning infant in crib within 24 hours of birth
3. Adhere to recommended schedule for follow-up postpartum visits
4. Presence and extent of perineal laceration

It is often helpful to use a formal approach for identifying clinical outcomes. It is assumed that the subject of the outcome is the client herself or some attribute of the client (e.g., a blood value, the position of the infant, blood loss). The client's behavior is the observable activity or measurement that the client will demonstrate at some future time. Things like drinking, walking, reporting, or the achievement of specific vital signs or lab values are examples of client behaviors. The criterion of performance sets the parameters for the behavior identified in the outcome (Murray & Atkinson, 2000). In clinical practice, the CNM may want the hemoglobin not to drop below 10.5 g/dL and weight gain not to exceed 35 lb. The time frame is a realistic estimate of when the client can reasonably be expected to achieve the outcome. Some outcomes are specific to the first trimester (e.g., taking supplements that include folic acid, avoiding medications that are possible teratogens); others begin at the first stage of labor (e.g., use of different techniques for relaxation, maintenance of hydration). Finally, a condition may be added if necessary. The CNM might specify the conditions under which the behavior specified in the outcome is to occur. Examples of such conditions: " . . . with the assistance of client's mother" or " . . . after 1 month of iron supplements" or " . . . using a food pyramid picture."

In clinical practice, when thinking of identifying client outcomes, it is important to emphasize that outcomes must be individualized for particular clients. Outcomes that are mutually established with clients are much more likely to be achieved than those that are solely determined by a CNM. There is also a cultural component to outcomes. What is desirable within one culture may be inappropriate in others. For example, in some cultures a grandmother plays a significant role in care of both the infant and the new mother. In such a case, the CNM needs to incorporate the grandmother, as a significant other, in any outcome measurement of the care process.

SCHEDULED MEASUREMENTS OF OUTCOMES

Essential to planning any outcome measurement study is a consideration of the measurement of the outcome. This is a major clinical consideration, requiring the knowledge of nurse-midwifery practice. One schema used by CNMs is to consider the following time periods: prenatal care (trimesters or weeks), intrapartum care (which may be further divided into stages of labor), and postpartum care (first 2 to 12 hours).

Another way to define time intervals might be to consider interim and discharge outcomes. At the completion of the childbirth process, there are some outcomes that signify the completion of the care process for that episode of care. The client may be independent in infant care and/or may have established a strong maternal–child bond and/or established new health-and-wellness patterns reflective of being a family. At this time, usually within 6 to 8 weeks postpartum, the CNM may discharge the client from the care relationship. While some women choose to remain in the CNM practice for primary care, the focus shifts from maternity care to well-woman care. Thus there is the completion of one phase of care and transition into another. Outcomes may then be classified as interim outcomes (all those occurring during the care process) and discharge outcomes (those at the completion of the care process). If discharge outcomes are not achieved, it may be an indication that there is a need for additional care. For example, if a mother appears to be experiencing postpartum depression, the CNM may consider a referral to a mental health professional.

VARIANCE FROM EXPECTED OUTCOMES

Variances occur when an expected outcome is not met at all, met later than expected, or even met ahead of the time defined for measurement (Murray & Atkinson, 2000). A rather standard classification system for variances has evolved in recent years. The system attempts to classify variances according to their cause. *System variances* are those that result from variations in the system, perhaps scheduling glitches or computer downtime (Murray & Atkinson, 2000). A patient may have failed to keep a scheduled appointment simply because the information was incorrectly entered into the computer and the client did not know the true date of her next appointment. If the clinical outcome being measured is rate of kept appointments, this will result in a variance.

Another type of variance is a *provider variance*. One CNM provider may choose not to do certain lab procedures, feeling that for this particular client it is duplicative or unnecessary. This may result in a variance in lab charges due to a provider variance.

The third kind of variance is *client variance*. One client may be physically active, within normal weight range, and accustomed to engaging in strenuous cardiovascular exercise 3 times per week. This client may experience fewer discomforts of pregnancy, less weight gain, a shorter labor, and a faster recovery than defined in clinical outcomes. This is also an example of a *positive variance* if weight gain and labor length still fall within normal ranges. It is important to understand that not all variances are negative. Variances can mean that the client *exceeded* the usual outcomes. It is equally important for CNMs to study both positive and negative outcomes in order to effectively change their clinical practice.

TOOLS FOR OUTCOME DATA COLLECTION

Before selecting and purchasing a data collection tool or designing a new data collection tool that might be duplicative or have limited use, it is important to first understand what tools and programs are available and their intended uses and applications. Currently, there are several tools available to assist CNMs in the collection of outcome data. The American Association of Birth Centers (AABC) developed the Uniform Data Set (UDS), an online data registry that collects comprehensive data on both the process and outcomes of the nurse-midwifery model of care. It is intended that the data set be used to simultaneously collect data from all providers in hospital, birth-center, and home-birth settings. Data from the UDS will be used in the AABC's National Study of Optimal Birth. Through the use of this outcome-data collection, this study has the potential to collect data on up to 200,000 midwifery births a year and continue the premiere nurse-midwifery research begun in the National Birth Center Study (Rooks, Wetherby, & Ernst, 1992, 1992a, 1992b). The UDS is stored on a password-protected secured site and is HIPPA-compliant. The UDS also supplies the provider with comprehensive statistical reports that include reports required for birth center accreditation, benchmarking reports for the ACNM Benchmarking project, registration logs, delivery logs, incomplete reports, and custom reports (American Association of Birth Centers, 2007). The ACNM has created the ACNM Data Set Series. This set consists of one-page data sets pertaining to antepartum care, intrapartal care, postpartum care, newborn care, and primary health care to women. Currently, two data sets (intrapartum and antepartum) are completed and available for use through the ACNM's website. Additional software programs are available both commercially and through the Centers for Disease Control and Prevention. These include word processing, epidemiological analysis, and data-management programs.

SOURCES OF OUTCOME DATA

Because outcome studies all involve some costs, it is useful to understand some of the existing sources of outcome data available for health care information. These sources may decrease effort and costs when assessing outcome data. These are selected sources; not all health care systems will have all of them:

1. *Routinely collected administrative data.* This typically includes vital statistics (births, deaths), payor source, Medicare/Medicaid,

and claims data (which includes principal diagnosis and procedure codes, complications, comorbidities, and records of adverse events). There may also be a case mix index (CMI), which is a measure of the resources used to treat a clinical population (Adams, 1996). CMI is useful as a tool for making comparisons among populations when there is not another tool to use to adjust for severity of illness. The clients of CNMs could be assumed to typically have a low CMI relative to other hospitalized patients.

2. *Birth logs.* Outcome data may also be gathered from birth logs. Hospitals and birth centers routinely keep concise data that usually include information such as place of birth, maternal age, gravity/parity, date of first prenatal visit, number of prenatal visits, total weight gain, significant prenatal events, significant intrapartum events, and infant data. Historically, birth logs have been kept in handwritten logs on birthing units.

3. *Data sets.* Data may also be gathered from existing data sets. Data may be collected from data sets such as the UDS or the ACNM Data Set Series. Many of these sets include comprehensive care and outcome data.

4. *Discharge summary.* Upon a patient's discharge, hospitals complete a discharge summary that consists of data extracted from the chart. This may include such data elements as: Social Security number, medical record number, name, admission and discharge dates, length of stay, disposition (home, nursing home, or subacute facility), total charges, employment status, and race. A cautionary note is that when race is included in this data set, it may be incomplete and unreliable on account of diversity within racial categories, the number of people with biracial identities, and differences in self-assignment to potential categories (Alvidrez, Azocar, & Miranda, 1996; Foster & Martinez, 1995).

5. *Obstetric discharge summary.* Obstetric units will typically have a department-specific form that will include additional data. This form includes such data elements as: intrapartum procedures; postpartum procedures; and data related to lacerations, infection, or phlebitis. These data may be entered into a computerized database that permits easy access and retrieval.

6. *Program-specific data collection.* Each health care system may collect data related to specific programs. For CNMs this may

include newborn screens for hearing loss, medications used during hospitalization, tests ordered, car seats distributed, teen births, and early discharge.

7. *Disease registration.* Some institutions participate in registries for various diseases. Programs of interest to CNMs might include sexually transmitted diseases, HIV/AIDS, or birth defects. Some of the registries are required by state law and reporting by providers is mandated.

8. *Critical pathways or clinical practice guidelines.* These are forms of a multidisciplinary plan of care and are used in many systems. Some perinatal clinical pathways are initiated at the first client visit and outline a plan of care concluding at discharge from the midwifery service. Most pathways contain outcomes that are evaluated at specified times.

One caution when collecting outcome data is the need to protect the confidentiality of the clinical record data. Most institutions maintain rigorous control over who may access data and for what purposes. If a CNM is considering an outcome study that has the potential to be published, the approval of a Human Subject Protection Committee or Institutional Review Board is necessary. This must be done before the initiation of such a study. Typically, the use of data for quality-improvement studies does not require such approval, but then the CNM must understand that no publication of results is possible. When in doubt, it is recommended to seek consultation with the chairperson of the Human Subject Protection Committee at the institution.

REVIEW OF NURSE-MIDWIFERY OUTCOME STUDIES

Discussion of several selected studies will illustrate approaches to outcome measurement within nurse-midwifery clinical practice. While the studies are largely from a research perspective rather than a quality-improvement focus, the measurement principles are the same.

The National Birth Center Study (Rooks, Wetherby, & Ernst, 1992, 1992a, 1992b) was a landmark investigation of 18,000 women who enrolled at 84 birth centers across the United States. A full report of the study included descriptions of the birth center clients, the birth center care providers, and the birth center care itself. The study measured clinical outcomes of birth centers and compared them to outcomes of low-risk hospital births. Client satisfaction and satisfaction with charges were also measured. Findings from this study led the researchers to conclude that there is no evidence that hospitals are a safer place than birthing centers for low-risk births. While a complete summary is beyond the scope of this chapter, the three articles that provide the complete report are essential reading for CNMs. Table 9.1 gives examples of some study outcomes and conclusions.

A second study (Paine & Tinker Dawkins, 1992) compared two types of bearing-down techniques as they related to the fetal and maternal outcomes of "arterial umbilical cord blood pH" and "length of the second stage of labor." In this group, the care process was either using the Valsalva maneuver or spontaneous pushing. Although the subject size was small, the authors concluded that the choice of bearing-down method does not have a negative effect on either the mother or the infant.

In another study, Oakley et al. (1996) compared the outcomes of women cared for by obstetricians and CNMs in a hospital-based setting. The authors reported that fiscal outcomes, specifically hospital charges and professional service fees, were significantly less for women in the nurse-midwife group. The lesser charges are especially interesting since the charges for obstetrician services and CNM services were the same in this institution. There was one bundled charge for all perinatal care, so the differences that existed between providers reflected charges beyond the usual and customary practice. Oakley also reported differences in clinical outcomes of infant–mother separation, extent of perineal laceration, and the number of maternal complications, with CNM providers being significantly lower on each outcome.

A study of macrosomic infant (birth weight > 4,000 grams) outcomes (Nixon, Avery, & Savik, 1998) asked specific research questions, such as: Is there a difference in Apgar scores, birth morbidity, and shoulder dystocias between infants with birth weights of 2,500 to 3,999 grams, 4,000 to 4,499 grams, and >4,500 grams? They also studied route of delivery, maternal position at birth, and antenatal variables that might predict poor infant outcomes. Shoulder dystocia occurred more frequently in large infants, but ICU admission rates did not. Apgar scores at 1 and 5 minutes were significantly higher for infants weighing > 4,500 grams. The Apgar differences were not clinically significant. The authors concluded that nurse-midwifery management of the labor

EXEMPLAR OUTCOME STUDIES FROM THE LITERATURE

Table 9.1

AUTHOR	NUMBER OF SUBJECTS	CLINICAL OUTCOMES	FISCAL OUTCOMES	CONCLUSIONS
Rooks et al. (1992)	18,000 low-risk women in 84 birth centers across the United States	***Selected infant outcomes:*** Fetal distress Shoulder dystocia Neonatal deaths 1-minute, 5-minute Apgar Low birth weight ***Selected maternal outcomes:*** Hypertension Maternal fever Abruptio placenta Breast-feeding four or more weeks Cesarean section	Average cost of usual delivery in a hospital delivery room Average cost of complete package of prenatal and intrapartum care provided in birth centers (Health Insurance Association of American, 1982, #290)	"There is no evidence that hospitals are safer (than birth centers)."
Paine & Tinker (1992)	13 Valsalva subjects 16 spontaneous subjects	Length of the second stage labor Arterial umbilical cord pH	None	"There is no relationship between the second stage bearing down method and arterial umbilical cord blood pH and length of the second stage of labor."

(Table 9.1 continued)

AUTHOR	NUMBER OF SUBJECTS	CLINICAL OUTCOMES	FISCAL OUTCOMES	CONCLUSIONS
MacDorman & Singh (1998)	All U.S. singleton vaginal births at 35–43 weeks gestation in 1991; Physician 2634550 CNM 153194	Infant, neonatal, and perinatal mortality Low birth weight Mean birth weight	None	"National data supports the findings of previous studies that CNM's have excellent birth outcomes . . . .CNM's provide a safe and viable alternative to maternity care in the U.S. particularly for low to moderate risk women."
Nixon, Avery, & Savik (1998)	322 infants of > 4,000 grams including those who were cared for by CNM and delivered by an MD	***Selected infant outcomes:*** 1-minute Apgar 5-minute Apgar Shoulder dystocia Intensive care admission rates Mean gestational age Cesarean section rate Forceps Vacuum extraction	None	"This study demonstrates that nurse-midwifery management of labors resulting in births of infants over 4,000 grams results in Apgar scores similar to those documented in the literature."
Sampselle & Hines (1999)	39 primiparous women who had spontaneous vaginal births	Intact perineum First-degree laceration Second-degree or episiotomy Third-degree laceration Perineal pain during first postpartum week	None	"To date, no harm to the mother or fetus has been linked to the use of spontaneous pushing and a growing body of evidence suggests that there are clear benefits."

(continued)

(Table 9.1 continued)

AUTHOR	NUMBER OF SUBJECTS	CLINICAL OUTCOMES	FISCAL OUTCOMES	CONCLUSIONS
Robinson, Norwitz, Cohen, & Lieberman (2000)	1,576 Singleton term, spontaneous vaginal delivery nulliparous Hospital Midwife 565 Faculty 192 Private 819	Rate of episiotomy Rate of third-degree lacerations Rate of fourth-degree lacerations	None	"The strongest factor associated with episiotomy at delivery was the category of obstetric provider . . . midwives performed episiotomy at lower rates than private practice and faculty MDs."
Jackson et al. (2003)	2,957 low-income pregnant women	Antepartum complications Intrapartum complications Neonatal complications	None	"For low-risk women both types of care result in safe outcomes for mothers, but there were fewer operative deliveries and less medical resources used in the collaborative care groups."

(Table 9.1 continued)

AUTHOR	NUMBER OF SUBJECTS	CLINICAL OUTCOMES	FISCAL OUTCOMES	CONCLUSIONS
Craigin & Kennedy (2006)	375 moderate-risk women giving birth at an urban hospital (196 CNM) (197 physician)	Optimality Index—U.S. scoring 40 care processes and outcomes across pregnancy, parturition, neonatal condition, and postpartum maternal condition, with higher average Optimality Index scores indicating more optimal balance between interventions and outcomes for a given health status	None	"Even among moderate risk patients, the midwifery model of care with its limited use of interventions can produce outcomes equivalent to or better than those of the biomedical model."
Hastings-Tolsam, Vincent, Emeis, & Francisco (2007)	510 singleton pregnancy with largely uncomplicated pregnancy in nurse midwifery faculty practice	Perineal trauma	None	"Side-lying position for birth and perineal support and compress use are important interventions for decreasing perineal trauma."

of these mothers, in consultation with physicians, produced outcomes similar to those reported in the medical literature.

A study (Sampselle & Hines, 1999) examined the perineal outcomes of 39 women who had spontaneous vaginal births. Chart data was examined for documentation of extent of episiotomy and/or laceration sustained. Findings indicated that women who used spontaneous pushing were more likely to have intact perineums and less likely to have episiotomies and second- or third-degree lacerations. Although the results of this study are consistent with previous findings in the literature, the authors cite the need for conclusive evidence to be gathered in randomized clinical trials.

One comparison study (Jackson et al., 2003) looked at outcomes, safety, and resource-utilization differences between traditional physician-based care and a collaborative (CNM/obstetricians) management birth center. This study included 2,957 low-income pregnant women and their infants who presented for prenatal care at several sites. Data from this study revealed that complications in both groups were similar while the collaborative care group had a greater number of spontaneous vaginal deliveries and less epidural anesthesia use. The study authors concluded that for low-risk women, both types of care result in safe outcomes for mothers, but there were fewer operative deliveries and less medical resources used in the collaborative care groups.

A recent comparison study (Craigin & Kennedy, 2006) looked at midwifery and medical care practices and measured optimal perinatal outcomes in 375 moderate-risk women. This pilot study used a new instrument (the Optimality Index—US) to compare nurse-midwife and physician care among women who were at moderate risk for poor pregnancy outcomes. The instrument consisted of scoring 40 care processes and outcomes across pregnancy, parturition, neonatal condition, and postpartum maternal condition, with higher average Optimality Index scores indicating more optimal balance between interventions and outcomes for a given health status. These data were collected from patient records. The authors of this study found that comparable groups of moderate-risk women cared for by nurse-midwives experienced less use of technology and health outcomes equal to or better than those of women cared for by physicians and had equally positive neonatal outcomes. The researchers acknowledge a limitation of this study was the use of a relatively small convenience sample and recommend additional similar studies using this tool with similar populations of women.

Finally, another study (Hastings-Tolsma, Vincent, Emesis, & Fransisco, 2007) examined factors related to perineal trauma in childbirth. This retrospective analysis used recorded birth data from the Nurse Midwifery Clinical Data Set from 510 singleton pregnancies with uncomplicated prenatal courses. Data revealed that for all women, laceration was more likely in lithotomy position for birth. Factors found to be protective of the perineum during birth included perineal massage, warm-compress use, manual support, and birthing in the left-lateral position. The authors concluded that side-lying position for birth perineal support and compress use are important interventions for decreasing perineal trauma during childbirth.

CONCLUSION

In 2005, CNMs attended 7.4% of all births and 10.6% of spontaneous vaginal births. This is a significant rise from 20 years prior, when CNM-attended births were noted to represent 0.6% of all births (Martin et al., 2007). As the number of births attended by nurse-midwives increases, it is important to assess outcomes in order to justify fiscal, quality, and safety goals for the care of women and babies. Nurse-midwives are poised to improve the quality of health care and to be change agents in the policy arena related to maternal care. This chapter has reviewed outcomes for nurse-midwifery practice. Suggested outcome classifications in midwifery practice, including examples of specific client and aggregate data, and outcomes studies regarding nurse-midwifery practice were presented. The definition of health care outcomes and the process of evaluating these in relation to nurse-midwifery practice have also been discussed.

Nurse-midwives should use the frameworks presented in this chapter to begin analyzing their practices and evaluating their own practice outcomes based on measurements used in previous studies. Evidence-based practice guidelines and protocols need to be evaluated and updated to reflect current clinical practice. Data demonstrating the safety, quality, and fiscal attributes provided by nurse-midwives need to be widely available for health care providers and consumers to evaluate when making decisions about maternal care. This information will increase the quality and safety of care provided to women and babies and increase the availability of nurse-midwifery services.

REFERENCES

Adams, T. P. (1996). Case mix index: Nursing's new management tool. *Nursing Management, 27*(9), 31–32.

Alvidrez, J., Azocar, F., & Miranda, J. (1996). Demystifying the concept of ethnicity for psychotherapy researchers. *Journal of Counseling and Clinical Psychology, 64* (5), 903–908.

American Association of Birth Centers. (2007). *American Association of Birth Centers.* Retrieved June 23, 2008, from http:///www.birthcenters.org/

American College of Nurse-Midwives. (2008). *Nurse-midwifery in 2008: Evidence-based practice. A summary of research on midwifery practice in the United States.* Retrieved July 7, 2008, from http://www.midwife.org/siteFiles/news/nurse_midwifery_in_2008.pdf

Breckinridge, M. (1981). *Wide neighborhoods: A story of the Frontier Nursing Service.* Lexington, KY: The University Press of Kentucky.

Cherry, J., & Foster, J. (1982). Comparison of hospital charges generated by certified nurse-midwives' and physicians' clients. *Journal of Nurse-Midwifery, 77,* 7–11.

Craigin, L., & Kennedy, P. (2006). Linking obstetric and midwifery practice with optimal outcomes. *The Association of Women's Health, Obstetric and Neonatal Nurses, 35,* 779–785.

Foster, S. L., & Martinez, C. R. (1995). Ethnicity: Conceptual and methodological issues in child clinical research. *Journal of Clinical Child Psychology, 24,* 214–226.

Governor's Health Reform Commission. (2007). *Roadmap for Virginia's health: A report of the Governor's Health Reform Commission.* Retrieved June 27, 2008, from http://www.hhr.virginia.gov/Initiatives/HealthReform/MeetingMats/ FullCouncil/Health_ReformComm_Draft_Report.pdf

Harris, M. D. (1991). Clinical and financial outcomes in patient care in a home health care agency. *Journal of Nursing Quality Assurance, 5,* 41–49.

Hastings-Tolsma, M., Vincent, D., Emesis, C., & Francisco, T. (2007, May/June). Getting through birth in one piece: Protecting the perineum. *Maternal Child Nursing,* 158–164.

Institute of Medicine [IOM]. (2001). *Crossing the quality chasm: A new health system for the 21st century.* Washington, DC: U.S. Government Printing Office. Retrieved January 19, 2004, from http://www.iom.edu

Jackson, D. J., Lang, J. M., Swartz, W. H., Ganiants, T. G., Fullerton, J., Ecker, J., et al. (2003). Outcomes, safety, and resource utilization in a collaborative care birth center program compared with traditional physician-based perinatal care. *American Journal of Public Health, 93,* 999–1006.

Lubic, R. (1981). Evaluation of an out-of-hospital maternity center for low-risk maternity patients. In L. Aiken (Ed.), *Health policy and nursing practice.* New York: McGraw-Hill.

Macdorman, M. F., & Singh, G. K. (1998). Midwifery care, social and medical risk factors and birth outcomes in the USA. *Epidemiology and Community Health, 52,* 310–317.

Martin, J. A., Hamilton, B. E., Sutton, P. D., Ventura, S. J., Menacker, F., Kirmeyer, S., et al. (2007). Births: Final data for 2005. *National Vital Statistics Reports, 56*

(6), 1–104. Retrieved October 15, 2008, from http://www.cdc.gov/nchs/data/nvsr/nvsr56/nvsr56_06.pdf

Murray, M. E., & Atkinson, L. D. (2000). *Understanding the nursing process in a changing care environment* (6th ed.). New York: McGraw-Hill.

Nixon, S. A., Avery, M. D., & Savik, K. (1998). Outcomes of macrosomic infants in a nurse-midwifery service. *Journal of Nurse Midwifery, 43,* 280–286.

Oakley, D., Murray, M. E., Murtland, T., Hayashi, R., Anderson, H. F., Mayes, F., & Rooks, J. (1996). Comparisons of outcomes of maternity care by obstetricians and certified nurse midwives. *Obstetrics and Gynecology, 88,* 823–829.

Paine, L. L., Dower, C. M., & O'Neil, E. H. (1999). Midwifery in the 21st century: Recommendations from the Pew Health Professions Commission/USSF Center for the Health Profession 1998 Taskforce on Midwifery. *Journal of Nurse Midwifery, 44,* 341–348.

Paine, L. L., & Tinker Dawkins, D. (1992). The effect of maternal bearing-down efforts on arterial umbilical cord pH and length of the second stage of labor. *Journal of Nurse-Midwifery, 37,* 61–63.

Reid, M., & Morris, J. (1979). Perinatal care and cost effectiveness: Changes in health expenditures and birth outcomes following the establishment of a nurse-midwife program. *Medical Care, 17,* 491–500.

Robinson, J., Norwitz, E., Cohen, A., & Lieberman, E. (2000). Predictors of episiotomy use at first spontaneous vaginal delivery. *Obstetrics and Gynecology, 96,* 214–218.

Rooks, J., Weatherby, N. L., & Ernst, E. K. M. (1992). The National Birth Center Study, Part I. Methodology and prenatal care and referrals. *Journal of Nurse Midwifery, 37,* 222–253.

Rooks, J., Weatherby, N. L., & Ernst, E. K. M. (1992a). The National Birth Center Study, Part II. Intrapartum and immediate postpartum and neonatal care. *Journal of Nurse Midwifery, 37,* 301–330.

Rooks, J., Weatherby, N. L., & Ernst, E. K. M. (1992b). The National Birth Center Study, Part III. Intrapartum and immediate postpartum and neonatal complications and transfers, postpartum and neonatal care, outcomes, and client satisfaction. *Journal of Nurse Midwifery, 37,* 361–397.

Sampselle, C., & Hines, S. (1999). Spontaneous pushing during birth: Relationship to perineal outcomes. *Journal of Nurse-Midwifery, 44,* 36–39.

Selwyn, B. J. (1990). The accuracy of obstetric risk assessment instruments for predicting mortality, low birth weight, and preterm birth. In J. Merkatz & J. Thompson (Eds.), *New perspectives on premature care.* New York: Elsevier.

Stewart, R., & Clark, L. (1982). Nurse-midwifery practice in an in-hospital birthing center. *Journal of Nurse-Midwifery, 27,* 21–26.

Tom, S. A. (1982, July/August). The evolution of nurse-midwifery: 1900-1960. *Journal of Nurse Midwifery, 27,* 4–13.

Tulman, L., & Fawcett, J. (1988). Return of functional ability after childbirth. *Nursing Research, 37,* 77–81.

Tulman, L., Fawcett, J., Groblewski, L., & Silverman, L. (1990). Changes in functional status after childbirth. *Nursing Research, 39,* 70–75.

10 Outcomes Assessment in Nurse Anesthesia

MICHAEL J. KREMER AND MARGARET FAUT-CALLAHAN

AN OVERVIEW OF OUTCOMES RESEARCH IN NURSE ANESTHESIA

Certified registered nurse anesthetists (CRNAs) have been providing anesthesia care to patients in the United States for more than 125 years. Some 37,000 CRNAs administer 30 million anesthetics annually in the United States (AANA, 2008a).

Assessing outcomes of nurse anesthesia care is an essential component of CRNA practice. Participating in quality assessment activities is among the *Standards for Accreditation* (2006) promulgated by the Council on Accreditation of Nurse Anesthesia Educational Programs (COA, C20, 2006) and in the *Scope and Standards for Nurse Anesthesia Practice* (AANA, 2008b). Recent studies have compared outcomes of care provided by various mixes of anesthesia providers (Pine, Holt, & Lou, 2003; Simonson, Ahern, & Hendryx, 2007), and have demonstrated satisfactory clinical outcomes with anesthesia provided by CRNAs. However, there is no ongoing prospective multicenter data collection related to anesthesia outcomes.

Methodological challenges in anesthesia outcomes research include the various mixes of anesthesia providers. CRNAs may be the sole anesthesia providers in rural and medically underserved areas, as well as in combat settings. Office-based anesthesia may be provided by a CRNA working collaboratively with a surgeon. In other settings, an anesthesiologist may work collaboratively with two to four CRNAs administering concurrent anesthetics.

The earliest outcomes research in nurse anesthesia was conducted by pioneering nurse anesthetist Alice Magaw. Miss Magaw published a paper in the *Northwestern Lancet* in 1899 on over 3,000 ether and chloroform anesthetics she administered without a fatality at the Mayo Clinic (Bankert, 1989). It has been suggested that subsequent legal challenges to nurse anesthesia practice were defeated through the documentation of safe, quality care by Miss Magaw (Bankert, 1989). Like Nightingale (McDonald, 2001), this leader in the specialty of nurse anesthesia recognized that, in addition to clinical excellence, maintenance of a clinical database and dissemination of research findings in peer-reviewed literature were requisites of professionalism.

STUDIES OF ANESTHESIA OUTCOMES

Municipal or state-level study commissions that examined anesthetic morbidity and mortality in the 1930s and 1940s were hampered by the unwillingness of anesthesia providers to share their data (Ruth, 1945). No concerted effort was made to track anesthetic outcomes until the 1950s.

The first large-scale study of anesthesia morbidity and mortality was conducted by Beecher and Todd (1954). Muscle relaxants were found to be significantly associated with anesthetic morbidity and mortality. Neuromuscular blockade was not routine and analyses of outcomes by providers were not conducted.

In the 1970s, a rapid increase in malpractice insurance premiums prompted a new research method for investigating anesthetic outcomes: analysis of closed malpractice claims. Pioneered by the National Association of Insurance Commissioners, this methodology was adopted by the American Society of Anesthesiologists (ASA), which has conducted the largest anesthesia closed claims study to date (ASA, 2008; Brunner, 1984), with over 7,000 cases reviewed. Numerous publications have emanated from this study, often with the focus of lessons learned in specific practice-related areas, such as equipment, airway management, and specialty practice areas (Bhananker et al., 2006; Caplan, Vistica, Posner, & Cheney, 1997; Caplan, Ward, Posner, & Cheney, 1988; Chadwick, Posner, Caplan, Ward, & Cheney, 1991; Cheney, 1999; Cheney, Domino, Caplan, & Posner, 1999; Cheney, Posner, Caplan, & Gild, 1994; Cheney, Posner, Lee, Caplan, & Domino, 2006; Domino, 2004; Domino, Posner, Caplan, & Cheney, 1999; Fitzgibbon et al., 2004; Gild, Posner, Caplan, & Cheney, 1992; Jiminez et al., 2007; Lee, Posner, Domino, Caplan, & Cheney, 2004; Peterson et al., 2005; Robbertze, Posner, & Domino, 2006).

The American Association of Nurse Anesthetists Foundation (AANAF) has also conducted a closed claims study that is methodologically similar to the ASA study. Peer-reviewed papers related to this study have also focused on lessons learned in specific areas, such as preinduction activities and the genesis of perioperative respiratory, peripheral nerve, and other injuries (Crawforth, 2002; Fritzlen, Kremer, & Biddle, 2003; Jordan, Kremer, Crawforth, & Shott, 2001; Larson & Jordan, 2001; MacRae, 2007; Moody & Kremer, 2001). Note that distinctions in outcomes between anesthesia providers related to adverse outcomes have not been described in these studies.

Research findings from both the AANAF and the ASA studies demonstrate that the process of care, rather than patient acuity or procedure complexity, is most frequently associated with outcomes that are not optimal (Caplan, Vistica, Posner, & Cheney, 1997; Jordan, Kremer, Crawforth, & Shott, 2001; Kremer, Faut-Callahan, & Hicks, 2002; Petty, Kremer, & Biddle, 2002). To foster improved decision making and reinforce principles of care to decrease the incidence of adverse outcomes, human patient simulation has been used as an instructional tool for clinicians and trainees.

The use of human patient simulation in the context of high-fidelity simulation labs provides trainees and practitioners the opportunity to develop crisis management skills in rarely occurring, potentially fatal scenarios (Blum et al., 2004; Cooper et al., 2008; Coopmans & Biddle, 2008; Gaba, 2004; Register, Graham-Garcia, & Haas, 2003; Smith, Jacob, Segura, Dilger, & Torsher, 2008). Human patient simulation has also been used for nurse anesthesia faculty development (Hartland, Biddle, & Fallacaro, 2003) and critically evaluated as an educational tool by nurse anesthesia educators (Hotchkiss, Biddle, & Fallacaro, 2002).

As noted earlier, a major methodological and design challenge for outcomes research is that anesthetic mortality occurs rarely today, approximately 1:200,000 cases (Jones, 2001; Lema, 2003). The Centers for Medicare and Medicaid Studies, the Centers for Disease Control and Prevention, the American Hospital Association, the American Society of Anesthesiologists, the American College of Surgeons, and the Veterans' Administration are collectively developing strategies to reduce surgical morbidity by 50% over a 5-year period. A desired outcome of this process is construction of a grid that prospectively compares surgical patient acuity and procedure complexity with outcomes, especially morbidity and mortality (Lema, 2003).

An estimated 40 million surgical procedures, most accompanied by anesthesia, are performed annually. Meaningful and accurate outcome data for the types of surgeries and anesthetics (with or without anesthesia providers) can be collected in a multiyear, multicenter prospective study. Costs associated with such a study would be offset by reductions in unnecessary surgery, risky surgery, poor health care providers, perioperative deaths, and delayed discharge times (Lema, 2003). To date, no such study has been designed or implemented. Political, logistical, and economical constraints may account for failure to implement such a study. Research findings reported by closed claims investigators provide information regarding the genesis of anesthetic morbidity and mortality, but do not provide epidemiologic data (e.g., a numerator and denominator) on anesthetic morbidity and mortality.

OUTCOMES IN RURAL SETTINGS

Nurse anesthetists are the primary anesthesia providers in rural America, which enables health care facilities in these medically underserved settings to offer obstetrical, surgical, and trauma-stabilization services. In some states, nurse anesthetists are the sole anesthesia providers in nearly 100% of the rural hospitals (AANA, 2008a). There is a paucity of outcomes research on anesthesia provided in rural America. Case mix and patient outcomes have not been studied relative to the rural anesthesia workforce (Orkin, 1998).

Rural CRNAs provide a broad range of anesthesia-related services within and outside of the operating room. A recent study found significant differences in the employment settings of medically directed and nonmedically-directed CRNAs, the availability of certain anesthetic agents and monitoring devices, and the representation of surgical specialists based on the size of the rural community and hospital. However, this study did not examine anesthetic or surgical outcomes (Monti Seibert, Alexander, & Lupien, 2004).

An analysis of cesarean section outcomes showed no difference in complication rates when anesthesia was provided by a CRNA or a CRNA-physician team. Since solo CRNAs often provide anesthesia in rural settings, these findings help to quantify outcomes of CRNA-provided anesthesia in rural settings (Simonson, Ahern, & Hendryx, 2007).

A rare prospective study of anesthesia outcomes in a rural hospital described data collected over a 25-year period on patients who underwent open (e.g., right subcostal incision, nonlaparoscopic approach) cholecystectomies. These patients were statistically compared with matched controls from urban medical centers. All the anesthetics were administered by the same CRNA. There were no statistically significant differences in outcomes, including postoperative complications, between the two data sets (Callaghan, 1995).

Another study of rural anesthesia services involved surveying hospital administrators regarding their satisfaction with anesthesia services in rural Washington and Montana (Dunbar, Mayer, Fordyce, et al., 1998). Survey respondents indicated that they were satisfied with the anesthesia services provided. The authors noted that "all the administrators rated the care provided in their anesthesia departments as either good or very good" (Dunbar et al., 1998, p. 805). A replication of this study was conducted with rural Illinois hospital administrators, which also demonstrated that the majority of respondent administrators rated anesthesia care in their facilities as "good or very good" (Stark & Kremer, 2001). The perceptions by hospital administrators about anesthesia care in their facilities are important, since administrators have access to data such as morbidity and mortality reports and patient satisfaction surveys.

OUTCOME MEASUREMENT IN NURSE ANESTHESIA

There have been national-level discussions of the need for outcomes research in nurse anesthesia for many years. One of the first initiatives to collect outcomes data that could be analyzed in aggregate was the AQ Plus program, initiated by the AANA in 1989 (Kraus, 1994). AQ Plus software included patient demographics, surgical procedures, anesthetic agents, and techniques used. The program did not have wide market penetration and the software was not suitable for aggregate data analysis. To date, there have not been products developed for practicing CRNAs to track their clinical outcomes.

Many nurse anesthesia programs utilize Web-supported clinical case-tracking applications. This type of software captures data such as patient demographics, procedures performed, types of agents administered, duration of the case, and so forth. The data can be entered using a handheld personal digital assistant (PDA) and later uploaded to a Web site. The data can be reviewed in aggregate on the Web site, or downloaded to a spreadsheet application for individual or aggregate analyses. Perhaps practitioners will increasingly employ such applications for quality-improvement processes, but there is likely concern that such data would be legally discoverable in the event of a medical malpractice action.

Automated anesthesia records are used in some practice settings. When this is the case, the system chosen may be able to capture data related to quality assurance and outcomes assessment. The availability of digital information on multiple patients permits analysis of patient characteristics or intraoperative events to clinical outcomes. It is clear that meaningful outcomes analysis of rarely occurring events, such as anesthetic mortality, requires large data sets. For some outcomes, a single facility may not have sufficient patient volume to conduct rigorous outcomes analyses. Databases in digital format can be shared among several institutions, increasing analytic power. Third-party payors are interested in patient outcomes. The availability of digital anesthesia outcomes information allows its integration into other hospital databases. When information about anesthesia care is incorporated into the medical record, the role of anesthesia in overall patient outcomes can be assessed. Individual provider variations in clinical practice can also be studied (Thys, 2007).

FAILURE TO RESCUE

"Failure to rescue" describes failure to prevent clinically important deterioration, such as death or permanent disability from a complication of an underlying disease or a complication of medical care. Failure to rescue provides a measure of the degree to which providers responded to adverse occurrences that developed on their watch. It may be related to the quality of monitoring or to the efficacy of actions taken once early complications are recognized, or both (AHRQ, 2008a).

Initial studies of surgical morbidity and mortality correlated with other quality measures. Rates of failure to rescue have been outcomes measures in studies on the impact of nurse-staffing ratios (Aiken et al., 2003).

The Agency for Health Research and Quality (AHRQ) technical report that developed the AHRQ Patient Safety Indicators (McDonald et al., 2002) reviews the evidence supporting failure to rescue as a measure of the quality and safety of hospital care. Although failure to rescue was included in the final set of approved indicators, the expert panels that reviewed each potential indicator identified some unresolved concerns about its use. For example, patients with advanced disease processes may be especially difficult to rescue from complications such as sepsis and cardiac arrest. Patients with advanced illness may not desire "rescue" from such complications (AHRQ, 2008a).

"Failure to rescue" methodology has been used to study anesthesia outcomes related to the anesthesia providers involved (Pine, Holt, & Lou, 2003; Silber et al., 2000). These two papers analyzed a Pennsylvania Medicare data set. Risk-adjusted mortality rates of Medicare patients undergoing carotid endarterectomy, cholecystectomy, herniorrhaphy, hysterectomy, knee replacement, laminectomy, mastectomy, or prostatectomy were compared for anesthesiologist-directed and non-anesthesiologist-directed cases and analyzed for a 3-year period. The result was a statistically insignificant difference in negative outcomes between anesthesiologist-directed and non-anesthesiologist-directed cases.

Clinicians and administrators have assessed the degree to which the "failure to rescue" indicator identifies true problems in the process of care at the individual or system level. Failure-to-rescue complications can be flagged through administrative data, and the clinical course of events then evaluated. Many factors influence whether a case is included in the measure, such as existing health problems, the presence of complex comorbidities, and variations in clinical documentation and coding practices (Talsma, Bahl, & Campbell, 2008). Therefore, studies that employ failure-to-rescue methodology need to rigorously assess multiple covariates and their potential association with a given outcome.

NURSE ANESTHESIA OUTCOME MEASURES AND PROJECTS

Anesthesia outcomes research focuses on what Lohr (1988) described as "the five D's: death, disease, disability, discomfort, and dissatisfaction." A shift toward outcomes studies focused on other aspects of health such as survival rates, states of physiological and psychological health, and satisfaction with care rendered was described by Lohr (1988), and papers on these topics verify that such a shift occurred (Minnick & Pabst, 1988).

The AANA Foundation (AANAF) funds research and professional development for nurse anesthetists. Outcomes studies have been among the top priorities of the AANAF research agenda for some time. The AANAF mission is "advancing the science of anesthesia through education and research" (AANA, 2008c). Current AANAF research-funding priorities include the following topics: cultural diversity, distance education, evidence-based practice, health care economics and disparities, and patient safety and outcomes (AANA, 2008d).

The thrust of AANAF nurse anesthesia outcomes research has been the ongoing study of closed malpractice claims (Jordan, Kremer, Crawforth, & Shott, 2001). The goal of this study has been to determine the causes of anesthesia-related patient injury or death, identify trends in adverse anesthetic outcomes, and compare research findings with current standards of practice. Results of this study have affected practice standards (MacRae, 2007). For example, current COA requirements for pediatric clinical experience were affected by data from the AANAF closed claims study.

Data for the AANAF closed claims study were collected with the permission of insurance carriers for CRNAs who need to obtain their own malpractice coverage, such as those nurse anesthetists who are not hospital- or group-employed. Ongoing data analysis has demonstrated results that mirror those of the ASA closed claims study: The most frequently represented patients in the database are relatively healthy patients who underwent elective surgical procedures. Monetary awards were directly related to the severity of the adverse outcome. When anesthesia care was determined to be inappropriate, the severity of the injury and monetary award were higher (Jordan, Kremer, Crawforth, & Shott, 2001).

These research findings resulted in recommendations to study nurse anesthesia educational curricula and continuing education offerings. For example, the challenging area of office-based surgery and related closed claims research findings influenced the development of AANA guidelines for office anesthesia (AANA, 2008e).

CRNAs are pursuing doctoral education in greater numbers, which bodes well for the future of the specialty and the generation of additional outcomes research. Funding initiatives for doctoral study and interviews with CRNA doctoral students and active researchers attest to the richness of discovery that is evident in this growing community of scholars. As noted earlier, an AANAF research priority area is evidence-based practice (EBP) (AANA, 2008d). A fertile area for investigation is the impact of EBP on clinical outcomes.

EVIDENCE-BASED PRACTICE

New clinical information is generated more quickly than practicing clinicians and trainees can assimilate it. Nurse anesthesia students, faculty, and practitioners need the most current information regarding health care and anesthesia practice. This information need is acute for student registered nurse anesthetists, since they must rapidly learn complex specialty-related content and use this information to justify clinical actions to their faculty (Pellegrini, 2006). Using EBP concepts helps balance the demand for current information with the exponentially increasing supply of specialty-related research information.

Evidence-based practice has been described as "the integration of individual clinical expertise with the best available external clinical evidence from systematic research" (Sackett, 1998). Health care professionals may believe that their practices have always reflected evidence-based underpinnings, but performance assessments indicate this is not the case (McGlynn et al., 2003). Current literature advocates increased adoption of EBP, but EBP implementation is inconsistent (Kavey, 2008).

The Institute of Medicine Committee on the Health Professions Education Summit suggested a paradigm shift for health professions education. The principal goal of this process is that "all health professionals will be educated to deliver patient-centric care as members of an interdisciplinary team, emphasizing evidence-based practice, quality improvement approaches and informatics" (Greiner & Knebel, 2003).

This paradigm shift would include movement of health care delivery away from the traditional physician-dominated practice toward the concept of the physician as team leader, seeking the best evidence for patient care. Ideally, such physicians and teams will have the ability and expectation to continuously learn and change, through utilization of evidence-based clinical decision support, informatics, and clinical data repositories. The potential scope of this initiative clearly includes all health professionals (Kavey, 2008).

Nurses may have the most experience in using EBP, with a record dating back to the time of Nightingale (McDonald, 2001). Nurses are the largest group of health care providers in the United States, numbering almost 3 million. There are significant workforce shortages of nurses (8.5% vacancy rate) and CRNAs (12.5% vacancy rate) (Merwin, Stern, & Jordan, 2007). A survey of 3,000 U.S. licensed nurses demonstrated that almost half of the respondents were unfamiliar with the term *evidence-based medicine*. More than half of these survey respondents had not identified a clinical problem that required research, and 43% "sometimes, rarely or never" read nursing journals or texts (Pravikoff, Tanner, & Pierce, 2005).

Significant information literacy and access to adequate information technology are needed for implementation of EBP with tools such as best-practice databases, clinical practice guidelines, electronic medical records, and computerized physician order entry. Nurses report that access to evidence-based information can be "extremely difficult." Fewer than 50% of respondents to Pravikoff's 2005 survey reported available workstation access to the Internet. This may be offset by increasing use of handheld PDAs with functional Web browsers. However, attitudes towards EBP are complex, with a majority of nurses identifying a colleague or supervisor as their primary information source rather than any independent literature source.

One suggested educational direction is to include EBP as a core competency throughout all levels of nursing curricula. Related competencies should include formation of PICOT questions, where P = patient population, I = intervention or area of interest, C = comparison intervention or comparison group, O = outcome, and T = time frame. Students and practitioners need to be able to search for the best evidence (specifically preappraised evidence and evidence-based clinical practice guidelines) and integrate the best evidence with their clinical expertise and patient preferences related to clinical decisions. Students also need to be able to assess outcomes based on EBP changes and participate in team EBP projects. Graduate students should be required to demonstrate facility with synthesizing a body of evidence to initiate and evaluate practice changes to improve the health of individuals, lead practice changes based on the best evidence for populations of patients, generate evidence through outcomes management, and mentor others in EBP (NLN, 2008).

It is difficult for practitioners and trainees to remain current with the relevant advances in their fields of interest. The major bibliographic databases cover less than half of the world's literature and are biased toward, English-language publications. Textbooks, editorials, and reviews that have not been systematically prepared may be unreliable. Much evidence is unpublished, and yet unpublished data may have clinical significance. More easily accessible research papers tend to exaggerate the benefits of interventions (Cochrane Collaboration, 2008).

The Cochrane Library consists of a regularly updated collection of EBP databases, including *The Cochrane Database of Systematic Reviews.* This database includes systematic reviews of health care interventions that are produced and disseminated by the Cochrane Collaboration. *The Cochrane Library* is published quarterly and is available on CD-ROM and the Internet. Abstracts of the reviews are available to browse and search without charge on this Web site (Cochrane, 2008). Anesthesia-related *Cochrane Reviews* topics include the bispectral index (Punjasawadwong, Bunchungmonogkol, & Pongschiewboon, 2008) and the evidence base behind modern preoperative fasting guidelines (Stuart, 2006).

A recent review described the implementation of EBP in anesthesiology and critical care. The authors found that outcomes research employing evidence-based approaches was seen in subspecialty areas such as pediatrics, obstetrics, and general anesthesia, as well as critical care. The integration of individual expertise with data from externally conducted systematic research was described as a benefit of EBP. While EBP has its origins in the treatment- and diagnosis-related competencies of primary care, its tenets are applicable to nontherapeutic specialties like anesthesia and critical care (Schulman, Schardt, & Erb, 2008).

NURSE ANESTHESIA COMPETENCIES, CURRICULAR MODELS, AND EVIDENCE-BASED PRACTICE

Organizations seek to identify the core capabilities, or competencies, that have sustainable value and wide applicability to the customers that they serve. Professional nursing organizations, which serve the interests of patients, generally identify role-related competencies that describe their vision of the skills and abilities the individual nurse must possess (Callahan, 1988). For example, in the *AANA Code of Ethics for the Certified Registered Nurse Anesthetist* (AANA, 2008f), competence includes engaging in lifelong professional educational activities, participating in continuous quality improvement initiatives, and maintaining licensure according to statutory and regulatory requirements for recertification.

In education, AANA has adopted master's-level educational competencies required of the CRNA for entry into practice. These are the acquired knowledge, skills, and competencies in patient safety, perianesthetic management, critical thinking, communication, and the professional role identified by the Council on Accreditation of Nurse Anesthesia Educational Programs *Standards for Accreditation of Nurse Anesthesia Educational Programs* (January, 2006) SIII: Program of Study Criterion 20. One of the related criteria in this standard is critical thinking, which "is demonstrated by the ability of the graduate to provide nurse anesthesia care based on sound principles and research evidence" (COA, 2006).

Movement of advanced practice nursing education to the practice doctorate level has mandated additional competencies to reflect this educational level. The *Competencies for the CRNA Practitioner at the Clinical Doctorate Level* may serve as the framework upon which the curricula of practice-focused doctoral education programs in nurse anesthesia will be based. The *Competencies for the CRNA Practitioner at the Clinical Doctorate Level* complement the *Practice Doctorate Nurse Practitioner Entry-Level Competencies 2006* (AANA, 2007).

Several of the identified competencies for doctorally prepared CRNAs speak to EBP. For example, the competency area of biological systems, homeostasis, and pathogenesis advocates use of "a systematic outcomes analysis approach in the translation of research evidence and data in the arts and sciences to demonstrate that will have the expected effects on nurse anesthesia practice" (AANA, 2007).

In the competency area of health care improvement, doctorally prepared CRNAs are expected to use "EBP to inform clinical decision making in nurse anesthesia." Regarding competencies in technology and informatics, a practice doctorate-prepared CRNA would use "information systems/technology to support and improve patient care and health care systems; design, select, and use information technology to evaluate programs of care and health systems, and critically evaluate clinical and research databases used as clinical decision support resources" (AANA, 2007).

Pellegrini (2006) noted that, as nurse anesthesia curricula and clinical practice evolve, instructional methods will need to reflect EBP. The paradigm of using clinical judgment and expertise as the basis for clinical decision making will shift to a structure that incorporates the best available evidence to formulate clinical decisions, as described above in the technology and informatics competency, along with clinical experience and expertise. Implementation of EBP principles into nurse anesthesia education will yield a well-informed student along with ensuring that students and faculty remain at the forefront of the latest evidence that is available in the literature (Pellegrini, 2006).

When one is presented with a clinical question, the EBP analysis is as follows:

1. Define the problem or question in terms of the patient or problem, the intervention or comparison interventions used to answer the question, and the findings of the research reviewed.
2. Outline the current steps in one's clinical practice to address the problem.
3. Use a ranking system to determine the quality of evidence available in the literature. This hierarchy, in descending order, consists of findings from systematic review of well-designed clinical studies (meta-analyses); results of one or more appropriately designed studies (randomized trials, cohort studies); results of large case series and case reports; editorials and opinion pieces; animal research; and in vitro research.
4. Identify the resources available to implement any proposed changes to practice, to differentiate which evidence is applicable to the current clinical setting.
5. Assess the validity of the research presented with a consistent rubric, to review clinical trials that includes these questions:

   a. Did the clinical trials studied include elements such as randomization of subjects, adequate sample size, and appropriate statistical analysis?
   b. Were the results relevant to clinical practice?
   c. Were the therapeutic interventions reported feasible for clinical practice?
   d. Were all research subjects accounted for at the end of the study?

The "pyramid of evidence" is central to EBP. This concept is depicted in Figure 10.1. Utilization of EBP in anesthesia practice is increasing. Longitudinal outcomes studies in practices where EBP is employed can determine if associations exist between the implementation of EBP and improved outcomes.

OUTCOMES ECONOMICS AND POLICY DEVELOPMENTS

One study estimated costs based on cases from four anesthesia services at four different hospitals: an academic medical center, a large and a medium-size community hospital, and a small community hospital. Labor cost projections for 10,000 anesthetics delivered annually showed that an all-CRNA anesthesia care model cost less than an all-physician model. The cost savings for a mixed model of physicians and CRNAs (in ratios ranging from 1:1 to 1:4) ranged from 33% to 41% of the total costs for an all-physician model (Cromwell & Snyder, 2000). There was not an explicit comparison of outcomes in this study, but other investigators have posited that the physician-CRNA model is cost-effective and safe (Abenstein & Warner, 1996).

   A 2001 Centers for Medicare & Medicaid Studies rule permitted states to opt out of the federal supervision requirement for anesthesiologist supervision of CRNAs. The rule amended the requirement in the Anesthesia Services Condition of Participation for hospitals, the Surgical Services Condition of Coverage for Ambulatory Surgical Centers, and the Surgical Services Condition of Participation for Critical Access Hospitals. To date, the governors of 14 states have opted out of this requirement (AANA, 2008g).

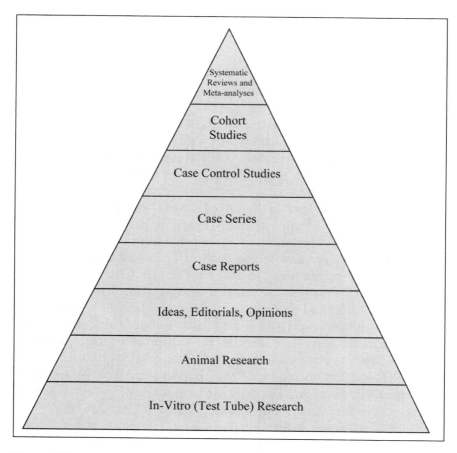

Figure 10.1 The pyramid of evidence.

For a state to "opt out" of the federal supervision requirement, the state's governor must send a letter to CMS that attests that: (1) the governor has consulted with the state's boards of medicine and nursing about issues related to access to and the quality of anesthesia services in the state; (2) it is in the best interest of the state's citizens to opt-out of the current federal physician-supervision requirement; and (3) the opt-out is consistent with state law (AANA, 2008g). This achievement would not have been possible without the outcomes achieved by

CRNAs, especially when providing care to citizens in rural and medically underserved areas.

CONCLUSIONS

Outcomes research seeks understanding of the end results of certain health care practices and interventions. End results include effects that people experience and care about, such as improvement in functional status and quality of life, as well as morbidity and mortality. Linkage of care provided to the attained outcomes is a function of outcomes research, which can lead to improved care. Outcomes research has altered the culture of clinical practice and health care research by changing how we assess the end results of health care services. Outcomes research is the key to knowing the quality of care that can be achieved, and how providers can move to that level of care (AHRQ, 2008b).

Issues that face advanced practice nursing related to justification of the use of APNs and measurement of the effects of APN services on patients and health care systems are similar to but distinct from those faced by individual APNs evaluating the outcomes of their particular practices. There is clearly a need for well-designed longitudinal assessments of how APNs, including CRNAs, impact clinical outcomes. Since reimbursement decisions are driven by evidence of provider performance, APNs who lack valid, reliable data to substantiate their "impactfulness" will struggle for equitable reimbursement (Ingersoll, 2008).

To address the need for addition of APN-sensitive outcome indicators requires development of electronic information systems that identify and track APN outcome data. This process requires national agreement on core outcome indicators germane to APNs and initiation of standards that support collection of APN-sensitive data. Health care organizations and third-party payers will be integral to the development of such systems (Ingersoll, 2008).

Outcomes measurement is interconnected with every other aspect of the APN role. Effective outcomes measurement and performance reviews related to outcomes criteria require APNs to work collaboratively with others, to plan and organize processes of care and assessment of quality in complex health-services environments, and to allow scrutiny of their individual practices by others. In the end, the quality and value of care will improve along with recognition by the community of the impact of the APN on outcomes of care (Ingersoll, 2008).

Nurses and APNs, including CRNAs, continue to be interested and involved in the area of outcomes to assure that patients are represented as more than a composite of physiologic variables or billing data. The use of outcomes measures has helped APNs articulate their unique value and contributions to the well-being of patients. Many health care outcomes measures do not identify or quantify the contributions of nurses. In anesthesia care, the role of CRNAs in patient outcomes has been at times diminished as a result of the economic competition between CRNAs and their physician counterparts.

Given the worsening mismatch between population health care needs and available resources, APNs and CRNAs must continue to demonstrate quality and cost-effectiveness. Historically, quality of care has been described using variables such as morbidity, mortality, length of stay, readmission, and cost. Methods have not been readily available to define quality in terms of the effect of health care delivery on the health of patients (Ditmyer et al., 1998). Combined administrative and health-related databases can demonstrate outcomes associated with nurse anesthesia practice.

Nurse anesthesia has made outcomes research an urgent priority. Development of methodologically sound outcomes research requires the preparation of more scholars within the specialty who have expertise in research design and measurement. Fortunately, more CRNAs are rising to the challenge of doctoral education.

Continuing to strive for the accurate measurement of nurse anesthesia outcome remains a goal of the nurse anesthesia specialty. With continued research, this goal can be attained.

REFERENCES

Abenstein, J., & Warner, M. (1996). Anesthesia providers, patient outcomes and costs. *Anesthesia & Analgesia, 82,* 1273–1283.

Agency for Healthcare Research and Quality [AHRQ]. (2008a). *AHRQ patient safety network—glossary.* Retrieved July 19, 2008, from http://psnet.ahrq.gov/glossary.asp-x#reffailuretorescue6

AHRQ. (2008b). *Outcomes research fact sheet.* Retrieved July 21, 2008, from http://www.ahrq.gov/clinic/outfact.htm

Aiken, L., Clarke, S., Cheung, R., Sloan, D., & Silber, J. (2003). Educational levels of hospital nurses and surgical patient mortality. *Journal of the American Medical Association, 290,* 1617–1623.

American Association of Nurse Anesthetists [AANA]. (2007). *Report of the Doctoral Task Force*. Park Ridge, IL: Author.

AANA. (2008a). *Certified registered nurse anesthetists (CRNAs) at a glance*. Retrieved July 19, 2008, from http://www.aana.com/aboutaana.aspx?ucNavMenu_TSMenu TargetID=179&u cNavMenu_TSMenuTargetType=4&ucNavMenu_TSMenuID= 6&id=265

AANA. (2008b). *The scope and standards for nurse anesthesia practice*. Retrieved July 20, 2008, from http://www.aana.com/Resources.aspx?ucNavMenu_TSMenuTarget ID=51&uc NavMenu_TSMenuTargetType=4&ucNavMenu_TSMenuID=6&id=785

AANA. (2008c). *The AANA Foundation*. Retrieved July 20, 2008, from http://www.aana. com/ProfessionalDevelopment.aspx?ucNavMenu_TSMenu TargetID=44&ucNav Menu_TSMenuTargetType=4&ucNavMenu_TSMenuID=6&id= 182

AANA. (2008d). *AANA Foundation Research Grants Program. Research funding priorities*. Retrieved July 20, 2008, from http://www.aana.com/uploadedFiles/Professional_ Development/AANA_F oundation/Applications/research_grants_08.pdf

AANA. (2008e). *Standards for office-based anesthesia practice*. Retrieved July 20, 2008, from http://www.aana.com/Resources.aspx?ucNavMenu_TSMenuTargetID=51&uc NavMenu_TSMenuTargetType=4&ucNavMenu_TSMenuID=6&id=785

AANA. (2008f). *Code of ethics for the certified registered nurse anesthetist*. Retrieved July 20, 2008, from http://www.aana.com/resources.aspx?ucNavMenu_TSMenuTarget ID=51&uc NavMenu_TSMenuTargetType=4&ucNavMenu_TSMenuID=6&id=665

AANA. (2008g). *Fact sheet concerning state opt-outs and November 13, 2001 CMS Rule*. Retrieved July 21, 2008, from http://www.aana.com/Advocacy.aspx?ucNav Menu_TSMenuTargetID=49&ucN avMenu_TSMenuTargetType=4&ucNavMenu_ TSMenuID=6&id=2573

American Society of Anesthesiologists [ASA]. (2008). *ASA closed claims project*. Retrieved July 19, 2008, from http://depts.washington.edu/asaccp/index.shmtl

Bankert, M. (1989). *Watchful care—A history of America's nurse anesthetists* (p. 31). New York: Continuum.

Beecher, H., & Todd, D. (1954). A study of deaths associated with anesthesia and surgery. *Annals of Surgery, 140,* 2–25.

Bhananker, S., Posner, K., Cheney, F., Caplan, R., Lee, L., & Domino, K. (2006). Injury and liability associated with monitored anesthesia care: A closed claims analysis. *Anesthesiology, 104,* 228–234.

Blum, R., Raemer, D., Carroll, J., Sunder, N., Felstein, D., & Cooper, J. (2004). Crisis resource management training for an anaesthesia faculty: A new approach to continuing education. *Medical Education, 38,* 45–55.

Brunner, E. (1984). The national association of insurance commissioners closed claims study. *International Anesthesiology Clinics, 22,* 17–30.

Callaghan, J. (1995). Twenty-five years of gallbladder surgery in a small rural hospital. *American Journal of Surgery, 169,* 313–315.

Callahan, L. (1988). Competence models: From theory to practical application. *AANA Journal, 56,* 5.

Caplan, R., Vistica, M., Posner, K., & Cheney, F. (1997). Adverse anesthetic outcomes arising from gas delivery equipment: A closed claims analysis. *Anesthesiology, 87,* 741–748.

Caplan, R., Ward, R., Posner, K., & Cheney, F. (1988). Unexpected cardiac arrest during spinal anesthesia: A closed claims analysis of predisposing factors. *Anesthesiology, 68,* 5–11.

Chadwick, H., Posner, K., Caplan, R., Ward, R., & Cheney, F. (1991). A comparison of obstetric and nonobstetric malpractice claims. *Anesthesiology, 74,* 242–249.

Cheney, F. (1999). The American Society of Anesthesiologists Closed Claims Project: What have we learned, how has it affected practice, and how will it affect practice in the future? *Anesthesiology, 91,* 552–556.

Cheney, F., Domino, K., Caplan, R., & Posner, K. (1999). Nerve injury associated with anesthesia: A closed claims analysis. *Anesthesiology, 90,* 1062–1069.

Cheney, F., Posner, K., Caplan, R., & Gild, W. (1994). Burns from warming devices in anesthesia. *Anesthesiology, 80,* 806–810.

Cheney, F., Posner, K., Lee, L., Caplan, R., & Domino, K. (2006). Trends in anesthesia-related death and brain damage: A closed claims analysis. *Anesthesiology, 105,* 1081–1086.

The Cochrane Collaboration. (2008). *Cochrane reviews.* Retrieved July 20, 2008, from http://www.cochrane.org/reviews/clibintro.htm#library

Cooper, J., Blum, R., Carroll, J., Dershwitz, M., Feinstein, D., Gaba, D., et al. (2008). Differences in safety climate among hospital anesthesia departments and the effect of a realistic simulation-based training program. *Anesthesia and Analgesia, 106,* 574–584.

Coopmans, V., & Biddle, C. (2008). CRNA performance using a handheld, computerized, decision-making aid during critical events in a simulated environment: A methodologic Inquiry. *AANA Journal, 76,* 29–35.

Council on Accreditation of Nurse Anesthesia Educational Programs [COA]. (2006). *Standards for accreditation of nurse anesthesia educational programs.* Park Ridge, IL: Author.

Crawforth, K. (2002). The AANA Foundation Closed Malpractice Claims Study obstetric anesthesia. *AANA Journal, 70,* 97–104.

Cromwell, J., & Snyder, K. (2000). Alternate cost-effective anesthesia care teams. *Nursing Economic$, 18,* 185–193.

Ditmyer, S., Koespsell, B., Branum, V., Davis, P., & Lush, M. (1998). Developing a nursing outcomes measurement tool. *Journal of Nursing Administration, 28,* 1331–1361.

Domino, K., Bowdle, T., Posner, K., Spitellie, P., Lee, L., & Cheney, F. (2004). Injuries and liability related to central vascular catheters: A closed claims analysis. *Anesthesiology, 100,* 1411–1418.

Domino, K., Posner, K., Caplan, R., & Cheney, F. (1999). Awareness during anesthesia: A closed claims analysis. *Anesthesiology, 90,* 1053–1061.

Dunbar, P., Mayer, J., Fordyce, M., Lishner, D., Hagopian, A., Spanton, K., & Hart, L. (1998). Availability of anesthesia personnel in rural Washington and Montana. *Anesthesiology, 88,* 800–808.

Fitzgibbon, D., Posner, K., Domino, K., Caplan, R., Lee, L., & Cheney, F. (2004). Chronic pain management: American Society of Anesthesiologists Closed Claims Project. *Anesthesiology, 100,* 98–105.

Fritzlen, T., Kremer, M., & Biddle, C. (2003). The AANA Foundation Closed Malpractice Claims Study on nerve injuries during anesthesia care. *AANA Journal, 71,* 347–352.

Gaba, D. (2004, October 13). The future vision of simulation in health care. *Quality and Safety in Health Care,* Suppl. 1, i2–10.

Gild, W., Posner, K., Caplan, R., & Cheney, F. (1992). Eye injuries associated with anesthesia. *Anesthesiology, 76,* 204–208.

Greiner, A. C., & Knebel, E. (Eds.). (2003). *Health professions education: A bridge to quality.* Washington, DC: The National Academies Press. Retrieved July 20, 2008, from http://www.iom.edu/Object.File/Master/44/388/Health%20Professiona ls%20 Sector%20-%20formatted.pdf

Hartland, W., Biddle, C., & Fallacaro, M. (2003). Accessing the living laboratory: Trigger films as an aid to developing, enabling and assessing anesthesia clinical instructors. *AANA Journal, 71,* 287–291.

Hotchkiss, M., Biddle, C., & Fallacaro, M. (2002). Assessing the authenticity of the human simulation experience in anesthesiology. *AANA Journal, 70,* 470–473.

Ingersoll, G. (2008). Outcomes evaluation and performance improvement: An integrative review of research on advanced practice nursing (p. 724). In A. Hamric, J. Spross, & C. Hanson (Eds.), *Advanced practice nursing: An integrative approach.* St. Louis: Saunders Elsevier.

Jiminez, N., Posner, K., Cheney, F., Caplan, R., Lee, L., & Domino, K. (2007). An update on pediatric anesthesia liability: A closed claims analysis. *Anesthesia and Analgesia, 104,* 147–153.

Jones, R. (2001). Comparative mortality in anaesthesia. *British Journal of Anaesthesia, 87,* 813–815.

Jordan, L., Kremer, M., Crawforth, K., & Shott, S. (2001). Data-driven practice improvement: The AANA Foundation closed malpractice claims study. *AANA Journal, 69,* 301–311.

Kavey, R. (2008). *IOM roundtable on evidence-based medicine, health professions sector statement.* Retrieved July 20, 2008, from http://www.iom.edu/Object.File/Master/44/ 388/Health%20Professiona ls%20Sector%20-%20formatted.pdf

Kraus, G. (1994). Quality assessment and improvement in the 1990s. In S. Foster & L. Jordan (Eds.), *Professional aspects of nurse anesthesia practice* (pp. 291–306). Philadelphia: F. A. Davis.

Kremer, M., Faut-Callahan, M., & Hicks, F. (2002). A study of clinical decision making by certified registered nurse anesthetists. *AANA Journal, 70,* 391–397.

Larson, S., & Jordan, L. (2001). Preventable adverse patient outcomes: A closed claims analysis of respiratory incidents. *AANA Journal, 69,* 386–392.

Lee, L., Posner, K., Domino, K., Caplan, R., & Cheney, F. (2004). Injuries associated with regional anesthesia in the 1980s and 1990s: A closed claims analysis. *Anesthesiology, 101,* 143–152.

Lema, M. (2003). Safe anesthetic practice—fact, fantasy or folly? *ASA Newsletter, 67*(5). Retrieved July 19, 2008, from http://www.asahq.org/Newsletters/2003/06_03/ ventilations06_03.html

Lohr, K. (1988). Outcomes measurement: Concepts and questions. *Inquiry, 25*(1), 37–50.

MacRae, M. (2007). Closed claims studies in anesthesia: A literature review and implications for practice. *AANA Journal, 75,* 267–275.

McDonald, K., Romano, P., Geppert, J., et al. (2002). *Measures of patient safety based on hospital administrative data—The patient safety indicators.* Rockville, MD: Agency for Healthcare Research and Quality. Publication No. 02-0038. Retrieved July 20, 2008, from http://www.ahrq.gov/clinic/evrptfiles.htm#psi

McDonald, L. (2001). Florence Nightingale and the early origins of evidence-based nursing. *Evidence-Based Nursing, 4,* 68–69.

McGlynn, E., Asch, S., Adams, J., et al. (2003). The quality of healthcare delivered to adults in the United States. *New England Journal of Medicine, 348,* 2635–2645.

Merwin, E., Stern, S., & Jordan, L. (2007). *Executive summary of AANA Foundation Faculty Workforce Study.* Park Ridge, IL: AANA Foundation.

Minnick, A., & Pabst, M. (1988). Improving the ability to detect the impact of labor on patient outcomes. *Journal of Nursing Administration, 28*(12), 17–21.

Monti Seibert, E., Alexander, J., & Lupien, A. (2004). Rural nurse anesthesia practice: A pilot study. *AANA Journal, 72,* 181–189.

Moody, M., & Kremer, M. (2001). Preinduction activities: A closed malpractice claims perspective. *AANA Journal, 69,* 461–465.

National League for Nursing [NLN]. (2008). *Transforming nursing education: Position statement, May 9, 2005.* Retrieved June 2, 2008, from www.nln.org/aboutnln/Positionstatements/transforming022005

Orkin, F. (1998). Rural realities. *Anesthesiology, 88,* 568–571.

Pellegrini, J. (2006). Using evidence-based practice in nurse anesthesia programs. *AANA Journal, 74,* 269–273.

Peterson, G., Domino, K., Caplan, R., Posner, K., Lee, L., & Cheney, F. (2005). Management of the difficult airway: A closed claims analysis. *Anesthesiology, 103,* 33–39.

Petty, W., Kremer, M., & Biddle, C. (2002). A synthesis of the Australian Patient Safety Incident Monitoring Study, the American Society of Anesthesiologists Closed Claims Project, and the American Association of Nurse Anesthetists Closed Claims Study. *AANA Journal, 70,* 193–202.

Pine, M., Holt, K., & Lou, Y. (2003). Surgical mortality and type of anesthesia provider. *AANA Journal, 71,* 109–116.

Pravikoff, D., Tanner, A., & Pierce, S. (2005). Readiness of U.S. nurses for evidence-based practice. *American Journal of Nursing, 105,* 45–51.

Punjasawadwong, Y., Bunchungmongkol, N., & Pongchiewboon, A. (2008). *Bispectral index for improving anaesthetic delivery and postoperative recovery.* Retrieved June 8, 2008, from http://www.cochrane.org/colloquia/abstracts/ottawa/P-118.htm

Register, M., Graham-Garcia, J., & Haas, R. (2003). The use of simulation to demonstrate hemodynamic response to varying degrees of intrapulmonary shunt. *AANA Journal, 71,* 277–284.

Robbertze, R., Posner, K., & Domino, K. (2006). Closed claims review of anesthesia for procedures outside the operating room. *Current Opinion in Anesthesiology, 19,* 436–442.

Ruth, H. (1945). Anesthesia study commissions. *Journal of the American Medical Association, 127,* 514–524.

Sackett, D. (1998). Evidence-based medicine [Editorial]. *Spine, 23,* 1085–1086.

Schulman, S., Schardt, C., & Erb, T. (2008). *Evidence-based medicine in anesthesiology.* Retrieved June 20, 2008, from http://www.ncbi.nlm.nih.gov/pubmed/17019268?ordinalpos=68&itool=EntrezSystem2.PEntrez.Pubmed.Pubmed_ResultsPanel.Pubmed_RVDocSum

Silber, J., Kennedy, S., Even-Shoshan, O., Chen, W., Koziol, L., Sowan, M., Longnecker, D., et al. (2000). Anesthesiologist direction and patient outcomes. *Anesthesiology, 93,* 152–163.

Simonson, D., Ahern, N., & Hendryx, M. (2007). Anesthesia staffing and anesthetic complications during cesarean delivery: A retrospective analysis. *Nursing Research, 56,* 9–17.

Smith, H., Jacob, A., Segura, L., Dilger, J., & Torsher, L. (2008). Simulation education in anesthesia training: A case report of successful resuscitation of bupivacaine-induced cardiac arrest linked to recent simulation training. *Anesthesia and Analgesia, 106,* 1581–1584.

Stark, P., & Kremer, M. (2001, August). *Perioperative care in rural Illinois.* Poster presentation, American Association of Nurse Anesthetists 68th Annual Meeting.

Stuart, P. (2006). The evidence behind modern fasting guidelines. *Best Practice Research in Clinical Anaesthesiology, 20,* 457–469. Retrieved June 20, 2008, from http://www.ncbi.nlm.nih.gov/pubmed/17080696?ordinalpos=61&itool=EntrezSystem2.PEntrez.Pubmed.Pubmed_ResultsPanel.Pubmed_RVDocSum

Talsma, A., Bahl, V., & Campbell, D. (2008). Exploratory analyses of the "failure to rescue" measure: Evaluation through medical record review. *Journal of Nursing Care Quality, 23,* 202–210.

Thys, D. (2007). *The role of information systems in anesthesia.* Retrieved July 19, 2008, from http://www.apsf.org/resource_center/newsletter/2001/summer/03Info sys.htmn

11

Resources to Facilitate APN Outcomes Research

DENISE BRYANT-LUKOSIUS, JULIE VOHRA, AND
ALBA DiCENSO

Assessing the outcomes of advanced practice nursing (APN) roles is an international area of focus. This chapter reviews work being done in Canada to further APN outcomes research, including the establishment of three key resources: a nationally funded APN Research Chair, a framework for conducting evaluations of APN roles, and an APN Research Data Collection Toolkit. An overview of these research resources will be provided and their application to promote high-quality outcome assessments of APN roles will be examined.

RESEARCH CHAIR IN ADVANCED PRACTICE NURSING

In 2000–2001, the Canadian Health Services Research Foundation (CHSRF), a foundation established by the Canadian government, and the Canadian Institutes of Health Research (CIHR), the federal government's health research funding agency, partnered to create a number of nursing and health services chairs, each funded for 10 years. These chairs were created primarily to provide a mentoring and teaching resource for graduate and postgraduate students and junior faculty in applied health services and nursing research. Unlike traditional research chairs, the focus of the CHSRF/CIHR chairs is on mentoring and education, so as to build a capacity of new researchers who can independently contribute to applied health services and nursing research issues. Central to each chair's activities are partnerships with relevant decision-making organizations, so that policy-relevant research may be undertaken and its findings disseminated and, thus, contribute directly to the evidence base used in decision making.

One of these chairs was awarded to a co-author of this chapter (A.D.) and focuses on APN. The goal of this chair program is to increase Canada's pool of nurse researchers who will conduct applied APN-related research that will serve the needs of clinicians, managers, and policy makers in the health sector. Activities designed to achieve this goal focus on (a) the education of nurse researchers at the graduate level, (b) linkage and exchange with decision makers to ensure policy relevance and the dissemination and uptake of research results, (c) mentoring of junior faculty and postdoctoral fellows to launch an APN-related research program, and (d) the conduct of research that will inform the practice of APN across Canada.

Annually, through a competitive process, a maximum of three graduate students (initially both Master's and PhD level, but more recently only PhD) enrolled in any university in Canada and planning to conduct APN-related health services research are accepted into the Chair Program and are awarded a $10,000 bursary. In addition to the university requirements for completion of the PhD, the Chair Program requires that all participating students (a) enroll in a graduate course on "Research Issues in the Introduction and Evaluation of APN Roles" specifically developed for APN Chair students and available via "distance learning," (b) write an APN-related commentary for the journal *Evidence-Based Nursing*, (c) complete a 90-hour practicum in a policy setting and a 90-hour research internship with a senior research team, (d) identify an interdisciplinary thesis committee to oversee an APN-related health services research study, (e) partner with a decision maker to identify a policy-informing thesis topic, and (f) attend monthly meetings of Chair Program students via remote technology. Chair funding permits graduate students from across the country to enroll in the APN-related graduate course by covering travel and accommodation costs for face-to-face classes at the beginning and end of the course, with

Table 11.1

SAMPLE THESIS TOPICS OF APN CHAIR PROGRAM STUDENTS

- Nurse practitioner (NP) plus physician (MD) collaborative service delivery models in long-term care
- Facilitators and barriers to the implementation of an NP role in public health
- Psychometric testing of the NP–MD collaborative practice questionnaire: a measure of collaboration between NPs and MDs in primary care
- Delineation of the clinical nurse specialist (CNS) role in First Nations and Inuit communities
- Practice patterns of CNSs working with First Nations and Inuit communities
- Effectiveness of an APN role in secondary prevention of myocardial infarction
- Development of an APN supportive care role in advanced prostate cancer
- Participatory action research with primary health care NPs: relevance of interprofessional collaboration to NP integration
- Job satisfaction of primary care NPs
- Development of an instrument to measure interprofessional collaboration
- A case study of the implementation of the NP role in a regional health authority
- Team perceptions of the effectiveness of the cardiology acute care NP role

teleconferencing and Web-based communication for the remainder of the course.

Between 2001 and 2008, the Chair Program accepted 23 graduate students from across Canada (6 MSc and 17 PhD), seven of whom have completed their degrees and Chair Program requirements (5 MSc and 2 PhD). Those who complete their PhDs are eligible to compete for a junior faculty position funded and supervised by the Chair Program, the objective of which is to secure postdoctoral funding. Junior faculty and postdoctoral fellows continue to be part of the Chair Program and, when these training experiences are completed, they become affiliate faculty in the program. To date, three junior faculty have been funded through the Chair Program, two of whom have applied and successfully competed for postdoctoral fellowships. In addition to the graduate students, numerous APN practitioners from across Canada are enrolling in the graduate course on "Research Issues in the Introduction and Evaluation of APN Roles." To date, 42 practicing advanced practice nurses, in addition to the Chair Program graduate students, have completed the course. The final assignment for this course is the preparation of a research proposal related to the development, implementation, or evaluation of an APN role. Table 11.1 illustrates some of the student thesis topics of Chair Program graduate students. More information about the Chair Program can be found at http://www.apnnursingchair. mcmaster.ca/.

During her doctoral and postdoctoral studies with the APN Chair Program, the first author of this chapter (D.B.L.) developed the PEPPA Framework to guide the development and evaluation of APN roles. PEPPA is an acronym for a Participatory, Evidence-Informed, Patient-Centered Process for Advanced Practice Nursing (APN) Role Development, Implementation, and Evaluation (Bryant-Lukosius & DiCenso, 2004). This framework guides the research of the APN Chair students. As the Chair Program students have planned and conducted their research, they have used a number of existing data-collection tools and have developed a variety of instruments. Having become widely known across the country over the past seven years, the APN Chair Program is often approached by researchers and decision makers for information about the availability of APN-related research data collection tools. As a result, the Chair Program has created an APN Research Data Collection Toolkit. Researchers conducting APN outcomes research may find both these resources, the PEPPA Framework and the APN Research Data Collection Toolkit, useful. The remainder of this chapter will briefly describe these two resources.

THE PEPPA FRAMEWORK

The PEPPA Framework was developed to provide APN researchers, health care providers, administrators, and policy makers with a guide to promoting the optimal development and deployment of APN roles. A critical feature of this framework is that strategies to support meaningful outcome evaluations of APN roles are incorporated throughout role planning and implementation.

The underlying premise of the PEPPA Framework is that *the mandate of all APN roles is to maximize, maintain, or restore patient health through innovation in nursing practice and in the delivery of health services* (Canadian Nurses Association, 2008; Davies & Hughes, 2002; Hamric, 2000; McGee & Castledine, 2003). This mandate is consistent with international views of advanced nursing practice. There is a heightened demand worldwide for advanced practice nurses, as clinical experts, leaders, and change agents, to assist organizations in developing sustainable

Table 11.2

COMMON PROBLEMS ASSOCIATED WITH APN ROLE IMPLEMENTATION

- Stakeholder confusion about APN terminology
- Lack of clearly defined roles and their goals or outcomes
- Role emphasis on physician replacement or support
- Underutilization of APN scope of practice and expertise in all role dimensions
- Failure to address role implementation barriers
- Limited use of evidence-based approaches to guide role development, implementation, and evaluation

Source: Adapted from Bryant-Lukosius et al. (2004).

models of health care (Bryant-Lukosius, DiCenso, Browne, & Pinelli, 2004).

There is also a growing body of high-quality research documenting the positive impact of APN roles on patient, provider, and health-system outcomes for a variety of patient populations (Brooten et al., 2002; Horrocks, Anderson, & Salisbury, 2002; McCorkle et al., 2000; Moore et al., 2002). These studies indicate that the value-added component of these roles is central to the underlying purpose and characteristics of advanced nursing practice. These characteristics include the provision of coordinated, integrated, holistic, and patient-centered care focused on maximizing health, quality of life, and functional capacity (Bryant-Lukosius, DiCenso, Browne, & Pinelli, 2004). Opportunities for innovation and improved patient and health-system outcomes are more likely to occur when the introduction of APN roles represents a complementary addition to the model of care rather than a transfer or substitution of role functions between health care providers.

A review of the international literature identified six frequently reported barriers that were common to the effective implementation of various types of APN roles (Bryant-Lukosius, DiCenso, Browne, & Pinelli, 2004). Many of these barriers could be avoided through improved planning and better stakeholder understanding of the roles (Table 11.2).

Our review of the literature also found that the costs associated with poor APN role implementation planning were high and justified

Table 11.3

THE COSTS OF POOR APN ROLE IMPLEMENTATION PLANNING

- Poor stakeholder acceptance of APN role
- Role conflict
- Role overload
- Poor APN job satisfaction
- Difficulty recruiting and retaining highly qualified APN practitioners
- Negative impact on the quality of patient care and patient safety
- Unrealized opportunity for innovation and to benefit from APN expertise for patients, health providers, and the health care system
- Ineffective use of limited health care resources
- Negative impact on long-term role sustainability

Source: Adapted from Bryant-Lukosius, DiCenso, Browne, & Pinelli (2004).

the need for more thoughtful, systematic approaches to role introduction (Table 11.3).

The PEPPA Framework builds on earlier models recommending steps for introducing new health providers (Spitzer, 1978) and specifically APN roles (Dunn & Nicklin, 1995; Mitchell-DiCenso, Pinelli, & Southwell, 1996), by incorporating additional steps and strategies to address known barriers to successful APN role implementation. The aims of the framework are to:

- Employ relevant data to support the need and identified goals for a clearly defined role.
- Support the development of advanced nursing practice characterized by patient-centered, health-focused, and holistic care.
- Promote the full integration and employment of APN knowledge, skills, and expertise from all role dimensions related to clinical practice, education, research, organizational leadership, and scholarly/professional practice (Canadian Association of Nurses in Oncology, 2001).
- Create practice environments that support APN role development by engaging stakeholders from the health care team, practice setting, and health care system in the role-planning process.
- Promote ongoing role development and model of care enhancement through continuous and rigorous evaluation of progress in achieving predetermined outcome-based goals.

Conceptual Foundations of the PEPPA Framework

The principles of participatory action research (PAR) informed the development of the framework. PAR is a democratic, systematic approach that involves individuals from organizations, education systems, and communities in promoting health and social change (Deshler & Ewert, 1995; Foote Whyte, 1991; Smith, Pyrch, & Lizardi, 1993). Key principles of PAR include: active participation in cycles of reflection and action; valuing what people know and believe by building on their current understanding; collective investigation, analysis, learning, and the conscious production of new knowledge; collective decision making and action in using new knowledge to address problems; and evaluating the impact of these actions (Bowling, 1997; Deshler & Ewert, 1995; Smith, 1997).

The principles of PAR are relevant to APN role development in several ways. First, PAR promotes the use of objective data in health care planning and decisions to develop, implement, and modify an APN role. Early pioneers in the development of APN roles have also emphasized the importance of good data to support the need for new health provider roles, in the same way that research evidence is used to support the introduction of new therapeutic interventions such as medications (Spitzer, 1978). Second, APN practitioners work collaboratively within interprofessional teams and in established relationships with other stakeholders in the health system. Stakeholder roles and relationships are influenced by their values, beliefs, experiences, and expectations. These relationships create the conditions that affect the effective delivery of health care services and can facilitate or obstruct the implementation of APN roles. Therefore, collective learning and consensus decision making in the health planning process, on the part of key stakeholders, are necessary for the effective implementation of APN roles.

The principles of PAR are consistent with research-based approaches recommended for the planning of nursing and health and human resources (Advisory Committee on Health Delivery and Human Resources, 2007; O'Brien-Pallas, Tomblin Murphy, Baumann, & Birch, 2001). These include the principles of collaborative decision making through involvement of appropriate stakeholders; ensuring that target population health care needs are foundational to any process; consideration of environmental trends and drivers (context); and a systems approach to ensure comprehensiveness in planning and in the assessment of outcomes.

The PEPPA Framework also draws on Donabedian's theory for evaluating the quality of health care by proposing a structure–process–outcome evaluation of the APN role (Donabedian, 1966, 1992). This approach is consistent with other structure-process-outcome models developed to evaluate APN roles (Byers & Brunell, 1998; Grimes & Garcia, 1997; Sidani & Irvine, 1999). *Structures* are factors that affect processes or determine how the APN role is implemented. Role structures may include characteristics of both APN and patient populations, APN education programs, practical and financial resources, nursing and health care policies, regulatory and credentialing mechanisms, the model of care, and the physical, cultural, and organizational environment in which the advanced practice nurse works (Bryant-Lukosius, DiCenso, Browne, & Pinelli, 2004). *Process* refers to what the advanced practice nurse does in the role. This includes the types of APN services and how these services are provided. To ensure maximal use of APN expertise and scope of practice, the PEPPA Framework recommends that role processes be considered across all dimensions of advanced nursing practice related to clinical practice, education, research, organizational leadership, and scholarly and professional development (CANO, 2001).

Outcomes are the results of APN role services and care and thus are affected by both structure and process factors. In the framework, outcomes may be evaluated from the perspectives of patients and families, the APN practitioner, other health care providers, the organization, and the broader health care system. Outcomes are determined by goals for improving the delivery of nursing and health care services established early in the APN role-planning process. A package of APN services and specific role activities for each dimension of advanced nursing practice are developed specifically to achieve these pre-established goals. Strategically linking APN role activities with pre-set goals and outcomes facilitates the selection of outcome measures that will be most sensitive to APN interventions (Burns, 2001; Minnick, 2001).

The ability to conduct meaningful evaluations of the APN role is further strengthened by linking role structures, processes, and outcomes in the early stages of role development. For example, in the PEPPA Framework the APN role is evaluated along with the model of care in which the role is situated. This strategy aids in determining how structures within the model of care such as other health provider roles, role relationships, and resources affect APN role processes and outcomes.

Finally, the PEPPA Framework posits that there is sufficient world-wide literature demonstrating that well-designed and sufficiently developed APN roles are effective in achieving positive outcomes for patients, providers, and the health care system (Bredin et al., 1999; Brooten et al., 2002; Carroll, Rankin, & Cooper, 2007; Fulton & Baldwin, 2004; Krichbaum, 2007; Mitchell-DiCenso et al., 1996; Naylor et al., 2004; Paez & Allen, 2006). Thus, important questions to address when evaluating APN roles are not "Are APN roles effective?" but "*How* are APN roles effective?" and "For *which* patient populations, under *which* conditions, and in *which* models of care delivery are APN roles *most* effective?"

Steps of the PEPPA Framework

The PEPPA Framework involves a nine-step process (see Figure 11.1). Steps 1 to 6 focus on establishing role structures. This includes health care decision making and planning about the need to develop and implement a new model of care that may require an APN role. Step 7 focuses on role processes and involves initiating the implementation plan and introduction of the APN role. Steps 8 and 9 include the short- and long-term evaluations of the APN role and the new model of care to assess progress and sustainability in achieving predetermined goals and outcomes.

Step 1: Define the Population and Describe the Current Model of Care

The purpose of Step 1 is to set some parameters or limits on the health care planning process. This includes identification of a priority patient population as the central focus of the process. Second, the scope of the process is determined by focusing on relationships and interactions from a team, organizational, and/or geographic perspective. Efforts are made to describe and understand the current model of care by identifying how and when patients interact with health care providers and services.

Step 2: Identify Stakeholders and Recruit Participants

In this step, key individuals who represent important stakeholder groups that are integral to the current model of care are identified and invited

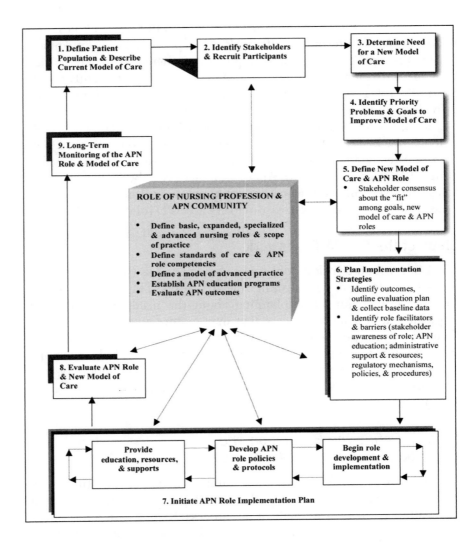

Figure 11.1 The PEPPA Framework: A Participatory, Evidence-Based, Patient-Centered Process for Advanced Practice Nursing (APN) Role Development, Implementation, and Evaluation.

Source: Adapted from Bryant-Lukosius & DiCenso (2004).

to participate in the health care redesign process. Strategies are employed to ensure a breadth of input from various stakeholders, including patients and families. The selection of participants also considers their roles and responsibilities within the model of care and their importance in facilitating the implementation of the new model of care and potential APN role.

Step 3: Determine the Need for a New Model of Care

In this step, the strengths and limitations of the current model of care for meeting patient health needs are assessed from a variety of stakeholder viewpoints. This involves conducting a needs assessment to collect and/or generate information about the extent, severity, and importance of unmet patient health needs and about the health care services required to meet these needs.

Step 4: Identify Priority Problems and Goals to Improve the Model of Care

In this step, participating stakeholders come to consensus regarding unmet patient health needs that are the most important to address. Priority problems associated with unmet health needs are identified, and outcome-based goals to improve the model of care delivery and patient health are established.

Step 5: Define the New Model of Care and APN Role

This step involves identifying strategies and solutions for achieving established goals. The need for new care practices and care delivery strategies is determined. The number, complement, and mix of health care providers required to implement the new model of care are examined. It is during this step that participants learn more about the purpose and types of various APN roles. The need for and the pros and cons of introducing an APN role rather than other nursing or health provider roles are considered. If an APN role is to be implemented, this step concludes with the development of a specific "job description" for an APN role within the new model of care.

Step 6: Plan Implementation Strategies

In this step, participants develop a plan to ensure system readiness for the role. This includes obtaining funding approval (if required) and identifying potential barriers to and facilitators of role implementation. Key factors to assess relate to APN and stakeholder education, marketing, recruitment and hiring, role-reporting structures, funding, and policy development. An important aspect of this stage is developing an evaluation plan and establishing timelines for role implementation and achievement of outcome-based goals.

Step 7: Initiate APN Role Implementation Plan

This step begins by initiating the role implementation plan developed in Step 6 and hiring an advanced practice nurse for the position. Full development and implementation of the APN role may take 3 to 5 years (Hamric & Taylor, 1989). During this period, efforts are made to monitor progress in role development and to modify or initiate strategies to support the implementation of the APN role. As Figure 11.1 illustrates, APN role implementation is a continuous process, in which the needs for new organizational policies and procedures and other types of role structures and supports are influenced by changes within the practice setting and stage of APN role development.

Step 8: Evaluate the APN Role and New Model of Care

In this step, formative evaluations that systematically evaluate APN role structures, processes, and outcomes are recommended as a strategy to promote ongoing role development. Several studies have demonstrated the importance of assessing APN role structures and processes to identify role barriers and facilitators (Guest et al., 2001; Read et al., 2001). In this type of evaluation, progress in achieving outcome-based goals is monitored and APN role structures and processes are examined to identify additional needs for supporting role development and implementation and further role enhancement.

Step 9: Monitor APN Role and Model of Care Over the Long Term

This step emphasizes the continuous and iterative process of ensuring that the APN role—and the model of care in which it is situated—

continue to be relevant, sustainable, and improved, based on new research and/or changes in the health care environment, patient needs, and treatment practices. Long-term monitoring of well-established roles is also helpful for maintaining a common vision for the role among key stakeholders (Seymour et al., 2002).

Current Applications of the PEPPA Framework

While development of the PEPPA Framework has been based on an extensive review of the APN literature (Bryant-Lukosius, DiCenso, Browne, & Pinelli, 2004) and other well-established models and theories, it has not been systematically evaluated. However, one recent study reports the positive effects of the framework when used to develop a unique model of NP practice in long-term care (McAiney et al., 2008). The framework's emphasis on stakeholder engagement to identify role priorities, establish a common vision of the NP role, and to participate in role planning was felt to contribute to the successful implementation of this new model of care. The NPs were found to improve staff confidence and reduce hospital admission rates by 39% to 43% (McAiney et al., 2008). The PEPPA Framework has also been used successfully to implement other advanced health provider roles, such as advanced physiotherapist roles designed to improve access to and the quality of care for patients undergoing hip and knee replacement surgery (Robarts et al., 2008).

A participatory action research project is currently under way to examine how the use of this framework affects the planning and implementation process for the introduction of oncology APN roles for underserved patient populations with cancer (Bryant-Lukosius et al., 2007). This study will also evaluate the effectiveness of a facilitator and the use of a toolkit designed to assist health care teams, health care planners, and administrators in applying the PEPPA Framework. Another toolkit, based in part on the PEPPA Framework, has also been developed by the Canadian Nurse Practitioner Initiative (2006) to support health care planners and administrators with the introduction of nurse practitioner roles, particularly in primary health care settings.

The framework is being used by large regional health authorities to implement new NP roles (Sawchenko, 2007) and to develop policies to support the successful implementation of NP and CNS roles in the regional health authority practice settings (Advanced Practice Nursing

Steering Committee, 2005; Avery, Hill-Carroll, Todoruk-Orchard, & DeLeon-Demare, 2006).

In Ontario, Canada, the PEPPA Framework is incorporated into the curricula of APN education programs for primary health care NPs, acute care NPs, and NPs as part of an anesthesia care team (Donald, 2008; University of Toronto, 2008). We have also used the framework as the basis for the graduate nursing course on "Research Issues in the Introduction and Evaluation of APN Roles" (McMaster University School of Nursing, 2008) and to develop systematic programs of research for APN roles in oncology (Bryant-Lukosius et al., 2007; Martelli-Reid et al., 2007) and in long-term care (Donald, 2008; Donald et al., 2007).

APN RESEARCH DATA COLLECTION TOOLKIT

In an effort to facilitate APN-related research, the APN Research Data Collection Toolkit has been developed and is fully accessible via the APN Chair Program Web site (http://www.apnnursingchair. mcmaster.ca). The objective of the toolkit is to identify instruments that could be used to facilitate data collection for monitoring and measuring APN role development, implementation, and evaluation. Focused on APN, the toolkit includes instruments that have been used in research related to CNSs as well as to primary and acute care NPs. The toolkit is an ongoing initiative to create a compendium of common instruments used in APN research. It was developed with the following users in mind: APN researchers, graduate students planning APN research, and decision makers who are seeking to evaluate one or more dimensions of APN care (e.g., patient satisfaction).

The steps involved in producing the toolkit include: (1) identifying and appraising measurement tools used in APN research; (2) compiling the results into a publicly accessible Web page; and (3) promoting the Web site, so that those introducing and evaluating APN roles can use the resource and contribute their own instruments to it. The first step taken to identify relevant measurement tools was to review the studies included in systematic reviews of APN-focused research (e.g., Horrocks, Anderson, & Salisbury, 2002) and in books focused on APN-related outcome measures (e.g., Kleinpell, 2001). Second, all APN-related research conducted through the APN Chair Program was reviewed and measurement tools extracted. Third, a systematic search of the literature focused on APN practitioners was conducted. These citations were reviewed by two APN researchers to identify relevant studies. Data collection instruments identified in any relevant studies were included in the toolkit.

Once a relevant measurement tool is identified, the primary author is contacted and asked to provide any additional information regarding the measurement instrument, an electronic copy of the instrument itself, and permission to post the tool on the APN Toolkit Web site. Figure 11.2 illustrates the type of information compiled for each instrument. The instruments are organized according to the steps of the PEPPA Framework, so that users of the Web site can link the instruments with the distinct steps described in this framework (e.g., needs assessment, describing the model of care, defining the APN role, role implementation and practice patterns, barriers to and facilitators of APN integration, outcomes evaluation). The summary developed for each instrument is sent to the instrument developer, who is asked to review it for accuracy.

The APN Toolkit Web site is housed on a secure server in the McMaster University domain area. Navigation of the Web page is available through a sidebar menu, as well as through the table of contents. To further facilitate ease of information retrieval, there is a keyword search function where users can enter a keyword to see if it is contained anywhere in the APN Toolkit Web site. Links to a PDF copy of the instrument are available to users, where permission has been granted by authors. Users are invited to submit references for instruments, updates, and corrections via a Web form. Users are also invited to submit any tools they have created that are not yet in the toolkit.

The APN Toolkit is an ever-growing resource that currently houses summaries of over 100 instruments. This toolkit will be an important resource for those introducing and evaluating APN practice by making available existing instruments that have been used, for example, to conduct needs assessments, measure practice patterns, identify barriers and facilitators, and evaluate provider and patient outcomes related to APN.

In summary, the establishment of a nationally funded research chair has facilitated the training of the next generation of Canadian nurse researchers who will continue to expand our knowledge about the effective development and deployment of APN roles for meeting patient, provider, and health system outcomes. Through the CHRSF/CIHR Chair

Misener Nurse Practitioner Job Satisfaction Scale (MNPJSS)

Original citation: Misener, T. R., & Cox, D. L. (2001). Development of the Misener Nurse Practitioner Job Satisfaction Scale. *Journal of Nursing Measurement,* *9*(1), 91–108.

Contact information:
Please see website for details.

Price & availability: Published in original citation. Contact author for permission to use.

Brief description of instrument: Assessment of job satisfaction of primary care NPs.

Scale format: 44 items, each measured using a 6-point Likert scale. Response options: "Very Satisfied" = 6; "Satisfied" = 5; "Minimally Satisfied" = 4; "Minimally Dissatisfied" = 3; "Dissatisfied" = 2; "Very Dissatisfied" = 1 point. One item for global satisfaction measured on a 10-point scale, 10 being the highest level of job satisfaction.

Administration technique: Self-administered questionnaire.

Scoring and interpretation: Total score is obtained by summing all 44 items. Subscale score is obtained by summing the subscale items.

Factors and norms: 6 factors, determined by factor analysis: (1) Intrapractice partnership/collegiality; (2) Challenge/autonomy; (3) Professional, social and community interaction; (4) Professional growth; (5) Time; (6) Benefits. Item mean (SD) reported in original citation.

Internal consistency: Cronbach's alpha on entire scale: 0.96; Cronbach's alphas on subscales range from 0.79 to 0.94.

Content & face validity: Instrument development based on literature review, review of existing instruments, and input from numerous NP experts.

Strengths: Easy to administer and score; covers a wide variety of previously published factors associated with job satisfaction.

Limitations: Relies heavily on factor analysis results to justify subscale, lacking theoretical rationale.

Published APN studies using instrument: See original citation.

PEPPA Framework step: 8.

Figure 11.2 An example of an APN-related data collection tool as summarized in the APN data collection toolkit.

in APN, these and other researchers, educators, health providers, and decision makers will have access to critically appraised tools for conducting APN-related research. As a relatively new resource, the PEPPA Framework has demonstrated wide applicability for APN role development. The framework can be employed to inform APN curricula, guide role implementation and policy formulation in support of APN, establish systematic approaches for role evaluation, and develop APN-focused programs of research.

REFERENCES

Advanced Practice Nursing Steering Committee, Winnipeg Regional Health Authority. (2005). *A guide to the implementation of the nurse practitioner role in your health care setting.* Retrieved January 21, 2008, from http://www.wrha.mb.ca/staff/nursing/files/np_toolkit_000.pdf

Advisory Committee on Health Delivery and Human Resources (ACHDHR). (2007). *A framework for collaborative pan-Canadian health human resources planning.* Ottawa: Author.

Avery, L., Hill-Carroll, C., Todoruk-Orchard, M., & DeLeon-Demare, K. (2006). *Improve patient care and outcomes: Adding a clinical nurse specialist to your team. A guide for successful integration.* Winnipeg Regional Health Authority. Retrieved January 21, 2008, from http://www.wrha.mb.ca/staff/nursing/files/cns_toolkit.pdf

Bowling, A. (1997). *Research methods in health: Investigating health and health services.* Philadelphia: Open University Press.

Bredin, M., Corner, J., Krishnasamy, M., Plant, H., Bailey, C., & A'Hern, R. (1999). Multicentre randomised controlled trial of nursing interventions for breathlessness in patients with lung cancer. *British Medical Journal, 318,* 901–904.

Brooten, D., Naylor, M. D., York, R., Brown, L. P., Hazard Munro, B., Hollingsworth, A. O., et al. (2002). Lessons learned from testing the quality cost model of advanced practice nursing (APN) transitional care. *Journal of Nursing Scholarship, 34,* 369–375.

Bryant-Lukosius, D., & DiCenso, A. (2004). A framework for the introduction and evaluation of advanced practice nursing roles. *Journal of Advanced Nursing, 48,* 530–540.

Bryant-Lukosius, D., DiCenso, A., Browne, G., & Pinelli, J. (2004). Advanced practice Inursing roles: Issues affecting role development, implementation, and evaluation. *Journal of Advanced Nursing, 48,* 519–529.

Bryant-Lukosius, D., Green, E., Bakker, D., Paulse, B., Wiernikowski, J., Snider, A., et al. (2007). *Increasing capacity for the effective implementation of oncology APN roles for under-serviced populations: A collaborative, facilitative approach.* A project of the Change Foundation & the Nursing Secretariat of the Ontario Ministry of Health and Long-Term Care, Toronto, ON. Retrieved July 10, 2008, from http://www.changefoundation.ca/nursingawards.html

Burns, S. M. (2001). Selecting advanced practice nurse outcome measures. In R. M. Kleinpell (Ed.), *Outcome assessment in advanced practice nursing* (1st ed., pp. 73–90). New York: Springer Publishing Company.

Byers, J., & Brunell, M. (1998). Demonstrating the value of the advanced practice nurse: An evaluation model. *AACN Clinical Issues, 9,* 296–305.

Canadian Association of Nurses in Oncology (CANO). (2001). *Standards of care, roles in oncology nursing, role competencies.* Kanata, ON: Author.

Canadian Nurse Practitioner Initiative. (2006). *Implementation and evaluation toolkit for nurse practitioners in Canada.* Retrieved October 16, 2008, from http://206.191.29.104/documents/pdf/Toolkit_Implementation_Evaluation_NP_e.pdf

Canadian Nurses Association (CNA). (2008). *Advanced nursing practice—A national framework.* Ottawa: Author.

Carroll, D. L., Rankin, S. H., & Cooper, B. A. (2007). The effects of a collaborative peer advisor/advanced practice nurse intervention. *Journal of Cardiovascular Nursing, 22,* 313–319.

Davies, B., & Hughes, A. M. (2002). Clarification of advanced nursing practice: Characteristics and competencies. *Clinical Nurse Specialist, 16,* 147–152.

Deshler, D., & Ewert, M. (1995). *Participatory action research: Traditions and major assumptions.* Retrieved November 19, 2001, from www.oac.uoguelph.ca/~pi/pdrc/articles/article.1

Donabedian, A. (1966). Evaluating the quality of medical care. *Milbank Memorial Quarterly, 44,* 166–203.

Donabedian, A. (1992, November). Commentary: The role of outcomes in quality assessment and assurance. *Quality Review Bulletin,* 356–360.

Donald, F. (2007). *Collaborative practice by nurse practitioners and physicians in long-term care homes: A mixed method study.* Unpublished doctoral thesis, McMaster University.

Donald, F. (2008). *The Ontario Primary Health Care Nurse Practitioner Program.* (Integrative practicum, provincial course professor; personal communication.)

Donald, F., Martin Misener, R., Ahktar-Danesh, N., Brazil, K., Bryant-Lukosius, D., Carter, N., DiCenso, A., Dobbins, M., Kaasalainen, S., Mcainey, C., Ploeg, J., Schindel Martin, L., Stolee, P., & Tanaguichi, A. (2007). *Understanding organizational and systems factors influencing the integration of the nurse practitioner role in long term care settings in Canada.* Research grant funded by the Canadian Institute of Health Research.

Dunn, K., & Nicklin, W. (1995, January–February). The status of advanced nursing roles in Canadian teaching hospitals. *Canadian Journal of Nursing Administration,* 111–135.

Foote Whyte, W. (1991). *Participatory action research.* London: Sage.

Fulton, J. S., & Baldwin, K. (2004). An annotated bibliography reflecting CNS practice and outcomes. *Clinical Nurse Specialist, 18*(4), 21–39.

Grimes, D. E., & Garcia, M. K. (1997). Advanced practice nursing and work site primary care: Challenges for outcomes evaluation. *Advanced Practice Nurse Quarterly, 3,* 19–28.

Guest, D., Peccei, R., Rosenthal, P., Montgomery, J., Redfern, S., Young, C., Wilson-Barnett, J., Dewe, P., Evans, A., Oakley, P., et al. (2001). *Preliminary evaluation of the establishment of nurse, midwife and health visitor consultants. Report to the Department of Health.* University of London, Kings College.

Hamric, A. (2000). A definition of advanced nursing practice. In A. B. Hamric, J. A. Spross, & C. M. Hanson (Eds.), *Advanced nursing practice: An integrative approach* (pp. 53–73). Philadelphia: W. B. Saunders.

Hamric, A. B., & Taylor, J. W. (1989). Role development of the CNS. In A. B. Hamric & J. Spross (Eds.), *The clinical nurse specialist in theory and practice* (2nd ed., pp. 41–82). Philadelphia: W. B. Saunders.

Horrocks, S., Anderson, E., & Salisbury, C. (2002). Systematic review of whether nurse practitioners working in primary care can provide equivalent care to doctors. *British Medical Journal, 324,* 819–823.

Kleinpell, R. (Ed.). (2001). *Outcome assessment in advanced practice nursing* (1st ed.). New York: Springer Publishing Company.

Krichbaum, K. (2007). APN post-acute care coordination improves hip fracture outcomes. *Western Journal of Nursing Research, 29,* 523–544.

Martelli-Reid, L., Bryant-Lukosius, D., Arnold, A., Ellis, P., Goffin, J., Okawara, G., Akhtar-Danesh, N., & Hapke, S. (2007). *A model of interprofessional research to support the development of an advanced practice nursing role in cancer care.* Poster presentation at the Canadian Association of Nurses in Oncology Conference, Vancouver, BC.

McAiney, C. A., Haughton, D., Jennings, J., Farr, D., Hillier, L., & Morden, P. (2008). A unique practice model for nurse practitioners in long-term care homes. *Journal of Advanced Nursing, 62,* 562–571.

McCorkle, R., Strumpf, N. D., Nuamah, I. E., et al. (2000). In older patients with late stage cancer, specialized home care by nurses improved survival after surgery. *Journal of the American Geriatrics Society, 48,* 1707–1713.

McGee, P., & Castledine, G. (2003). A definition of advanced practice for the UK. In P. McGee & G. Castledine (Eds.), *Advanced nursing practice* (2nd ed., pp. 17–30). Oxford, UK: Blackwell Publishing.

McMaster University School of Nursing, Health Sciences Library. (2008). *Finding resources for Nursing 706: Research issues in the introduction and evaluation of advanced practice nursing roles.* Last updated, March 18, 2008. Retrieved July 10, 2008, from http://hsl.mcmaster.ca/education/nursing/706.htm

Minnick, A. (2001). General design and implementation challenges in outcomes assessment. In R. M. Kleinpell (Ed.), *Outcome assessment in advanced practice nursing* (1st ed., pp. 91–102). New York: Springer Publishing Company.

Mitchell-DiCenso, A., Guyatt, G., Marrin, M., Goeree, R., Willan, A., Southwell, D., et al. (1996). A controlled trial of nurse practitioners in neonatal intensive care. *Pediatrics, 98,* 1143–1148.

Mitchell-DiCenso, A., Pinelli, J., & Southwell, D. (1996). Introduction and evaluation of an advanced nursing practice role in neonatal intensive care. In K. Kelly (Ed.), *Outcomes of effective management practice* (pp. 171–186). Thousand Oaks, CA: Sage.

Moore, S., Corner, J., Haviland, J., Wells, M., Salman, E., Normand, C., Brada, M., O'Brien, M., & Smith, I. (2002). Nurse led follow up and conventional medical follow up in management of patients with lung cancer: Randomized trial. *British Medical Journal, 325*(7373), 1145–1151.

Naylor, M. D., Brooten, D. A., Campbell, R. L., Maislin, G., McCauley, K. M., & Schwartz, J. S. (2004). Transitional care of older adults hospitalized with heart failure: A randomized controlled trial. *Journal of the American Geriatrics Society, 52,* 675–684.

O'Brien-Pallas, L., Tomblin Murphy, G., Baumann, A., & Birch, S. (2001). Framework for analyzing health human resources. In *Canadian Institute for Health Information. Future Development of Information to Support the Management of Nursing Resources: Recommendations.* Ottawa: Canadian Institute for Health Information.

Paez, K., & Allen, J. K. (2006). Cost-effectiveness of nurse practitioner management of hypercholesterolemia following coronary revascularization. *Journal of the American Academy of Nurse Practitioners, 18,* 436–444.

Read, S., Jones, M. L., Collins, K., McDonnell, A., Jones, R., Doyal, L., Cameron, A., Masterson, A., Dowling, S., Vaughan, B., Furlong, S., & Scholes, J. (2001). *Exploring new roles in practice (ENRIP) final report.* Sheffield: University of Sheffield. Retrieved March 8, 2003, from http://www.shef.ac.uk/content/1/c6/01/33/98/enrip.pdf

Robarts, S., Kennedy, D., MacLeod, A. M., Findlay, H., & Gollish, J. (2008). A framework for the development and implementation of an advanced practice role for physiotherapists that improves access and quality care for patients. *Healthcare Quarterly, 11*(2), 67–75.

Sawchenko, L. (2007). An evidence-informed approach to the introduction of nurse practitioners in British Columbia's Interior Health Authority. *Links, 10*(3), 4. Retrieved July 10, 2008, from http://www.chsrf.ca/other_documents/newsletter/pdf/links_v10n3_e.pdf

Seymour, J., Clark, D., Hughes, P., Bath, P., Beech, N., Corner, J., Douglas, H., Halliday, D., Haviland, J., Marples, R., Normand, C., Skilbeck, J., & Webb, T. (2002). Clinical nurse specialists in palliative care. Part 3. Issues for the Macmillan Nurse role. *Palliative Medicine, 16,* 386–394.

Sidani, S., & Irvine, D. (1999). A conceptual framework for evaluating the nurse practitioner role in acute care settings. *Journal of Advanced Nursing, 30*(1), 58–66.

Smith, S. E. (1997). Deepening participatory action-research. In S. E. Smith & D. G. Willms (Eds.), *Nurtured by knowledge: Learning to do participatory action-research* (pp. 173–264). New York: Apex Press.

Smith, S. E., Pyrch, T., & Lizardi, A. (1993). Participatory action-research for health. *World Health Forum, 14,* 319–324.

Spitzer, W. O. (1978). Evidence that justifies the introduction of new health professionals. In P. Slayton & M. J. Trebilcock (Eds.), *The professions and public policy* (pp. 211–236). Toronto: University of Toronto Press.

University of Toronto, Lawrence S. Bloomberg Faculty of Nursing. (2008). *Nurse Practitioner in Anesthesia Care Program. Course outlines.* Retrieved July 10, 2008, from http://www.nursing.utoronto.ca/Assets/Continuing+Education/Anesthesia+Courses+All.pdf

Vohra, J. U., & DiCenso, A. (2008). *Advanced Practice Nursing (APN) Toolkit* Web site. Retrieved October 31, 2008, from http://apntoolkit.mcmaster.ca

Index

R

Recruitment of nursing personnel,
savings through, 220
Referrals, documentation of, 214
Research Chair Programs
Canadian Health Services Research
Foundation Research Chair,
277–280
Canadian Institutes of Health
Research Research Chair,
277–280
Research Data Collection Toolkit,
Advanced Practice Nursing,
280, 290–293
*Research Issues in the Introduction and
Evaluation of APN Roles,*
278–279
graduate course, 279
Research resources, 2–5, 277–296
APN Research Data Collection
Toolkit, 280, 290–293
Canadian Health Services Research
Foundation, 277–280
Canadian Institutes of Health
Research, 277–278
education, 277–280
mentoring, 277–280
PEPPA Framework, 280–290
applications, 289–290
conceptual foundations of, 283–285
steps, 285–289
*Research Issues in the Introduction and
Evaluation of APN Roles,* 278
graduate course, 279
thesis topics, Advanced Practice
Nursing Chair Program
Students, 279
Researcher, clinical nurse specialist role
as, 202
Responsibility agreement form, warfarin
patient, 185–186
Retention of nursing personnel, savings
through, 220
Revenue generation, analysis of cost-
benefit, 221
Risk-management data review, 214

Role activities measurement, outcome
measurement, distinguished,
202–203
Role of clinical nurse specialist, 202–205
Role-sensitive outcome measure
selection, 89–95
Rural settings, nurse anesthesia
outcomes in, 258–259

S

Satisfaction measures, 95–96
Search examples, 123–126
Selection of outcome measures, 2–6,
89–105
aggregate data, 92–95
categories of outcome data, 95–100
aggregate data, 99–100
benchmark data, 99–100
clinical outcome measures, 96–97
efficiency, 97–98
financial outcomes, 98
satisfaction, 95–96
clinical nurse specialist, 91–92
control charts, 92–93
evidence-based practice, 91
LOS data, 99
medical acute care floor, acute care
nurse practitioner, 8, 90
outcomes manager, 98
quality assurance, 91
role-sensitive outcome measure
selection, 89–95
roles/outcome measures, 100–104
cardiac cath lab acute care nurse
practitioners, 100–101
congestive heart failure acute care
nurse practitioner, 101
lung transplant coordinators, 103
neuroscience outcomes managers,
103–104
pulmonary outcomes manager,
101–102
surgical service coordinators,
102–103
service line designation by discharge
unit, 99

Women's Health Care in Advanced Practice

Catherine Ingram Fogel, PhD, RNC, FAAN
Nancy Fugate Woods, PhD, RN, FAAN, Editors

This book is the ideal tool to help graduate level nursing students expand their understanding of women's health care and wellness issues. For easy reference, *Women's Health Care in Advanced Practice Nursing* is organized into four parts:

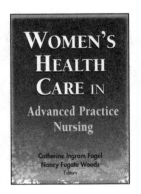

- Women and Their Lives, covering connections between women's lives and their health
- Frameworks for Practice, addressing health care practice with women
- Health Promotion, covering ways for women to promote their health and prevent many chronic diseases
- Threats to Health and Health Problems, addressing problems unique to women, diseases more prevalent in women, and those in which there are different risk factors

Key features include:

- The most recently available data on selected social characteristics of women with a focus on changing population demographics
- Separate chapters on health issues of adolescent/young adult, midlife, and older women
- Chapters on preconceptional and prenatal care
- Chapters covering cardiovascular disease, chronic disease, sexually transmitted infections and other common infections, HIV/AIDS, and women with disabilities
- Lesbian health care content, which is integrated throughout

2008 · 736 pp · Hardcover · 978-08261-0235-5

11 West 42nd Street, New York, NY 10036-8002 • Fax: 212-941-7842
Order Toll-Free: 877-687-7476 • Order Online: www.springerpub.com

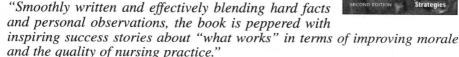

Assessing and Measuring Caring in Nursing and Health Science

Second Edition

Jean Watson, RN, PhD, HNC, FAAN, Editor

"As in the first edition, the author has done a magnifi-cent job compiling these instruments and providing important information that the reader can use to evalu-ate their usefulness."

—Ora Lea Strickland, RN, PhD, FAAN
(From the Foreword)

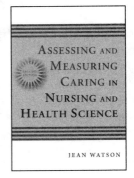

ASSESSING AND
MEASURING
CARING IN
NURSING AND
HEALTH SCIENCE

JEAN WATSON

This book provides all the essential research tools for assessing and measuring caring for those in the caring professions. Watson's text is the only comprehensive and accessible collection of instruments for care measure-ment in clinical and educational nursing research. The measurements address quality of care, patient, client, and nurse perceptions of caring, and caring behaviors, abilities, and efficacy.

Newly updated, this edition also contains three new chapters, which document the most effective caring language and provide innovative methods of selecting appropriate tools for measurement based on validity and reliability.

Key features of new edition:

- A chapter providing a comprehensive literature review of the research and measurement of caring
- A chapter entitled "Caring Factor Survey," which presents a new scale based on Watson's original theory of human caring
- Chapters outlining instruments for care measurement, including Holistic Caring Inventory, Peer Group Caring Interaction Scale, and many more
- New instruments focused on assessing caring at the administrative-relational caring level
- An updated section dedicated to challenges and future directions of the measurement of caring

September 2008 · 368 pp · Softcover · 978-0-8261-2196-7

11 West 42nd Street, New York, NY 10036-8002 • Fax: 212-941-7842
Order Toll-Free: 877-687-7476 • Order Online: www.springerpub.com